Foundations of Epidemiology

SECOND EDITION

Abraham M. Lilienfeld, M.D., M.P.H., D.Sc. (Hon.)
UNIVERSITY DISTINGUISHED SERVICE PROFESSOR OF EPIDEMIOLOGY
THE JOHNS HOPKINS UNIVERSITY
SCHOOL OF HYGIENE AND PUBLIC HEALTH

David E. Lilienfeld, A.B., M.S. Eng.
MINNESOTA DEPARTMENT OF HEALTH
DIVISION OF DISEASE PREVENTION AND CONTROL

New York   Oxford
OXFORD UNIVERSITY PRESS
1980

Library of Congress Cataloging in Publication Data

Lilienfeld, Abraham M
  Foundations of epidemiology.

  Bibliography: p.
  Includes index.
    1. Epidemiology. I. Lilienfeld, David E., joint
author. II. Title. [DNLM: 1. Epidemiologic methods.
2. Epidemiology. WA100 L728f]
  RA651.L54 1980 614.4 80-11840
  ISBN 0-19-502722-1 ISBN 0-19-502723-X (pbk.)

15 14 13 12 11 10

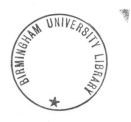

For Lorraine, Julia, and Saul

Preface

The purpose of this book is to present the concepts and methods of epidemiology as they are applied to a variety of disease problems. The broad scope of epidemiology is liberally illustrated with studies of specific diseases. Emphasis is placed on the integration of biological and statistical elements in the sequence of epidemiologic reasoning that derives inferences about the etiology of disease from population data. The epidemiologist's role in integrating knowledge obtained from a variety of scientific disciplines is described.

A knowledge of biostatistics is indispensable in the conduct of epidemiologic studies and the analysis of their results. This information can be found in many textbooks of biostatistics. To provide the minimal background necessary for understanding the epidemiologic methods that are discussed, however, we have added a new appendix of selected statistical procedures used frequently by epidemiologists.

This book has been designed as a text for introductory courses in epidemiology wherever they are offered. Thus, it can be used in schools of medicine, public health, allied health sciences, dentistry, nursing, and veterinary medicine, as well as in environmental health sciences and other programs offered by colleges of arts and sciences.

The text can be divided into four parts. Chapters 1 to 3 review the historical background and conceptual basis of epidemiology. Chapters 4 to 7 discuss demographic studies, including mortality and morbidity, and their application to epidemiologic problems.

The next four chapters, 8 to 11, consider the epidemiologic study, both observational and experimental. The last chapter illustrates the ways and means by which the types of data obtained from the various studies are integrated into a conceptual whole and focused on the derivation of biologic inferences.

Though several changes have been made in this edition, the book's structure remains basically the same. Many chapters have been extensively revised to include findings from recent epidemiologic studies. These chapters have been expanded, using many new examples from a greater variety of epidemiologic problems. New chapters on clinical and community trials have been added to strengthen the discussion of experimental epidemiology. The chapter on theoretical epidemiology has been modified and placed in an appendix.

To enhance the teaching value of the book, sets of study problems have been added to all appropriate chapters. These problems are not limited to reviewing topics discussed in the same chapter in which they appear. Rather, they cumulatively review material from preceding chapters, helping readers to integrate this material. The problems give students an opportunity to apply the methods and reasoning patterns that constitute epidemiology. Some of them invite broad consideration of various epidemiologic issues and viewpoints.

Some Comments on Terminology. The terms we have used to describe the different types of demographic and epidemiologic studies and their resultant measures are unchanged from those of the previous edition. During the past several years, however, the number of terms in use has proliferated considerably, causing much confusion, particularly to students. To remedy this problem, several committees have been constituted in an attempt to standardize epidemiologic terminology.

Here we should like to list some synonyms for several of the more frequently used terms; others are noted in the text. This list is by no means complete:

1. *Retrospective studies,* in addition to being called "case-control" studies, are also referred to as "case-referent" studies.
2. *Prospective studies* are also termed "longitudinal" studies, as well as "cohort" studies. What we call "non-concurrent prospective" studies are also referred to as "historical cohort,"

"retrospective cohort," "retrospective longitudinal" and "historical prospective" studies.
3. *Relative risk* is also termed the "risk ratio."
4. *Attributable risk,* as it is used in the book, is sometimes called "population attributable risk."

Acknowledgments

The development of the ideas and mode of their presentation in this book owe much to my students, from whom I have learned and continue to learn a great deal, and to many colleagues in epidemiology with whom I have collaborated over the years in various types of studies. I am particularly grateful for the influential role of Dr. Jacob Yerushalmy, Dr. Alexander Langmuir, Dr. Leonard Schuman, Dr. Milton Terris, and Dr. Warren Winkelstein. The exchange of ideas and collaboration with many colleagues in the fields of epidemiology, biostatistics, biology, and sociology, as well as with my colleagues in the Department of Epidemiology over many years, have been a continuing and enjoyable source of stimulation.

A.M.L.

The communication of ideas is the essence of teaching. I am indebted to my teachers for transmitting to me the tenets and philosophy of epidemiology. Dr. Cedric Garagliano and Dr. David Pyne have contributed much time and effort toward this end. I am also grateful for the helpful discussions with and encouragement from Dr. Samuel Greenhouse, Dr. Lloyd Stevenson, Dr. Ralph Paffenbarger, and Dr. George Comstock. Finally, thanks need to be given to the past and present authors of many epidemiologic studies, reports, and articles for their instruction in the methods of epidemiology.

D.E.L.

We would like to acknowledge the editorial advice and encouragement of Jeffrey House at Oxford University Press, who helped considerably in bringing this book to its completion. Much of its readability is the direct result of his studious review of the text. Special thanks go to Mrs. Eileen Eckels and Mary Lou Eisenhart, who typed the seemingly infinite number of drafts of the manuscript and to Jack Mandel and Joseph McLaughlin for having read the entire manuscript and suggested many improvements; to Paul Fine and I. D. Hill for many helpful suggestions; to many readers who have sent us their comments on specific points; and to Mr. Steven Balter for many of the illustrations. We are grateful to those authors and publishers who graciously permitted publication of their material.

Lastly, much credit must be given to members of our family, who have tolerated many dreary evenings and weekends of silence during the writing of this book. This work was supported, in part, by Research Career Award No. 5K06-GM13901 to Abraham Lilienfeld from the National Institute of General Medical Sciences, National Institutes of Health, Bethesda, Maryland.

A. M. L.
D. E. L.

Pikesville, Maryland
January 1980

Contents

Foundations of Epidemiology

1 Laying the Foundations: The Epidemiologic Approach to Disease

Epidemiology is concerned with the patterns of disease occurrence in human populations and of the factors that influence these patterns. The epidemiologist is primarily interested in the occurrence of disease by time, place, and persons. He tries to determine whether there has been an increase or decrease of the disease over the years; whether one geographical area has a higher frequency of the disease than another; and whether the characteristics of persons with a particular disease or condition distinguish them from those without it.

The personal characteristics with which the epidemiologist is concerned are the following:

1. Demographic characteristics such as age, sex, color, ethnic group.
2. Biological characteristics such as blood levels of antibodies, chemicals, enzymes; cellular constituents of the blood; measurements of physiological function of different organ systems of the body.
3. Social and economic factors such as socioeconomic status, educational background, occupation, nativity.
4. Personal habits such as tobacco and drug use, diet, physical exercise.
5. Genetic characteristics such as blood groups.

These areas of endeavor are well described by Hirsch's definition of historical and geographical pathology as a science which . . . will give, firstly, a picture of the occurrence, the distribution and the types of the diseases of mankind, in distinct epochs of time and at various points of the earth's surface; and secondly, will render an account of the relations of these diseases to the external conditions surrounding the individual and determining his manner of life. (12, 14)

This statement has commonly served as a base for defining epidemiology as "the study of the distribution of a disease or a physiological condition in human populations and of the factors that influence this distribution" (16). A more inclusive description was given by Wade Hampton Frost, one of the architects of modern epidemiology, who noted that "epidemiology is essentially an inductive science, concerned not merely with describing the distribution of disease, but equally or more with fitting it into a consistent philosophy" (12). Thus, epidemiology can be regarded as a sequence of reasoning concerned with biological inferences derived from observations of disease occurrence and related phenomena in human population groups. To this we can add that epidemiology is an integrative, eclectic discipline deriving concepts and methods from other disciplines, such as statistics, sociology, and biology, for the study of disease in populations.

A. GENERAL PURPOSES OF EPIDEMIOLOGIC STUDIES

The information obtained from an epidemiologic study can be utilized in several ways:

1. To elucidate the etiology of a specific disease or group of diseases by combining epidemiologic data with information from other disciplines such as genetics, biochemistry, and microbiology.
2. To evaluate the consistency of epidemiologic data with etiological hypotheses developed either clinically (at the bedside) or experimentally (in the laboratory).
3. To provide the basis for developing and evaluating preventive procedures and public health practices.

Examples of each of these three general purposes will be presented.

Etiological Studies of Disease

A simple example of the use of epidemiologic data to determine etiological factors would be the investigation of an outbreak of food poisoning to determine which food was contaminated with the microorganism or chemical responsible for the epidemic. Another example would be the study of a disease that occurs with higher frequency among workers in occupations exposing them to particular chemicals, as illustrated by the study of arsenic and cancer by Mabuchi (18). In this study, lists were obtained of all men who had been employed in a pesticide plant. The workers were divided into those who had been predominantly exposed to arsenical compounds and those whose major exposure was to nonarsenical chemicals. Approximately 87 percent of 1,050 male and 67 percent of 343 female employees were traced to determine their mortality experience. The observed numbers of deaths from specific causes were then compared with those expected based on the death rates of the community in which the plant was located. A significantly larger number of deaths from lung cancer was found to have occurred in the group exposed to arsenic than would have been expected; further, this relationship between lung cancer and exposure to arsenic indicated a dose-response effect, i.e., the longer an employee was exposed to arsenical compounds, the greater was his or her chance of dying from lung cancer. The investigators concluded that a causal relationship existed between exposure to arsenical compounds and lung cancer.

Only occasionally do investigators find that the increased exposure of individuals to certain agents results in a decreased frequency of disease. A classical example of this kind of relationship is that between the presence of fluorides in the water supply and dental caries. The investigation of this relationship is worth recounting, as it illustrates in concise form how a sequence of studies can be conducted to develop a preventive measure for a disease.

By the late 1930s, it had been recognized that mottled enamel of teeth was due to the use of a water supply with a high fluoride concentration (5, 7, 8). Earlier, a practicing dentist had formed a clinical impression that persons with mottled teeth had less caries than usual (2, 21, 22). This led the Public Health Service to conduct surveys of children 12–14 years of age in thirteen cities in four states where the fluoride concentration in the water supply varied considerably (6). The results indicated that dental caries decreased

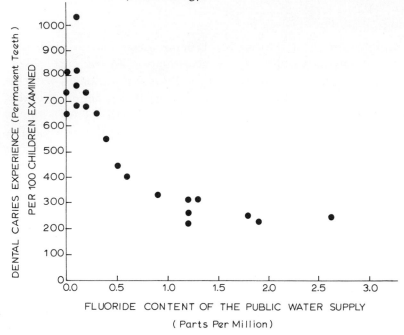

Figure 1–1. Relationship between the amount of dental caries in permanent teeth and fluoride content in the public water supply

Source: Dean, Arnold, and Elvove (6).

with increasing content of fluoride in the water, thus suggesting that the addition of fluorides to the water supply should decrease the frequency of dental caries (Fig. 1–1). This could best be demonstrated by a comparative experiment, where fluorides were added to the water supply of one community and the water supply remained untouched in a comparable community where the fluoride concentration was naturally low. The dental caries experience of school children in these communities could then be determined by periodic examinations over a number of years, and compared. Several such studies were initiated, including one comparing Kingston and Newburgh, New York (Table 1–1) (1). In the town with fluorides in the water supply, the index of dental caries (DMF) was found to be lower than in the one without fluorides. In this instance, a clinical impression led to both an epidemiologic survey and a comparative experiment, both of which demonstrated the relationship between a population characteristic, fluoride consumption, and a disease, dental caries.

Table 1–1. DMF* Teeth per 100 Children, Ages 6–16, Based on Clinical and Roentgenographic Examinations—Newburgh and Kingston, New York, 1954–1955

Age‡	Number of Children with Permanent Teeth		Number of DMF Teeth		DMF Teeth per 100 Children with Permanent Teeth§		
	Newburgh	Kingston	Newburgh	Kingston	Newburgh	Kingston	Percent Difference K–N
6–9‖	708	913	672	2,134	98.4	233.7	−57.9
10–12	521	640	1,711	4,471	328.1	698.6	−53.0
13–14	263	441	1,579	5,161	610.1	1,170.3	−47.9
15–16	109	119	1,063	1,962	975.2	1,648.7	−40.9

* DMF includes permanent teeth decayed, missing (lost subsequent to eruption), or filled.
† Sodium fluoride was added to Newburgh's water supply beginning May 2, 1945.
‡ Age at last birthday at time of examination.
§ Adjusted to age distribution of children examined in Kingston who had permanent teeth in the 1954–1955 examination.
‖ Newburgh children of this age group were exposed to fluoridated water from the time of birth.

Source: Ast and Schlesinger (1).

Table 1–2. Oral Contraceptive Practice Among Women Aged 40–44 Years Who Died from Myocardial Infarction (MI), and Controls

Oral Contraceptive Practice	Patients with Myocardial Infarction		Controls	
	No.	Percent	No.	Percent
Never used	78	73.6	86	84.3
Current users (used during month before death or during same calendar period for controls)	18	17.0 } 28 (26.4%)	7	6.9 } 16 (15.7%)
Ex-users (used only more than one month before death or during same calendar period for controls)	10	9.4	9	8.8
Total	106	100.0	102	100.0
Not known	2		8	
Comparison between users and women not currently using oral contraceptives	$\chi^2 = 4.35$; $P < 0.05$			

Source: Mann et al. (20).

Consistency with Etiological Hypotheses

The investigator attempts to determine whether an etiological hypothesis developed clinically, experimentally, or from other epidemiologic studies is consistent with the epidemiologic characteristics of the disease in a human population group(s). Many studies of the relationship between oral contraceptive use and various forms of cardiovascular disease illustrate this approach. Over a period of years, epidemiologic studies had shown a relationship between oral contraceptive use and both venous thromboembolism and thrombotic stroke (4, 27). Soon after these studies started to appear, the first of a series of case reports associated oral contraceptive use with myocardial infarction (3). This stimulated several investigators to conduct epidemiologic studies of this issue (19, 20). The statistically significant results of one recent study by Mann, Inman, and Thorogood for women aged 40–44 who died from myocardial infarction are presented in Table 1–2 (20).

Table 1–3. Frequency of Diabetes among Siblings and Parents of Diabetic Patients Admitted to the Mayo Clinic

Diabetes Status of Parents	Number Families	Siblings		
		Total	Diabetes	
			Number	Percent
Both diabetic	22	100	16	16.0
One diabetic	370	1,620	185	11.4
Neither diabetic	1,589	6,664	311	4.7
Total families	1,981	8,384	512	6.1

Source: Steinberg and Wilder (26). Reprinted by permission of The University of Chicago Press. Copyright © 1952, The American Society of Human Genetics, Waverly Press, Inc.

Basis for Preventive and Public Health Services

Perhaps the simplest example of this objective is the epidemiologic evaluation of vaccines in controlled trials in human populations, such as the national study that was conducted to establish the effectiveness of the Salk vaccine in the prevention of poliomyelitis (11). In addition to controlled trials and the other types of epidemiologic studies already mentioned, information on the population distribution of a disease in itself provides the basis for developing certain aspects of community disease control programs. Knowledge of specific etiological factors is not essential for this purpose. For example, epidemiologic data on those persons with a higher frequency of a disease or a higher risk of developing one are useful to the physician or public health administrator in indicating those segments of the population where his activities should be focused.

The familial aggregation of diabetes mellitus illustrates this point. In a study of diabetic patients admitted to the Mayo Clinic, Steinberg and Wilder obtained a history of the presence or absence of diabetes among their parents and siblings (Table 1–3) (26). Whether one hypothesizes a genetic etiological mechanism or environmental factors common to family members as an explanation for the observed familial aggregation, the higher-than-usual frequency of the disease in certain families suggests to the physician that the examination of parents and siblings of known diabetic patients will provide for the early detection of diabetes in a high-risk group of the population.

B. CONTENT OF EPIDEMIOLOGIC ACTIVITIES

Epidemiologists engage in four broad areas of study, each involving different methods: observations, "natural experiments," experimental epidemiology, and theoretical model construction.

Observational Epidemiology

This refers to the observation and analysis of the occurrence of disease in human population groups and to the inferences that can be derived about etiological factors that influence this occurrence. Appropriate methods for selecting specific groups in the population and for analyzing information obtained from them have been developed. Much of what the epidemiologist does falls into this category and, therefore, several of the later chapters as well as Appendix 1 deal with it. The studies of arsenic-exposed employees, dental caries, oral contraceptives, and familial aggregation of diabetes already cited are examples of observational investigations.

"Natural Experiments"

Occasionally, the investigator is fortunate enough to observe the occurrence of a disease under natural conditions so closely approximating a planned, controlled experiment that it is categorized as a "natural experiment." Any inferences about etiological factors derived from such situations are considerably stronger than if they had been derived solely from an observational study. The studies by Doll, Hill, and Peto in England of the relationship between tobacco use and lung cancer illustrate this approach (9, 10, 23). In 1951, these investigators ascertained the smoking habits of British male physicians, aged thirty-five and over, and followed them to determine their mortality from different causes, in particular, lung cancer. Initially, this study indicated that physicians who smoked cigarettes had a mortality rate from lung cancer that was about ten times that of nonsmoking physicians (9). Questionnaires were sent to these physicians again to determine their cigarette smoking

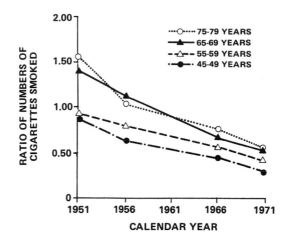

Figure 1–2. Trend in ratio of numbers of cigarettes smoked by male physicians to numbers smoked by British men of same ages, by age groups, 1951–1971

Source: Doll and Peto (10).

habits in 1956, 1966 and 1971 (10, 23). The findings of these surveys in terms of the ratio of number of cigarettes smoked by the male physicians to the numbers smoked by all British men in the same age group is shown in Figure 1–2. There was about a 50 percent decline in cigarette smoking among these male physicians. During this same period of time, the investigators continued to obtain information on the mortality experience of the physicians, comparing it with the mortality among all British men (10, 23). Figure 1–3 presents the trend of the physicians' mortality experience from lung cancer and from all other cancer as a percentage of national mortality. There was approximately a 40 percent decline in mortality from lung cancer with essentially no change in all other cancer deaths.

Experimental Epidemiology

In planned experiments, the investigator has control over the population groups he or she is studying (either human or animal) by deciding which groups are exposed to a possible etiological factor or preventive measure. The Newburgh-Kingston dental caries study, for instance, was a planned, controlled experiment. An important

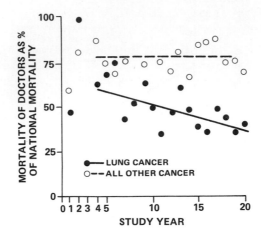

Figure 1–3. Trend in mortality of male doctors as percent of national mortality of same ages for lung cancer and all other cancer, 1951–1971

Source: Doll and Peto (10).

feature of many experiments is that the investigator can randomly allocate subjects to experimental and control groups. This method is discussed in greater detail in Chapters 10 and 11.

Theoretical Epidemiology

This involves the development of mathematical/statistical models to explain different aspects of the occurrence of a variety of diseases. With some infectious diseases, models have been generated to elucidate the reasons for outbreaks of disease, that is, epidemics. Computer usage has broadened the scope of such model building to include the simulation of epidemics. For example, the Reed-Frost model was developed to explain the relationship of various biological and social factors to the occurrence of epidemics. Other models have been devised to interpret the age distribution of cancer. Appendix 2 further explores this area.

Development and Evaluation of Study Methods

As the scope of epidemiology has been broadened to include new and/or different types of diseases, epidemiologists have had to develop new methods of study. In some cases these methods have been adapted from other disciplines, such as sociology, statistics, biology and demography. However, the appropriateness of such new methods for particular epidemiologic situations is not necessarily always apparent. Therefore, these methods need to be evaluated for different epidemiologic circumstances to determine their utility.

One often hears the statement that there are "two epidemiologies," one for infectious diseases and the other for noninfectious diseases. This is a misconception. In general, the methods used and the inferences derived are the same for both disease groups; this will be illustrated throughout our discussions. The reader should note that epidemiology is essentially a *comparative* discipline. It is mainly concerned with studying diseases and related phenomena at different time periods, in different places and among different types of people (i.e., "time, place, and persons") and then comparing them. This approach is used for all categories of disease, infectious and noninfectious alike (17).

C. THE SEQUENCE OF EPIDEMIOLOGIC REASONING

Epidemiology was defined at the beginning of this chapter in terms of a reasoning process. The observational study, one of the major tools of epidemiology, affords an excellent view of the reasoning process by which one achieves the objective of elucidating etiological factors of a disease. Basically, the epidemiologist uses a two-stage sequence of reasoning:

1. The determination of a statistical association between a characteristic and a disease.
2. The derivation of biological inferences from such a pattern of statistical associations.

The methods used to determine the statistical associations fall into one of two broadly defined categories:

a) Associations based on group characteristics.
b) Associations based on individual characteristics.

Although there is a certain degree of overlap between these two groups, their distinction has proved to be extremely useful.

In studying *group* characteristics, the epidemiologist concentrates on the comparison of the mortality and/or morbidity experience from a given disease in different population groups in the hope that any observed differences can be related to differences in the local environment, in personal living habits, or even in the genetic composition of these groups. In these studies, information on the characteristics of the individual members of the population groups is not usually obtained. Generally, existing mortality and morbidity statistics are utilized. For example, let us assume that Community A has a higher mortality rate from cancer of the liver than Community B. Furthermore, Community A is engaged primarily in mining, while Community B is engaged in agriculture. The comparison would suggest that mining may be of etiological importance in liver cancer. Usually, the results of such studies provide *clues* to etiological hypotheses and serve as a basis for more detailed investigations. Such an observed relationship, generally termed an "ecological correlation," may suffer from an **"ecological fallacy,"** that is, the two communities differ in many other factors, and one or more of those may be the underlying reason for the differences in their observed mortality or morbidity experience (13, 24, 25). The various types of studies of group characteristics will be discussed in Chapters 4–7.

After an association has been established in either a study of group characteristics, or when a lead has been developed from either clinical studies of patients, experimental work, or other sources, the investigator will attempt to determine whether this association is also present within *individuals*. He will seek answers to such questions as:

1. Do persons with the disease have the characteristic more frequently than those without the disease?
2. Do persons with the characteristic develop the disease more frequently than those who do not have the characteristic?

Such associations are established by cross-sectional, retrospective, and prospective studies, which will be discussed in Chapters 8 and 9.

These two general methods of determining statistical associations —those between groups and those within individuals—must be distinguished, since a relationship derived from a study of individuals is less likely to result from an ecological fallacy and is, therefore, more likely to be biologically significant than one derived from a study of group characteristics. Conversely, an association derived from studies of groups has a greater likelihood of being the result of a third common factor.

D. AN EXAMPLE OF THE EPIDEMIOLOGIC APPROACH

The essentials of the epidemiologic approach in determining the specific etiological agent of a disease are perhaps best demonstrated by the investigation of the origin of a food poisoning outbreak. This usually includes ascertaining whether a statistical association is found between the consumption of a specific food at some event and the specific form of the disease. This is accomplished by computing food-specific attack rates, defined as follows:

$$\text{Food-specific attack rate} = \frac{\text{Number of persons who ate a specific food and became ill}}{\text{Total number of persons who ate the specific food}},$$

and comparing them with attack rates for those who had not eaten the specific food. The report of a salmonellosis outbreak caused by the bacteria, *Salmonella infantis, Salmonella agona,* and *Salmonella schwarzengrund* illustrates this approach (15).

The events investigated were a picnic sponsored by a local business firm, catered by a bar-restaurant, and a smorgasbord catered by the same bar-restaurant, which were attended by a total of 173 persons. A number of people who had attended either or both of these events developed salmonellosis. On September 14, 1973, shortly after the events, eight of these people were hospitalized. The physician for seven of those hospitalized thought that the symptoms were suspicious and notified local and state health officials, who then initiated an epidemiologic investigation.

The food preparers were interviewed regarding both these meals and who ate them. From the business firm, the bar-restaurant owner and the attendees themselves, it was determined who had eaten food at the picnic and the smorgasbord. All of the 40 persons who ate only at the picnic, 71 of the 118 who ate only at the smorgasbord, and 10 of the 15 who ate at both events were questioned. A crude attack rate was computed:

$$\text{Crude attack rate} = \frac{\text{Number of persons ill with disease}}{\text{Number of persons attending the event}}.$$

Of the 121 persons interviewed, 90 had become ill; however, 5 of those ill became ill before the meal, and therefore were removed from both the numerator and denominator. Since not all the attendees at each of the events were interviewed, one must assume that those interviewed are a representative *sample* of all those who had attended that event. Hence, one can estimate the number who became ill among those who attended each of both events; this is shown in Table 1–4. Since the total estimated number of ill persons was 129, the overall crude attack rate is 129/173 or 75 percent. Food-specific attack rates were also computed for each event (Tables 1–5 and 1–6). These tabulations show a definite statistical association between salmonellosis and potato salad at the picnic and salmonellosis and potato salad and/or chicken dressing at the smorgasbord. Additional analysis of the attack rates at the smorgasbord showed very high rates for those who consumed the chicken dressing (88 percent), the potato salad (88 percent), or both (90 percent), while those who consumed neither of these foods had a very low attack rate (20 percent). Since all but one person interviewed ate chicken at each event, one cannot rule out chicken as another vehicle of transmission. This additional analysis strengthened the inference that there was an etiological relationship between chicken dressing and/or potato salad consumption and salmonellosis.

Clinical and laboratory investigations were conducted to identify the specific forms of salmonellosis. The major clinical symptoms were diarrhea, abdominal pains or cramps, chills, and fever; headache and nausea or vomiting were reported less frequently. Symptoms lasted from two to eight days. The time of onset for those who ate only one meal ranged from 6 to 66 hours from the time of eating, with a median period (the "incubation period") of 23 hours.

Laboratory examinations were carried out on stool specimens obtained from 11 persons who were hospitalized. *Salmonella infantis* was cultured from stools of nine patients, *S. agona* from the stools of five of the same patients, and *S. schwarzengrund* from the stool of one of these five patients. Among ten others who were ill but not hospitalized, *S. infantis* was isolated from the stools of nine; and *S. schwarzengrund* from one of these five.

These data showed that the consumption of chicken and potato salad was associated with three separate organisms leading to the

Table 1-4. Estimation of Number of Ill Persons for Calculation of Crude Attack Rate

	Number of Persons at the Event (1)	Number Interviewed (2)	Number Excluded (became ill before meal) (3)	Adjusted Number Interviewed (4)	Number Ill Among Those Interviewed (5)	Attack Rate (5)/(4) = (6)	Estimated Number of Ill Persons (1) × (6) = (7)
Ate at picnic only	40	40	1	39	25	64%	26
Ate at smorgasbord only	118	71	4	67	50	75%	88
Ate at both meals	15	10	0	10	10	100%	15

Total estimated number of ill persons = 26 + 88 + 15 = 129

Source: Adapted from Levy et al. (15).

Table 1–5. Food-specific Attack Rates for Picnic (No. = 41: 27 ill, 14 not ill)*

Food Items Served	Persons Who Ate Specified Food				Persons Who Did Not Eat Specified Food				Difference in Attack Rates
	Ill (1)	Not Ill (2)	Total (3)	Attack Rate (%) (4)	Ill (5)	Not Ill (6)	Total (7)	Attack Rate (%) (8)	(4) − (8) = (9)†
Chicken	27	14	41	66	0	0	0	–	–
Potato salad	23	5	28	82	3	9	12	25	57%‡
Beets	1	0	1	100	25	10	35	71	29%
Cole slaw	17	7	24	71	5	5	10	50	21%
Baked beans	19	8	27	70	4	4	8	50	20%
Coffee	16	7	23	70	11	7	18	61	9%
Butter	20	10	30	67	5	2	7	71	−4%
Bread	14	7	21	67	12	5	17	71	−4%
Olives	7	4	11	64	19	8	27	70	−6%

* The total of those who ate and did not eat a specific food item does not always equal 41 because those not sure of having eaten a specific food item were excluded from this table.

† The difference in attack rates ranged from −14% to −74% for corn, beer, tomatoes, green beans, ham, and cucumbers and are not shown here.

‡ The difference between attack rates of those who ate potato salad and those who did not is statistically significant (P < .001) by Fisher's exact test. All other differences are not statistically significant.

Source: Levy et al. (15).

Table 1-6. Food-specific Attack Rates for Smorgasbord (No. = 67: 50 ill, 17 not ill)*

Food Items Served	Persons Who Ate Specified Food				Persons Who Did Not Eat Specified Food				Difference in Attack Rate
	Ill (1)	Not Ill (2)	Total (3)	Attack Rate (%) (4)	Ill (5)	Not Ill (6)	Total (7)	Attack Rate (%) (8)	(4) − (8) = (9)†
Chicken	49	16	65	75	0	1	1	0	75%
Chicken dressing	37	5	42	88	11	11	22	50	38%‡
Potato salad	37	5	42	88	11	9	20	55	33%‡
Coffee	32	7	39	82	16	9	25	64	18%
Bean salad	15	3	18	83	30	14	44	68	15%
Cole slaw	27	7	34	79	17	9	26	65	14%
Rigatoni	30	8	38	79	18	9	27	67	12%
Olives	15	4	19	79	32	12	44	73	6%
Scalloped potatoes	21	7	28	75	23	9	32	72	3%
Baked beans	21	7	28	75	27	10	37	73	2%
Cucumbers	14	5	19	74	32	12	44	73	1%
Ham	39	14	53	74	9	3	12	75	−1%

* The total of those who ate and did not eat a specific food does not equal 67 because those not sure of having eaten a specific food item were excluded from this table.

† The difference in attack rates ranged from −3% to −35% for bread, butter, tomatoes, tossed salad with french dressing, pickles, fruit gelatin, pickled beets and apple ring and are not shown in table.

‡ The differences between attack rates of those who ate chicken dressing and those who did not and between attack rates of those who ate potato salad and those who did not are each statistically significant (P <.01 for each) by chi-square tests. All other differences are not statistically significant.

Source: Levy et al. (15).

19

development of salmonellosis. It appears that the potato salad was contaminated by being placed in a pan in which the chicken had been prepared earlier. The association was strengthened by the results of an environmental investigation of the chicken farm co-operative that supplied the poultry. The chickens used for both events were traced to three farms in the cooperative (Farms A, B, and C). One feed sample from Farm A grew *S. cubana,* and one of the four composite pellet feed samples from Farm B grew *S. typhimurium.* Although the salmonella serotypes in the feed samples differed from those isolated in the outbreak, the outbreak serotypes might have been isolated from the feed if the chicken farms had been investigated immediately after the outbreak.

In summary, the findings were:

1. Chickens at Farms A, B, and/or C were fed with salmonella-contaminated feed;
2. The chicken dressing probably became contaminated with salmonella when it was prepared in plastic pans from which raw chicken pieces (from Farms A, B, and/or C) had recently been removed;
3. The chicken dressing was not properly heated prior to the picnic; and
4. The potato salad became contaminated when it was placed in a container that had also held contaminated chicken pieces.

The pattern of statistical associations and the events surrounding the preparation of the food clearly implicated the chicken dressing and potato salad, contaminated with *Salmonellae,* as the cause of this epidemic.

STUDY PROBLEMS

1. What is the epidemiologic significance of the expression "time, place, persons"?
2. What is an "ecological fallacy"? Why is it important to the epidemiologist?
3. Wade Hampton Frost stated in 1936:

Epidemiology at any given time is something more than the total of its established facts. It includes their orderly arrangement into chains of inference which extend more or less beyond the bounds of direct observation.

What did Frost mean by this statement?

4. What is the difference between the crude attack rate, food-specific attack rate, and salmonellosis attack rate? What is the general form of an attack rate?
5. Why should the epidemiologist be interested in population-based statistics, such as mortality rates? Why should he also be cautious in their use?
6. What is an incubation period? Do diseases commonly known as "noninfectious diseases," such as cancer and stroke, have an incubation period?

REFERENCES

1. Ast, D.B., and Schlesinger, E.R. 1956. "The conclusion of a ten-year study of water fluoridation." *Amer. J. Pub. Health* 46:265–271.
2. Black, G.V., and McKay, F.S. 1916. "Mottled teeth: An endemic developmental imperfection of the teeth, heretofore unknown in the literature of dentistry." *Dent. Cosmos* 58:129–156.
3. Boyce, J., Fawcett, J.W., and Neal, E.W.P. 1963. "Coronary thrombosis and conovid." *Lancet* 1:111.
4. Collaborative Group for the Study of Stroke in Young Women. 1973. "Oral contraception and increased risk of cerebral ischemia or thrombosis." *N. Engl. J. Med.* 288:871–878.
5. Dean, H.T. 1938. "Endemic fluorosis and its relation to dental caries." *Publ. Health Reps.* 54:1443–1452.
6. ———, Arnold, F.A., Jr., and Elvove, E. 1942. "Domestic water and dental caries. V. Additional studies of the relation of fluoride domestic waters to dental caries experience in 4,425 white children, aged 12 to 14 years, of 13 cities in 4 states." *Pub. Health Reps.* 57:1155–1179.
7. ———, and Elvove, E. 1936. "Some epidemiological aspects of chronic endemic dental fluorosis." *Amer. J. Pub. Health* 26:567–575.
8. ———, Jay, P., Arnold, F.A., Jr., McClure, F.J., and Elvove, E. 1939. "Domestic water and dental caries, including certain epidemiological aspects of oral L. acidophilus." *Pub. Health Reps.* 54:862–888.
9. Doll, R., and Hill, A.B. 1950. "Smoking and carcinoma of the lung: Preliminary report." *Brit. Med. J.* 2:739–748.
10. ———, and Peto, R. 1976. "Mortality in relation to smoking: 20 years' observations on male British doctors." *Brit. Med. J.* 2:1525–1536.
11. Francis, T., Jr., Korns, R.F., Voight, R.B., Boisen, M., Hemphill, F.M., Napier, J.A., and Tolchinsky, E. 1955. "An evaluation of the 1954 poliomyelitis vaccine trials: Summary report." *Amer. J. Pub. Health* 45:1–63.
12. Frost, W.H., 1941. "Epidemiology." In *Papers of Wade Hampton Frost, M.D.* K. E. Maxcy, ed., New York: The Commonwealth Fund, pp. 493–542.

13. Goodman, L.A. 1953. "Ecological regressions and behavior of individuals." *Amer. Soc. Rev.* 18:663–664.
14. Hirsch, A. 1883. *Handbook of Geographical and Historical Pathology, Vol. I.* London: New Sydenham Society.
15. Levy, B.S., McIntire, W., Damsky, L., Lashbrook, R., Hawk, J., Jacobsen, G.S., and Newton, B. 1975. "The Middleton outbreak: 125 cases of food-borne salmonellosis resulting from cross-contaminated food items served at a picnic and a smorgasbord." *Amer. J. Epid.* 101:502–511.
16. Lilienfeld, D.E. 1978. "Definitions of epidemiology." *Amer. J. Epidemiol.* 107:87–90.
17. Lilienfeld, A.M. 1973. "Epidemiology of infectious and non-infectious disease: Some comparisons." *Amer. J. Epid.* 97:135–147.
18. Mabuchi, K. 1978. Occupational exposure to arsenic and cancer: A study in pesticide workers. Dr.P.H. Dissertation, Baltimore, Md.: The Johns Hopkins University.
19. Mann, J.I., Doll, R., Thorogood, M., Vessey, M.P., and Waters, W.E. 1976. "Risk factors for myocardial infarction in young women." *Brit. J. Prev. and Soc. Med.* 30:94–100.
20. ———, Inman, W.H., and Thorogood, M. 1976. "Oral contraceptive use in older women and fatal myocardial infarction." *Brit. Med. J.* 2:445–447.
21. McKay, F.S. 1925. "Mottled enamel: A fundamental problem in dentistry." *Dent. Cosmos* 67:847–860.
22. ———, and Black, G.V. 1916. "An investigation of mottled teeth." *Dent. Cosmos* 58:477–484.
23. Report of the Royal College of Physicians. 1971. *Smoking and Health Now.* London: Pitman Medical and Scientific Publishing Co.
24. Robinson, W.S. 1950. "Ecological correlations and the behavior of individuals." *Amer. Soc. Rev.* 15:351–357.
25. Selvin, H.C. 1958. "Durkeim's suicide and problems of empirical research." *Amer. J. Soc.* 63:607–619.
26. Steinberg, A.G., and Wilder, R.M. 1952. "A study of the genetics of diabetes mellitus." *Amer. J. Human Genet.* 4:113–135.
27. Vessey, M.P., and Mann, J.I. 1978. "Female sex hormones and thrombosis. Epidemiological aspects." *Brit. Med. Bull.* 34:157–162.

2 Threads of Epidemiologic History

> The more extensive a man's knowledge of what has been done, the greater will be his power of knowing what to do.
>
> BENJAMIN DISRAELI

The development of epidemiology has spanned many centuries. As an eclectic discipline, epidemiology has borrowed from sociology, demography, and statistics, as well as other fields of study. Hence, the reader should not be surprised to learn that its history is interwoven with that of other scientific disciplines. It was not until the nineteenth century that the fabric of epidemiology was finally woven into a distinct discipline with its own philosophy, concepts, and methods.

This chapter will focus on the growth of two major components of epidemiology's conceptual framework: 1) the idea that the environment (with its biological, chemical, physical, and social components) plays a significant role in determining the occurrence of disease and 2) the epidemiologic study.

A. THE ENVIRONMENT

The general concept that the environment influences disease occurrence had its origin in antiquity, and so did a more specific idea that many diseases are contagious.

The first is stated in the Hippocratic work *On Airs, Waters, and Places,* which stresses the importance of considering the variety of environmental influences on diseases in humans (25):

Whoever wishes to investigate medicine properly, should proceed thus: in the first place to consider the seasons of the year, and what effects each of them produces (for they are not all alike, but differ much from themselves in regard to their changes). Then the winds, the hot and the cold, especially such as are common to all countries, and then such as are peculiar to each locality. We must also consider the qualities of the waters, for as they differ from one another in taste and weight, so also do they differ much in their qualities. In the same manner, when one comes into a city to which he is a stranger, he ought to consider its situation, how it lies as to the winds and the rising of the sun; for its influence is not the same whether it lies to the north or the south, to the rising or to the setting sun. These things one ought to consider most attentively, and concerning the waters which the inhabitants use, whether they be marshy and soft, or hard, and running from elevated and rocky situations, and then if saltish and unfit for cooking; and the ground, whether it be naked and deficient in water, or wooded and well watered, and whether it lies in a hollow, confined situation, or is elevated and cold; and the mode in which the inhabitants live, and what are their pursuits, whether they are fond of drinking and eating to excess, and given to indolence, or are fond of exercise and labor, and not given to excess in eating and drinking. Copyright © 1939, Williams and Wilkins Co., Baltimore.

The idea that disease is caused by a contagium vivum (a living contagion) necessarily depended upon the development of two other concepts: the specificity of both diseases and their causes, and the existence of microscopic organisms. Though the germ theory is relatively modern (it was definitely established only about a century ago), some practices commonly associated with it are truly ancient in their origin; for example, the custom of isolating people with contagious diseases is recorded in the Bible and was continued by the Catholic Church during the Middle Ages. Girolamo Fracastoro (1478–1553), an Italian, is usually credited with being the first to state explicitly that specific diseases directly result from specific contagions (17, 57). His *De Contagione* (1546) presented the first general theory of contagion for epidemic diseases (17). Fracastoro, however, did not have any notion of microorganisms (3, 47, 51). Several of his contemporaries expressed similar ideas, and one of them, Girolamo Cardano, stated in 1557 that "the seeds of disease were minute animals, capable of reproducing their kind" (52).

Early in the seventeenth century, the microscope was invented. Almost 20 years before Leeuwenhoek discovered microorganisms in 1683 by using the microscope, Kircher generalized Cardano's concept into a theory of contagium vivum for epidemic diseases (47, 57). In *Scrutinium Pestis* (1658), Kircher referred to "true latent germs" and claimed to have seen living microorganisms in the blood of victims of the bubonic plague (it is only *now* believed that he saw only red blood cells) (57). His ideas attracted widespread support in other publications and were accepted by such prominent physicians as William Harvey (51, 52).

During the early 1700s, an alternative explanation for the origin of epidemics, "the miasma theory," developed; this idea was based on the notion that when the air was of a "bad quality" (a state that was not precisely defined but was supposedly due to decaying organic matter), the persons breathing that air would become ill; "malaria" means "bad air." It is commonly believed that the acceptance of the miasma theory led to the total abandonment of the contagium vivum idea. However, the contagium vivum theory was still very much alive during the eighteenth century; Plenciz was its principal, though not its sole, proponent (47). Its strength is indicated both by the belief that there was an incubation period for diseases and by the widespread practice of smallpox inoculation (3, 51, 54). Neither the idea of an incubation period nor the use of smallpox inoculation was as consistent with the miasma theory as with the contagium vivum theory.

Cogressi used the contagium vivum concept in 1714 to explain the bovine epizootic then afflicting Italian herds (4). In *LaNuova Idea Del Mal Contagiosos de Boui,* he alluded to Leeuwenhoek's discovery, while also speculating on mechanisms of immunity and transmission. Corte and many other Italians adopted the contagium vivum doctrine after the Marseilles plague epidemic in 1720. It appeared to be the only scientifically consistent explanation for the epidemic. Several of Corte's contemporaries supported the contagium vivum doctrine, and in 1726 one of them, Boile, gave "public microscopic demonstrations" of specific disease-causing "animalcules" in Paris (4).

The leading eighteenth century American exponent of contagium vivum was a New England clergyman, Cotton Mather, an early advocate of smallpox inoculation. Proposing in *The Angel of Bethesda* that smallpox was caused by "animalcula," he used his knowledge of the work of Kircher, Leeuwenhoek, and others to infer the concept of a germ theory of disease (41, 51). *The Angel of Bethesda* was not published; however, other publications, including some of Mather's other writings, suggest that the idea was widely accepted (3). Indeed, Benjamin Rush, one of the eighteenth century's leading physicians, generally viewed as a staunch miasmatist, was originally a contagionist; he adopted the miasma theory only when the contagium vivum hypothesis, as it had then been developed, failed to account for the seemingly bizarre yellow fever epidemics that plagued North America (58).

After 1800, in the pre-Pasteur era, significant contributions to the contagium vivum theory were made by Agostino Bassi, an Italian lawyer, Pierre-François Bretonneau, a French physician, and Jacob Henle, a German anatomist. Bassi "proved by careful experimentation that disease could be produced by small organisms growing within the host" (39). In his studies of muscardine, a silkworm disease, Bassi reasoned in 1816 that (39):

> Not having succeeded with so many and different methods in producing in silkworms the disease muscardine, except with the use of true calcined (diseased) worm, I decided that it did not develop spontaneously in this insect, and therefore, there must be an extraneous germ which, entering from without, grows; and I decided to follow the traces of this fatal thing; and to discover its true nature and its habits and all the ways by which it is introduced into the silkworm causing in it this terrible disease.

Bassi discovered this "fatal thing" to be a fungus and was honored for his discovery by the European scientific community (30). In *Des Inflammations Spéciales du Tissue Muqueux* (1826), Pierre-François Bretonneau demonstrated a "clear concept that communicable diseases are specific and that this specificity is determined in large measure by the nature of the disease cause" (47). In 1840, Henle summarized the complete doctrine of contagium vivum, presenting for the first time all of the scientific evidence for and against the doctrine (46).

In 1851, the *Lancet* published excerpts of a paper presented to the London Epidemiological Society by John Grove, "On the Nature of Epidemics," in which he stated (22): "Whether we examine an epidemic or infectious disease of plants, of animals, or of man, we find that the essence of the affection is something which has the power of reproducing its own species." He viewed this faculty of reproduction as "indicating the existence of a germ and classed the agents of disease among living things deducing the impossibility of accounting for epidemics and infections upon the chemical basis, seeing that in no purely chemical process was there any multiplication of the agents" (22). In an 1853 paper, "On Contagion and Infection in Relation to Epidemic Diseases," Grove stated: "Wherever the agents of communicable diseases have been demonstrated, they have uniformly been shown to depend upon some form of cell-life" (23).

Thus, by the mid-1800s, almost 25 years before Pasteur, the contagium vivum doctrine was espoused by many European scientists (30). Indeed, there is evidence that it was the scientific basis for the initiation of the filtration of part of the London water supply in 1829 (30). During the "Greening of Epidemiology," in the mid-1800s, the contagium vivum theory and the evolving epidemiologic study merged; thus began the current era of epidemiology (33).

B. THE EPIDEMIOLOGIC STUDY

As noted in Chapter 1 (p. 13), the essence of the epidemiologic study is the comparison of groups of people with regard to a characteristic of interest. The earliest recorded account of such a comparison is, interestingly enough, found in the Old Testament in the first chapter of the Book of Daniel (53):

1. In the third year of the reign of Jehoiakim king of Judah came Nebuchadnezzar king of Babylon unto Jerusalem, and besieged it. . . .
3. And the king spoke unto Ashpenaz his chief officer, that he should bring in certain of the children of Israel, and of the seed royal, and of the nobles. . . .
5. And the king appointed for them a daily portion of the king's food, and of the wine which he drank that they should be nourished for three years. . . .
8. But Daniel purposed in his heart that he would not defile himself with the king's food, nor with the wine which he drank; therefore he requested of the chief of the officers that he might not defile himself. . . .
10. And, the chief of officers said unto Daniel: "I fear my lord the king who hath appointed your food and your drink; for why should he see your faces sad in comparison with the youths of your own age?" . . .

11. Then said Daniel to the steward. . . .

12. Try thy servants, I beseech thee, ten days; and let them give us pulse (leguminous plants) to eat and water to drink. . . .

13. Then let our countenances be looked upon before thee, and the countenances of the youths that eat of the king's food. . . .

14. So, he hearkened unto them and tried them in this matter, and tried them ten days. . . .

15. And at the end of ten days their countenances appeared fairer, and they were fatter in the flesh, than all the youths that did eat of the king's food.

The underlying logic for the modern form of the epidemiologic study evolved from the Scientific Revolution of the 1600s, which indicated that the orderly behavior of the physical universe could be expressed in terms of mathematical relationships (40). During this period, Francis Bacon developed the basis of inductive logic and, with it, the concept of "inductive laws" (11). Many seventeenth century scientists reasoned that if mathematical relationships could be found to *describe, analyze,* and *understand* the physical universe, then similar relationships, known as *"laws of mortality,"* must exist in the biological world (33, 42). Laws of mortality were considered to be generalized statements about the relationships between disease (as manifested by mortality) and man. These laws formed the basis of the life table (see below), which attempted to both quantitate and express them mathematically. From this philosophical base, the epidemiologic study evolved.

For specific aspects of disease, such as epidemics, attempts were made to formulate "laws of epidemics." In fact, the contagium vivum theory was regarded in a like manner. It was a generalization of the observed facts that several diseases (smallpox, measles, cholera) were thought to be caused by contagia viva.

Inspired by Bacon's writings, the Royal Society of London was founded in 1662. Its initial members included Robert Boyle, the formulator of Boyle's Law, William Petty, one of the founders of economics, and John Graunt, a tradesman who was a close friend of Petty and one of the Society's financial patrons. That same year, Graunt published his *Natural and Political Observations Mentioned in a Following Index and Made Upon the Bills of Mortality,* a pioneering work in the comparative study of mortality and morbidity in human populations (20, 36).

An intellectually curious man, Graunt collected the Bills of Mor-

Table 2–1. Life Table of Deaths in London Adapted from Graunt's "Observations"

Exact Age	Deaths	Survivors
0	—	100
6	36	64
16	24	40
26	15	25
36	9	16
46	6	10
56	4	6
66	3	3
76	2	1
80	1	0

Source: Graunt (20).

tality, which had been initiated in 1603 by the parish clerks, in London and in a parish town of Hampshire. After organizing the published Bills, he derived from them inferences about mortality and fertility in the human population, noting the usual excess of male births, the high infant mortality, and the seasonal variation in mortality. Graunt attempted to distinguish two broad causes of mortality, the acute and the "chronical diseases," and to discern urban-rural differences in mortality. From collected data, he constructed the first known life table, summarizing the mortality experience in terms of the number, percent, or probability of living or dying over a lifetime, a truly outstanding achievement (Table 2–1). Further, Graunt noted that one could attempt to formulate a law of mortality from such tables; he proposed that each country should prepare similar tables so that they could be compared to construct a general law of mortality (36). Reviewing Graunt's work at the tercentenary of the publication of his *Observations,* D.V. Glass said (19):

> But, whatever the particular and varying emphases, demographers in general would agree that probably the most outstanding qualities of Graunt's work are first, the search for regularities and configurations in mortality and fertility; and secondly, the attention given—and usually shown explicitly—to the errors and ambiguities of the inadequate data used in that search. Graunt did not wait for better statistics; he did what he could with what was available to him. And by

so doing, he also produced a much stronger case for supplying better data.

As mathematical principles developed during the late 1600s and early 1700s, Graunt's ideas were refined and extended. During this period, the idea of using comparative groups in studies also began to emerge. The control group was initially viewed as another group in which a law of mortality, formulated from a different ("experimental" or "study") group, could be tested. In light of this development, it is not surprising that two noteworthy epidemiologic papers, each the first of its kind, appeared in the middle of the eighteenth century.

The first, a report of an experiment, was published in 1747 by James Lind, who had developed certain hypotheses from epidemiologic observations regarding the etiology and treatment of scurvy (35). He decided to evaluate these hypotheses in the following way:

On the 20th of May, 1747, I took twelve patients in the scurvey, on board the SALISBURY at sea. Their cases were as similiar as I could have them. They all in general had putrid gums, the spots and lassitude, with weakness of their knees. They lay together in one place, being a proper apartment for the sick in the fore-hold; and had one diet common to all, viz., water-gruel sweetened with sugar in the morning; fresh mutton broth often times for dinner; at other times puddings, boiled biscuit with sugar, etc.; and for supper, barley and raisins, rice and currents, sago and wine, or the like. Two of these were ordered each a quart of cyder a day. Two others took twenty-five gutts of elixir vitriol three times a day, upon an empty stomach; using a gargle strongly acidulated with it for their mouths. Two others took two spoonsful of vinegar three times a day, upon an empty stomach; having their gruels and their other food well acidulated with it, as also the gargle for their mouth. Two of the worst patients, with the tendons in the ham rigid (a symptom none of the rest had), were put under a course of sea water. Of this, they drank half a pint every day, and sometimes more or less as it operated by way of a gentle physic. Two others had each two oranges and one lemon given them every day. These they eat with greediness, at different times, upon an empty stomach. They continued but six days under this course, having consumed the quantity that could be spared. The two remaining patients took the bigness of a nutmeg three times a day, of an electuary recommended by a hospital-surgeon, made of garlic, mustard seed, rad raphan, balsam of Peru, and gum myrrh;

using for common drink, barley-water well acidulated with tamarinds; by a decoction of which, with the addition of cremor tartar, they were gently purged three or four times during the course.

The consequence was, that the most sudden and visible good effects were perceived from the use of the oranges and lemons; one of those who had taken them being at the end of six days fit for duty. The spots were not indeed at that time quite off his body, nor his gums sound; but without any other medicine, than a gargarism of elixir vitriol, he became quite healthy before we came into Plymouth, which was on the 16th of June. The other was the best recovered of any in his condition; and being now deemed pretty well, was appointed nurse to the rest of the sick.

From these results, Lind inferred that citric acid fruits cured the scurvy and that this would also provide a means of prevention. The British Navy eventually accepted his analysis, requiring the inclusion of limes or lime juice in the diet on ships from 1795; hence, the nicknaming of British seamen as "limeys."

The other paper, an epidemiologic analysis, was published in 1760 by Daniel Bernoulli, a member of the noted European family of mathematicians (5). Having evaluated the available evidence, Bernoulli concluded that inoculation protected against smallpox and conferred life-long immunity. Using a life table, not unlike those of today, he determined that inoculation at birth would increase life expectancy.

The French Revolution at the end of the eighteenth century had a far-reaching influence on epidemiology. It stimulated an interest in public health and preventive medicine, thereby facilitating the development of the epidemiologic approach to disease. Furthermore, it permitted several individuals from the lower classes to assume positions of leadership in medicine. One such person was Pierre Charles-Alexandre Louis, one of the first modern epidemiologists. Louis was very much aware of the need for discovering laws of nature in medicine, as he indicated in a letter dated March 22, 1833 (6, 27):

Think for a moment, Sir, of the position in which we physicians are placed. We have no legislative chambers to enact laws for us. We are our own lawgivers; or rather we must discover the laws on which our profession rests. We must *discover* them and not invent them; for the laws of nature are not to be invented.

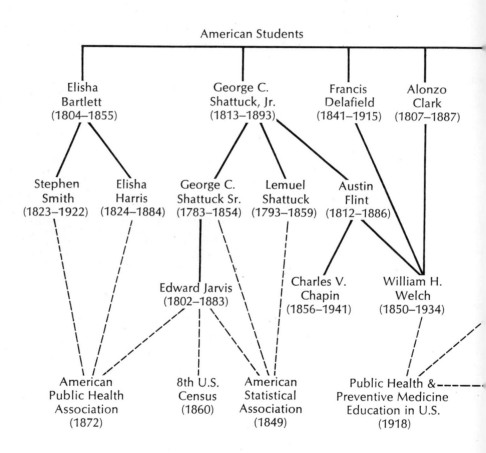

Daniel Bernoulli
(1700–1782)

Simeon D. Poisson
(1781–1840)

American Students

Elisha
Bartlett
(1804–1855)

George C.
Shattuck, Jr.
(1813–1893)

Francis
Delafield
(1841–1915)

Alonzo
Clark
(1807–1887)

Stephen
Smith
(1823–1922)

Elisha
Harris
(1824–1884)

George C.
Shattuck Sr.
(1783–1854)

Lemuel
Shattuck
(1793–1859)

Austin
Flint
(1812–1886)

Edward Jarvis
(1802–1883)

Charles V.
Chapin
(1856–1941)

William H.
Welch
(1850–1934)

American
Public Health
Association
(1872)

8th U.S.
Census
(1860)

American
Statistical
Association
(1849)

Public Health &
Preventive Medicine
Education in U.S.
(1918)

Epidemiology, Statistics, and Public Health in the United States

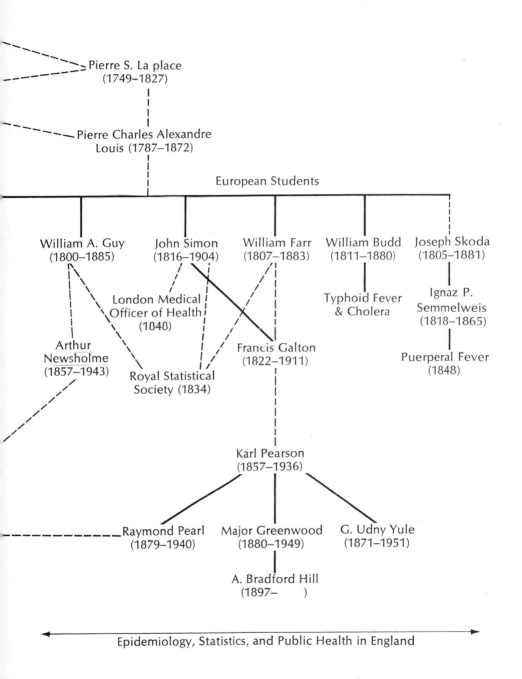

Figure 2–1. Influence of Louis on the Development of Epidemiology, Statistics, and Public Health in Europe and the United States.

Table 2–2. Examples of William Farr's Understanding of Epidemiologic Concepts

Epidemiologic Concept	Farr's Statement
Scope of epidemiology	"The causes that make the rates of mortality vary may be considered under two heads— (1) Causes inherent in the population itself, such, for example, as *sex* and *age*. (2) Causes outside the population, such as air, water, food, clothing, dwellings, or such groups of causes as are involved in residence, and relation of the several parts to each other in time and space."
Person-years	"A year of life is the lifetime unit. It is represented by one person living through a year; or by two persons living through half a year."
Relationship of death rate and probability of dying (or living)	"The rate of mortality serves to give the probability of living a year."
Standardized mortality rate	"[If] the number of boys under 5 years of age was 147,390, the annual rate of mortality in the healthy districts [the standard population] was .04348; . . . 6367 deaths which would have happened in London . . . continuing the process . . . the mortality in London should [be] 15 in 1,000."
Dose-response effect	"The effects are in some regulated proportion to the intensity of the causes."

Louis conducted several observational studies, the most famous of which demonstrated that bloodletting was not efficacious in the treatment of disease and, thus, helped reverse a trend toward its increasing use in medical practice (37). His approach to epidemiology is illustrated by a comment, in 1836, on the question of the inheritance of phthisis (tuberculosis) (38): "To determine the question satisfactorily, tables of mortality [life tables] would be necessary, comparing an equal number of persons born of phthisical parents with those in an opposite condition." Louis was not the first to use statistical methods in medicine, which he termed "la méthode numerique," but he pioneered in emphasizing their importance in medicine (29, 33, 50).

Louis was a well-known teacher with students from both England and the United States. His influence was international, and had an astounding impact on the growth of epidemiology that extends

Table 2–2 cont.

Epidemiologic Concept	Farr's Statement
Need for large numbers of population and biological inferences	"When the number of cases is considerable the relative mortality is most correctly expressed and . . . slight differences deserve little attention."
Herd immunity	"The small-pox would be . . . sometimes arrested, by vaccination which protected a part of the population."
Prevalence = incidence × duration	"In estimating the prevalence of disease, two things must be distinctly considered; the relative frequency of their attacks, and the relative proportion of sick-time they produce. The first may be determined at once, by a comparison of the number of attacks with the numbers living; the second by enumerating several times the living and the actually sick of each disease, and thence deducing the mean proportion suffering constantly. Time is here taken into account: and the sick-time, if the attacks of two diseases be equal, will vary as their duration varies, and whatever the number of attacks may be, multiplying them by the mean duration of each disease will give the sick-time."
Retrospective and prospective studies	"Is your inquiry to be retrospective or prospective? If the former the replies will be general, vague, and I fear of little value."

Source: Lilienfeld and Lilienfeld (32).

even to the present (31–34) (Fig. 2–1). Two of Louis's students, William Augustus Guy and William Farr, were instrumental in the development of epidemiology in England in the mid-1800s. They became intimately associated with the relatively young Statistical Society of London, predecessor of the present Royal Statistical Society and eventually both were to serve as its President (33). Guy became Dean of the King's College Medical School and was among the pioneers in the public health movement in England (8, 34). Farr, as the first Compiler of Abstracts of the Registrar General's Office, organized the first modern vital statistics system (15). His understanding of epidemiologic ideas was outstanding (Table 2–2) (33). Farr was frequently consulted by Francis Galton, who credited him with stimulating his own interest in biometrics (18). John Simon, the first Medical Officer of Health in England, was associated with Farr in the first known epidemiologic society, the London Epidemiological Society (LES), which was organized in 1850. Among its founding members were John Simon, Thomas Watson, Thomas Addison, who described Addison's disease, and Richard Bright, who described Bright's disease (12). The influence of Louis on the Society is readily apparent in the inaugural remarks of the Society's first President (13): "Statistics, too, have supplied us with a new and powerful means of testing medical truth, and we learn from the labours of the accurate Louis how appropriately they may be brought to bear upon the subject of epidemic disease."

The initial purpose of the London Epidemiological Society was to determine the etiology of cholera, but its activities quickly expanded. Its report on smallpox vaccination in 1853, for example, was the major reason for the passage of the Vaccination Act of 1853, mandating vaccination on a nationwide basis. One of the Society's founding members, John Snow, conducted a series of classical studies of cholera (55). Snow, who was known for his administration of chloroform to Queen Victoria during childbirth, investigated the occurrence of cholera in London during 1848–1854 in addition to reviewing reports of epidemics occurring aboard ships and in Europe.

In London, several water companies were responsible for supplying water to different parts of the city. In 1849, Snow noted that the cholera rates were particularly high in those areas of London that were supplied by the Lambeth Company and the Southwark and Vauxhall Company, both of whom obtained their water from the Thames River at a point heavily polluted with sewage. Between 1849 and 1854 the Lambeth Company had its source of water relocated to a less contaminated part of the Thames. In 1854, when another epidemic of cholera occurred, an area consisting of two-thirds of London's resident population south of the Thames was being served by both companies. In this area, the two companies had their water mains laid out in an interpenetrating manner, so that houses on the same street were receiving their water from different sources. Snow ascertained the total number of houses supplied by each water company, calculated cholera death rates per 10,000 houses for the first seven weeks of the epidemic and compared them with those for the rest of London; the data were supplied to Snow by Farr (Table 2–3). His findings were indisputably

Table 2–3. Deaths from Cholera per 10,000 Houses by Source of Water Supply, London, 1854

Water Supply	Number of Houses	Deaths from Cholera	Deaths in Each 10,000 Houses
Southwark and Vauxhall Company	40,046	1,263	315
Lambeth Company	26,107	98	37
Rest of London	256,423	1,422	59

Source: Snow (55).

clear, the mortality rates in the houses supplied by the Southwark and Vauxhall Company were between eight and nine times greater than those in homes supplied by the Lambeth Company. From these findings, integrated with his investigation of the Broad Street Pump cholera outbreak and his assessment of other characteristics of cholera epidemics, Snow inferred the existence of a "cholera poison" transmitted by polluted water.

John Snow's achievement was based on his logical organization of observations, his recognition of a natural experiment, and his quantitative approach in analyzing the occurrence of a disease in a human population. The influence of his report was more widespread than has been realized. It led to legislation mandating that *all* of the water companies in London filter their water by 1857, only two years after the report's publication. (It was not until 1883 that Robert Koch identified the cholera vibrio.)

Snow's biographer and close friend, Sir Benjamin Ward Richardson, was a leading member of the LES, as well as a pioneer of the Sanitary Movement. One of epidemiology's leaders in the nineteenth century, Richardson was among the first to attempt to develop a disease-reporting system and to propose the teaching of preventive medicine in medical schools (31).

A somewhat different approach to the epidemiologic study of disease is embodied in William Budd's studies of typhoid fever, which were published during the years 1857–1873 (9). Budd, an active member of the LES and a student of Louis, practiced medicine in his native village of North Tawton, a remote rural community in England. From his observations of the environmental conditions of the village, he argued against the miasmatic origin of typhoid fever:

Much there was, as I can myself testify, offensive to the nose, but [typhoid] fever there was none. It could not be said that the atmospheric conditions necessary to [typhoid] fever was wanting, because while this village remained exempt, many neighbouring villages suffered severely from the pest. . . . Meanwhile privies, pigstyes, and dungheaps continued, year after year, to exhale ill odours, without any specific effect on the public health. . . . I ascertained by an inquiry conducted with the most scrupulous care that for fifteen years there had been no severe outbreak of this disorder, and that for nearly ten years there had been but a single case. For the development of this fever a more specific element was needed than either the swine, the dungheaps, or the privies were, in the common course of things, able to furnish.

From his epidemiologic observations of an outbreak of typhoid fever that occurred in North Tawton between July 11 and November 1839, Budd inferred that it was a contagious disease. During this period, he saw more than eighty patients with typhoid fever. Noting instances of three or four successive cases occurring in the same household, he ascribed these to contagion. Considerably more important was his observation that three individuals who left the village during the epidemic for other villages spread the disease to some of their new contacts. He traced specific instances of person-to-person contact that resulted in the appearance of typhoid fever in villages previously free of the disease despite environmental conditions similar to North Tawton. Budd concluded that typhoid fever is a "contagious, or self-propagating fever," that the intestinal disturbance is its distinctive manifestation, and that "the contagious matter by which the fever is propagated is cast off, chiefly, in the discharges from the diseased intestine." It was not until 1880 that the typhoid fever bacillus was described.

In his monograph on typhoid fever, Budd included a testimony to the value of Louis's work (9):

Louis, who on all points relating to the natural history of this fever is the greatest of authorities, living or dead—whose monograph on it is unique in medicine as a model of elaborate research—and whose conscientious accuracy is only paralleled by his slowness of belief, declares himself to the same effect in language which is the more striking from the contrast it presents to the caution with which he expresses himself on most subjects.

Louis's work had an influence on other physicians in European medical centers. Skoda, a leading internist in the Vienna Medical School, used and taught Louis's numerical method (28). A student of Skoda, Semmelweiss, conducted one of the most sophisticated epidemiologic studies (28, 48). He noted the changing trends of maternal mortality from puerperal fever in two maternity wards of the large university hospital, the Allgemeines Krankenhaus in Vienna, in which midwifery and medical students and physicians were trained in obstetrics. During 1833–1840, midwifery students, medical students, and physicians were equally distributed between these two wards, which did not differ in their maternal mortality. In 1840, the training system was changed, and one ward was used for training midwives and the other for medical students and physicians. A difference in maternal mortality between these two wards then appeared and continued for the period 1841–1846; the maternal mortality rate was 9.9 percent in the ward used by medical students and physicians in contrast to that of 3.9 percent in the ward used by midwifery students. Having observed that the medical students and physicians performed autopsies prior to their attendance in the maternity wards and the midwifery students did not, Semmelweis hypothesized that the high maternal mortality resulted from the transmission of infectious material from the autopsy room to the maternity clinic by the physicians and medical students. In 1847 he instituted the practice of having the physicians and medical students wash with chlorinated solutions before performing deliveries, and the death rate fell to 1.3 percent in 1848, equaling that in the ward used by the midwifery students.

Such comparative experimentation did not become part of the armamentarium of the clinician and epidemiologist until the twentieth century, when its role in determining the etiology of a disease was most extensively demonstrated by Goldberger. In a series of both observational and experimental studies, to be further discussed in Chapter 11, Goldberger demonstrated that pellagra was not an infectious disease—the prevailing concept—but rather a result of a dietary deficiency of a vitamin, later determined to be nicotinic acid, part of the vitamin B complex. This method has become a major tool of investigation in all branches of medicine and epidemiology, as will be discussed in Chapters 10 and 11.

Another example of an epidemiologic study at this time comes from Denmark (44). A cabinetmaker from Copenhagen landed in the Faroe Islands on March 28, 1846, and developed symptoms of measles early in April. The population of the Faroes at the time numbered 7864; 6100 came down with measles between the end of April and October and 170 deaths occurred. The islanders had experienced measles in the past, but there had been no cases between 1781 and 1846.

The Danish government sent a twenty-six-year-old physician, P.L. Panum, to deal with the epidemic situation; to his observations, we owe much of our knowledge of measles. Panum personally visited fifty-two villages and made observations on several thousand cases of measles of which he personally treated 1000. He obtained information on "the circumstances and dates of their exposure to infection, the dates on which the exanthem [rash] appeared on them and the time that elapsed thereafter before other residents broke out with the exanthem." From these observations, he concluded that the period from exposure to development of the rash (the incubation period) is usually thirteen to fourteen days and that the patient is infectious at the time that the rash is breaking out, or had just broken out, and possibly for a few days prior to the eruption, although he was not certain about this. He did not find the disease to be transmissible during the period of desquamation (when the rash disappears with shedding of the skin), which was the prevalent view at the time. From these observations on personal contacts, he concluded that measles can be transmitted only by direct contact between infected and susceptible individuals. It is not conveyed by miasma nor does it arise spontaneously, at least not in the Faroe Islands. He also suggested that one attack of measles conferred lifelong immunity, since none of the ninety-eight inhabitants who had had measles before 1781 developed the disease in 1846. His hypothesis was validated when the Faroes had another measles epidemic in 1875 and only persons under thirty years of age became ill.

In England it is seen (Fig. 2–1) that through his students, Louis's ideas were transmitted to Francis Galton, who would later derive the correlation coefficient. Galton, in turn, was a close colleague of Karl Pearson, discoverer of the chi-square distribution and one of the founders of the British School of Biometry. One of Pearson's contemporaries, Arthur Newsholme, who became one of the leading British Medical Officers of Health of the early 1900s, was clearly influenced by the work of Guy, Farr, and Richardson (43). He was later recruited by William Henry Welch, the first Dean of the

Johns Hopkins School of Medicine and organizer of the Johns Hopkins School of Hygiene and Public Health, to teach public health administration at the latter institution. Pearson later directed Galton's Eugenics Laboratory and attracted Major Greenwood, G. Udny Yule, and Raymond Pearl as students. Greenwood became a leading English epidemiologist of the early 1900s; Yule, one of the leading English statisticians; and Pearl was recruited by Welch to teach biostatistics at the Johns Hopkins University. One of Greenwood's students was A. Bradford Hill, who pioneered the application of epidemiologic methods to noninfectious diseases.

Louis's influence was not restricted to Europe, as many Americans came to Paris to study with him. They, in turn, transmitted his ideas to their students in the United States (24). One of these students was James Jackson, Jr., whose father was Professor of Medicine at Harvard. Jackson, who in 1832, conducted an epidemiologic study of cholera under Louis's supervision, noted that (37):

> M. Louis has not brought forward a new system of medicine; he has only proposed and pursued a *new method* in prosecuting the study of medicine. This is . . . the method of induction, the method of Bacon.

Both Henry I. Bowditch and Oliver Wendell Holmes, Sr., studied under Louis for several years prior to their becoming professors of medicine at Harvard. Bowditch played an important role in the hygienic movement of the United States. The relevance of the numerical method to such a development is briefly indicated by his statement that "Louis's use of the numerical method . . . is now adopted by some of the best minds as the basis of Public Hygiene" (7). Holmes, independently of Semmelweis, elucidated the contagious nature of puerperal fever (26). Members of the Shattuck family in Boston, of whom George C. Shattuck, Jr., studied under Louis, were among the founders of the American Statistical Association (ASA) in 1839 (1, 16, 33, 34). At the time the ASA was founded, George C. Shattuck, Sr., was chairman of the department of medicine at Harvard. Later he served as the second president of the ASA, during 1846–1852. A cousin, Lemuel Shattuck, one of the founders of the ASA, prepared the landmark report in 1850 that outlined the basis for a public health organization (49). It contained detailed recommendations on vital statistics including a census, nomenclature for causes of disease and death, and the collection of data by age, race, sex, occupation, etc. One of George Shattuck, Sr.'s students, Edward Jarvis (also influenced by Louis's ideas) became the third President of the ASA. He was responsible for the reorganization of the eighth (1860) U.S. census so that it could be used by epidemiologists and biometricians (21).

Another group of Louis's students was present in New York City and had an important influence on the development of epidemiology and public health, directly or indirectly through their own students. Among these were Elisha Bartlett, Alonzo Clark, and Francis Delafield, all of whom taught at either Columbia University's College of Physicians and Surgeons or at the Bellevue Hospital Medical College. Bartlett was the first to provide an explicit rationale for a *control* group in an epidemiologic study (2, 29, 34). Among this group's students were Elisha Harris and Stephen Smith. Harris and Smith, together with Jarvis and Bowditch, were among the founders of the American Public Health Association in 1872 (45). Harris also became the first vital statistics registrar in New York City.

In Philadelphia, Louis's students included W. Gerhard and A. Stillé (24). Gerhard is recognized for his contribution to the differentiation of typhus from typhoid fever. Stillé, a leading American pathologist, held the Chair of Medicine at the University of Pennsylvania and became the first secretary of the American Medical Association, later its president. Although he did not study abroad, Austin Flint had studied at Harvard under Louis's students and Louis's work made a considerable impression on him; he taught at the Bellevue Hospital Medical College in the latter half of the nineteenth century (14). Clark, Delafield, and Flint all taught William Henry Welch, who played a major role in transmitting Louis's ideas to the epidemiologists of the early twentieth century (56) (Fig. 2–1). Another of Flint's students was Charles V. Chapin, who became a leading epidemiologist and a pioneer in the American public health movement (10). Chapin developed many epidemiologic techniques, the most widely known of which is the secondary attack rate (see Chap. 6, p. 141).

During the early part of the twentieth century, further developments in epidemiology in the United States were associated with the United States Public Health Service and its Hygienic Laboratory, founded in 1887. In these agencies there were such pioneers as

Milton Rosenau, Wade Hampton Frost, Kenneth Maxcy, and Joseph Goldberger.

C. THE EPIDEMIOLOGIC FABRIC

The epidemiologic fabric was woven together largely from the numerical (quantitative) method, the development of a vital statistics system, the stimulus of a hygienic or public health movement, and the concept of comparative studies. It has now matured as a scientific discipline so that its study is necessary for a full understanding of the etiology of human and other diseases as well as their prevention and treatment.

REFERENCES

1. American Statistical Association. 1940. "Historical exhibits: Minutes of the first six meetings." *J. Amer. Stat. Assn.* 35:298 308.
2. Bartlett, E. 1844. *An Essay on the Philosophy of Medical Science.* Philadelphia: Lea and Blanchard.
3. Bayne-Jones, S. 1968. *Evolution of Preventive Medicine in the United States Army, 1607–1939.* Washington, D.C.: U.S. Government Printing Office.
4. Belloni, L. 1960. *Le "Contagium Vivum" Avant Pasteur.* Paris: University of Paris.
5. Bernoulli, D. 1760. "Mathematical and physical memoirs, taken from the registers of the Royal Academy of Sciences for the year 1760: An attempt at a new analysis of the mortality caused by smallpox and of the advantages of inoculation to prevent it." In *Smallpox Inoculation: An Eighteenth Century Mathematical Controversy. Translation and Critical Commentary* by L. Bradley, 1971. Nottingham, England: University of Nottingham.
6. Bollet, A.J. 1973. "Piérre Louis: The numerical method and the foundation of quantitative medicine." *Amer. J. Med. Sci.* 266:92–101.
7. Bowditch, H.I. 1877. *Public Hygiene in America.* Boston: Little, Brown. Reprinted Edition. New York: Arno Press, 1972, p. 17.
8. Brockington, C.F. 1965. *Public Health in the Nineteenth Century.* Edinburgh: E. & S. Livingstone.
9. Budd, W. 1931. *Typhoid Fever: Its Nature, Mode of Spreading and Prevention.* Original publication 1873. New York: American Public Health Association.
10. Cassedy, J.H. 1962. *Charles V. Chapin and the Public Health Movement.* Cambridge: Harvard University Press.
11. Copleston, F. 1963. *A History of Philosophy, Vol. 3, Pt. II. Garden City,* N.Y.: Image Books.
12. Epidemiological Society of London. 1901. *Commemoration Volume. Transactions of the Epidemiological Society of London.* London: Shaw and Sons.
13. "Epidemiological Society." 1850. *Lancet* 2:641.

14. Evans, A.S. 1958. "Austin Flint and his contributions to medicine." *Bull. Hist. Med.* 32:224–241.
15. Farr, W. 1975. *Vital Statistics: A Memorial Volume of Selections from the Reports and Writings of William Farr.* Metushen, N.J.: New York Academy of Medicine.
16. FitzPatrick, P.J. 1958. "Leading American statisticians of the nineteenth century, II." *J. Amer. Stat. Assn.* 53:689–701.
17. Fracastoro, G. 1546. *De Sympathia et Antipathia Rerum Liber Unus de Contagione et Contagiosis Morbis et Curatione Libri III.* Venetiis.
18. Galton, F. 1908. *Memories of My Life.* London: Methuen and Co.
19. Glass, D.V. 1963. "John Graunt and his natural and political observations." *Proc. Roy. Soc. (Biology)* 159:2–37.
20. Graunt, J. 1662. *Natural and Political Observations Mentioned in a Following Index, and Made Upon the Bills of Mortality.* London. Reprinted, Baltimore: The Johns Hopkins Press, 1939.
21. Grob, G.N. 1976. "Edward Jarvis and the federal census: A chapter in the history of nineteenth-century American medicine." *Bull. Hist. Med.* 50:4–27.
22. Grove, J. 1851. "On the nature of epidemics." *Lancet* 2:146.
23. ———. 1853. "On contagion and infection in relation to epidemic diseases." *Lancet* 2:119.
24. Hinsdale, G. 1945. "The American medical argonauts: Pupils of Pierre Charles Alexandre Louis." Transact. and Studies of the College of Physicians of Philadelphia 13:37–43.
25. Hippocrates. 1939. *The Genuine Works of Hippocrates.* Translated from the Greek by Francis Adams. Baltimore: Williams and Wilkens, p. 19.
26. Holmes, O.W. 1891. "The Contagiousness of Puerperal Fever." In *Medical Essays 1842–1882.* Boston: Houghton, Mifflin, pp. 103–172.
27. Jackson, J. 1835. *A Memoir of James Jackson, Jr., M.D. with Extracts From His Letters to His Father; and Medical Cases, Collected by Him.* Boston: I.R. Butts. Reprinted edition, New York: Arno Press, 1972, p. 23.
28. Lesky, E. 1976. *The Vienna Medical School of the 19th Century.* Baltimore: The Johns Hopkins University Press, pp. 123, 181–192.
29. Lilienfeld, A.M., and Lilienfeld, D.E. 1979. "A century of case-control studies: Progress?" *J. Chron. Dis.* 32:5–13.
30. Lilienfeld, D.E. 1977. "Contagium vivum and the development of water filtration: The beginning of the sanitary movement." *Prev. Med.* 6:361–375.
31. ———, and Lilienfeld, A.M. 1977. "Teaching preventive medicine in medical schools: An historical vignette." *Prev. Med.* 6:469–471.
32. ———, and Lilienfeld, A.M. 1977. "Epidemiology: A retrospective study." *Amer. J. Epid.* 106:445–459.
33. ———. 1979. "The greening of epidemiology: Sanitary physicians and the London Epidemiological Society (1830–1870)." *Bull. Hist. Med.* 52:503–528.
34. ———, and Lilienfeld, A.M., 1980. "The French influence on the development of epidemiology." *Bull. Hist. Med.* (in press).
35. Lind, J. 1753. *A Treatise of the Scurvy.* Edinburgh: Sands, Murray, and Cochran.
36. Lorrimer, F. 1959. "The development of demography." In *The Study of Population.* P.M. Hauser and O.D. Duncan, eds. Chicago: University of Chicago Press, pp. 124–179.
37. Louis, P.C.–A. 1836. *Researches on the Effects of Bloodletting in Some Inflammatory Diseases, and on the Influence of Tartarized Antimony and*

Vesication in Pneumonitis. Translated by C. G. Putman with Preface and Appendix by James Jackson. Boston: Milliard, Gray and Co.

38. ———. 1837. "Pathological researches on phthisis." *Amer. J. Med. Sci.* 19:445–449.
39. Major, R.H. 1944. "Agostino Bassi and the parasitic theory of disease." *Bull. Hist. Med.* 16:97–107.
40. Mason, S.F. 1962. *A History of the Sciences.* New York: Collier Books.
41. Mather, C.C. 1972. *The Angel of Bethesda.* G.W. Jones, ed. Barre, Mass.: American Antiquarian Society and Barre Publishers.
42. Merz, J.T. 1976. *A History of European Scientific Thought in the Nineteenth Century, Vol. 2.* Gloucester, Mass.: Peter Smith.
43. Newsholme, A. 1935. *Fifty Years in Public Health. Vol. 1.* London: Allen and Unwin.
44. Panum, P.L. 1940. *Observations Made During the Epidemic of Measles on the Faroe Islands in the Year 1846.* New York: American Public Health Association.
45. Ravanel, M.P. 1921. *A Half Century in Public Health.* New York: American Public Health Association. Reprinted Edition, New York: Arno Press, 1970.
46. Rosen, G. 1937. "Social aspects of Jacob Henle's medical thought." *Bull. Hist. Med.* 5:509–537.
47. ———. 1958. *A History of Public Health.* New York: M.D. Publications.
48. Semmelweis, I.P. 1861. "The etiology, the concept and the prophylaxis of childbed fever." Translated by F.B. Murphy. 1941. *Med. Classics* 5:350–773.
49. Shattuck, L. 1850. *Report of a General Plan for the Promotion of Public and Personal Health devised, prepared and recommended by the Commissioners appointed under a Resolve of the Legislature of Massachusetts relating to a Sanitary Survey of the State.* Boston: Dutton and Wentworth. Reprinted, Cambridge: Harvard University Press, 1948.
50. Shyrock, R.H. 1947. *The Development of Modern Medicine.* New York: Knopf.
51. ———. 1972. "Germ theories in medicine prior to 1870: Further comments on continuity in science." *Clio Medica* 7:81–109.
52. Singer, C., and Singer, D. 1914. "The development of the doctrine of contagium vivum, 1500–1750." In *Section XXIII. History of Medicine, Proceedings of the 17th International Congress of Medicine, London.* 2:187–210.
53. Slotki, J.J. 1951. *Daniel, Ezra, Nehemiah. Hebrew Text and English Translation with Introductions and Commentary.* London: The Soncino Press, pp. 3–6.
54. Smillie, W.G. 1955. *Public Health: Its Promise for the Future.* New York: Macmillan.
55. Snow, J. 1936. "On the mode of communication of cholera." In *Snow on Cholera.* New York: The Commonwealth Fund, pp. 1–175.
56. Welch, W.H. 1920. *Papers and Addresses, Vol. 1.* Baltimore: The Johns Hopkins Press.
57. Winslow, C.-E.A. 1943. *The Conquest of Epidemic Diseases.* New York: Hafner Press.
58. Woodward, T.E. 1975. "Marylanders defeat Philadelphia: Yellow fever updated." Presented at the 99th Annual Meeting of the American Clinical and Climatological Association on October 27, 1975 at Tuckerstown, Bermuda, British West Indies.

3 Selected Epidemiologic Concepts of Disease

Many of the fundamental epidemiologic concepts have evolved from studies of infectious diseases, but they are equally applicable to noninfectious diseases and conditions. Only those that have been found to be of pragmatic value will be considered in this chapter.

A. AGENT, HOST, AND ENVIRONMENT

Essentially, the epidemiologic patterns of infectious diseases depend upon factors that influence the probability of contact between an infectious agent and a susceptible person known as the host. The presence of infectious material varies with the duration and extent of its excretion from an infected person, the climatic conditions affecting survival of the agent, the route of entry into the host, and the existence of alternative reservoirs or hosts of the agent. The availability of susceptible hosts depends upon the extent of mobility and interpersonal contact within the population group, and the degree and duration of immunity from previous infections with the same or related agents.

Relationships similar to those existing among infectious agents of disease, the human host and his environment, also exist among non-infectious etiological agents, host, and environment. For example, whether or not a person develops a specific form of cancer may depend upon the extent of his exposure to the carcinogenic agent, the dose of the agent, and his susceptibility, which may be influenced by genetic and/or immunological factors. A classification of agent, host, and environmental factors is presented in Table 3–1 as a frame of reference in the search for determinants of disease occurrence in a population.

It can be seen that a specific scientific discipline is usually concerned with a particular category of the factors listed in Table 3–1.

Table 3–1. A Classification of Agent, Host, and Environmental Factors Which Determine the Occurrence of Diseases in Human Populations

I. *Agents of Disease*—Etiological Factors.

Examples

A.	Nutritive elements	
	excesses	Cholesterol
	deficiencies	Vitamins, proteins
B.	Chemical agents	
	poisons	Carbon monoxide, carbon tetrachloride, drugs
	allergens	Ragweed, poison ivy, medications
C.	Physical agents	Ionizing radiation, mechanical
D.	Infectious agents	
	metazoa	Hookworm, schistosomiasis, onchocerciasis
	protozoa	Amoebae, malaria
	bacteria	Rheumatic fever, lobar pneumonia, typhoid, tuberculosis, syphilis
	fungi	Histoplasmosis, athlete's foot
	rickettsia	Rocky moutain spotted fever, typhus
	viruses	Measles, mumps, chickenpox, smallpox, poliomyelitis, rabies, yellow fever

II. *Host Factors* (Intrinsic Factors)—Influences Exposure, Susceptibility, or Response to Agents.

Examples

A.	Genetic	Sickle cell disease
B.	Age	—
C.	Sex	—
D.	Ethnic group	—
E.	Physiologic state	Fatigue, pregnancy, puberty, stress, nutritional state
F.	Prior immunologic experience	Hypersensitivity, protection
	active	Prior infection, immunization
	passive	Maternal antibodies, gamma globulin prophylaxis
G.	Intercurrent or preexisting disease	
H.	Human behavior	Personal hygiene, food handling, diet, interpersonal contact, occupation, recreation, utilization of health resources

III. *Environmental Factors* (Extrinsic Factors)—Influences Existence of the Agent, Exposure, or Susceptibility to Agent.

		Examples
A.	Physical environment	Geology, climate
B.	Biologic environment	
	human populations	Density
	flora	Sources of food, influence on vertebrates and arthropods, as a source of agents
	fauna	Food sources, vertebrate hosts, arthropod vectors
C.	Socioeconomic environment	
	occupation	Exposure to chemical agents
	urbanization and economic development	Urban crowding, tensions and pressures, cooperative efforts in health and education
	disruption	Wars, floods

The geneticist concentrates on genetic factors; the microbiologist on infectious agents; the physicist on physical agents; the sociologist on human behavior, ethnic groups, and socioeconomic environments. The epidemiologist, however, attempts to integrate the data necessary for his analysis of a particular disease from diverse disciplines. The need for evaluating the *interaction* of these factors relative to time, place, and persons is the main reason for viewing this frame of reference as primarily an epidemiologic concept.

B. CLASSIFICATION OF HUMAN INFECTIONS BY MODE OF TRANSMISSION

As is evident from Table 3–1, infectious diseases are usually classified by the etiological agent, such as a virus or bacterium. This classification, based on the biological features of the agent, is satisfactory from many points of view, including that of potential preventive measures. However, it is also possible to classify diseases by their epidemiologic features. In many instances, this may be more advantageous for applying preventive measures than an etiological classification. Infectious diseases, for example, can be divided according to the way they are spread through human populations:

1. *Common Vehicle Epidemics.* The etiological agent is transmitted by water, food, air, or inoculation (Table 3–2). Com-

Table 3–2. Classification of Human Infections by Selected Epidemiologic Features*

	Examples
I. *Dynamics of Spread through Human Populations:*	
A. Spread by a "common vehicle"	
ingestion with water, food or beverage	Salmonellosis
inhalation in air breathed	Q fever (in laboratory)
inoculation (intravenous, subcutaneous)	Serum hepatitis
B. Propagation by serial transfer from host to host	
respiratory route of transfer	Measles
anal-oral route	Shigellosis
genital route	Syphilis
II. *Portal of Entry (and Portal of Exit) in Human Host:*	
Upper respiratory tract	Diphtheria
Lower respiratory tract	Tuberculosis
Gastrointestinal tract	Typhoid fever
Genitourinary tract	Gonorrhea
Conjunctiva	Trachoma
Percutaneous	Leptospirosis
Percutaneous (bite of arthropod)	Yellow fever
III. *Principal Reservoir of Infection:*	
Man	Infectious hepatitis
Other vertebrates (zoonoses)	Tularemia
Agent free-living (?)	Histoplasmosis
IV. *Cycles of Infectious Agent in Nature:* (arrows designate transfer to occasional host)	
Man-man	Influenza
Man-arthropod-man	Malaria
Vertebrate-vertebrate ↘ man	Psittacosis
Vertebrate-arthropod-vetebrate ↘ man	Arthropod-borne Viral encephalitis

V. *Complex Cycles*—seen especially in certain helminth infections. For example, in paragonimiasis the cycle is as follows:

Ovum—miracidium—cercaria—adult—ovum
(in snail)　(in crab,　(in man)
crayfish)

The agent is free-living in fresh water during a part of its existence as ovum, miracidium, and cercaria.

* Diseases may be capable of being classified in more than one category in this classification: the most usual situation is given in the examples cited.

mon vehicle epidemics can result from a single exposure of a population group to the agent, from repeated multiple exposures, or from continued exposure over a period of time. They are usually characterized by explosiveness of onset and limitation or localization in time, place, and persons. This type of epidemic can be illustrated by a food poisoning outbreak, which is the result of a single source of exposure.

2. *Epidemics Propagated by Serial Transfer from Host to Host.* The agent is spread through contact between infected and susceptible individuals by means of the respiratory, anal, oral, genital, or other route; by dust; by insects and arthropods (vectors) (Table 3–2). The course of such an epidemic, in which the agent is transmitted by contact between individuals, is illustrated in Figure 3–1.

This simple division of infectious diseases by mode of transmission provides a basis for considering possible measures to prevent the occurrence of epidemics in the community. But several types of infections, particularly from viral and parasitic agents, may have more complicated modes of transmission, as categorized in Sections IV and V of Table 3–2. An example is given in Figure 3–2.

C. THE INCUBATION PERIOD

One important epidemiologic feature of a disease is the incubation period. This is the interval between the time of contact and/or entry of the agent and onset of illness. In infectious diseases, it is generally thought of as the time required for the multiplication of the microorganism within the host up to a threshold point where the parasitic population is large enough to produce symptoms in the host.

Each infectious disease has a characteristic incubation period, largely dependent upon the rate of growth of the organism in the host (3). For different diseases, other factors play a role, including the dosage of the infectious agent, its portal of entry, and the rate and degree of immune response by the host. An incubation period will vary among individuals; and, in a group of cases, its distribution will be asymmetrical, so that the part of the curve with the longer incubation periods has a longer "tail," that is, the curve is

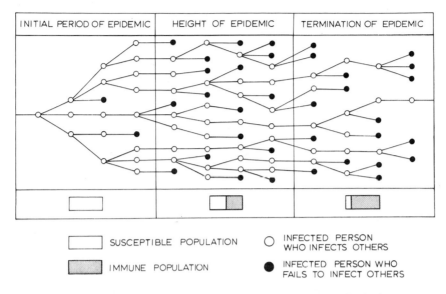

INITIAL PERIOD OF EPIDEMIC	HEIGHT OF EPIDEMIC	TERMINATION OF EPIDEMIC

SUSCEPTIBLE POPULATION

IMMUNE POPULATION

○ INFECTED PERSON
   WHO INFECTS OTHERS

● INFECTED PERSON WHO
   FAILS TO INFECT OTHERS

Figure 3-1.   Course of a typical propagated epidemic in which the agent is transmitted by contact between individuals

Source: Burnet and White (5).

"skewed to the right" (Fig. 3–3). Sartwell pointed out that this asymmetrical curve resembles a log-normal distribution. Indeed when one graphs the frequency of incubation periods against the logarithm of time, the skewness essentially disappears and the curve resembles a normal distribution (22, 23).

In a graph of a common vehicle epidemic from a single source, the curve resulting from plotting the times of onset of the disease also represents the distribution of incubation periods. Knowing the incubation period for a disease in a single source common vehicle epidemic enables one to estimate the time of exposure to the disease agent.

The only three factors necessary to describe this type of epidemic are:

1. Distribution of times of onset of illness, known as the epidemic curve.
2. The specific disease, which is characterized by its incubation period.
3. The time of exposure.

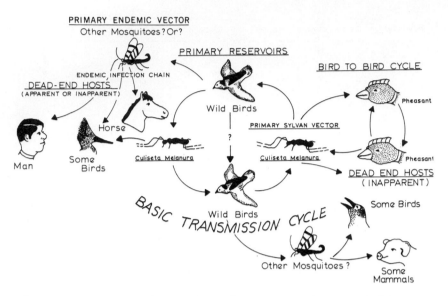

Figure 3–2.   Summer infection chains for eastern equine encephalitis

Source: Hess and Holden (16).

In practice, if only two of these factors are known, it is possible to deduce the third factor, as illustrated in Figure 3–4.

If one recognizes an infectious disease from its clinical characteristics, the incubation period is then also known. In a single-source common vehicle epidemic, the epidemic curve represents the distribution of incubation periods and the median point on the curve will represent the median incubation period. The median is preferred as a measure of central tendency because of the usual skewness of the distribution of incubation periods. Using the median incubation period, one can estimate the time of exposure to the etiological agent and then investigate the events that had occurred about that time, in order to determine the cause of the epidemic. Likewise, if sufficient information is available to construct the epidemic curve and the time of exposure is known, one can determine the type of infectious disease if the incubation period of that disease is already known.

Although the prototype for this kind of reasoning is the previously mentioned single-source food poisoning outbreak, it is also applicable to diseases caused by several, possibly different, etiological agents, one of which may be known. Cobb, Miller, and Wald

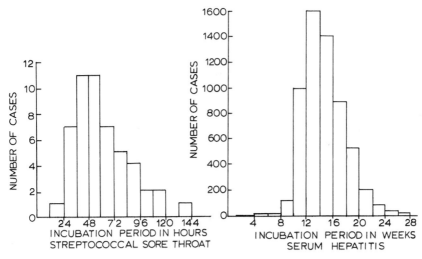

Figure 3–3. Distribution of incubation periods in an epidemic of food-borne streptococcal sore throat and a series of cases of serum hepatitis following administration of icterogenic lots of yellow fever vaccine

Source: Sartwell (22).

attempted to apply this approach to leukemia, where exposure to radiation is recognized as being one etiological factor for some forms of the disease (7). They analyzed the cases of leukemia that occurred after the 1945 atomic bomb explosion in Hiroshima, which can be regarded as a single exposure. Figure 3–5(A) compares the annual incidence of leukemia following explosion of the bomb for those who were located less than 1,000 meters (m) from the hypocenter at the time of the explosion with the incidence among those who were 2,000 m or more from the center, generally considered an unexposed group. The annual leukemia incidence rate proved to be higher for the first group, but interestingly, the peak incidence of leukemia occurred in 1951 or 1952, about six years after the radiation exposure. Admittedly, the data for the earlier years are probably incomplete, but, nonetheless, the shape of the curve resembles that of an epidemic curve observed in single-exposure common vehicle epidemics. The incidence pattern for those who were between 1,000 to 1,999 m at the time of the bomb is similar although their rates are lower (Fig. 3–5[B]). It should be added that continued follow-up of these survivors still shows an excessive rate of leukemia in the exposed group.

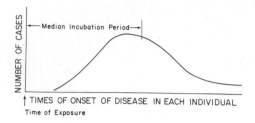

Figure 3–4. Distribution of times of onset of disease (the epidemic curve) and median incubation period in a single source common vehicle epidemic

Cobb, Miller, and Wald also collated several reports of ankylosing spondylitis patients who developed leukemia following radiation treatment either by a single exposure or multiple exposures over a number of years. In the latter case, they determined the central point of the exposure period and adjusted for the size of the administered dose. Assuming the interval between the time of exposure and onset of leukemia to be the incubation period, they obtained the results presented in Figure 3–6. These results show that the peak of the curve is present at about four years after exposure to radiation and that 90 percent of the cases have occurred within nine years of such exposure.

If one is willing to assume from these data that the incubation period of leukemia patients induced by unknown factors is similar to those caused by radiation, it would suggest that the search for etiological factors of leukemia should focus on the ten-year period prior to the onset of the disease in adults. However, new data obtained in further studies may change these estimates. It is also of interest that the distribution of leukemia cases is skewed to the right, similar to that observed in single-source common vehicle epidemics of infectious diseases. The skewness in the ankylosing spondylitis data may partially reflect the number of patients who had multiple exposures over a period of several years.

An example of similar reasoning is the analysis of the changing pattern of mortality from leukemia among children under five years of age in England and Wales between 1931 and 1953 (17). Hewitt noted the similarity between the shape of the mortality curve and the curves usually observed in incubation periods of infectious diseases. He also noted an increasing peak of mortality during this period at about three to four years of age (Fig. 3–7). Among the possible factors that might have produced this increase, he postu-

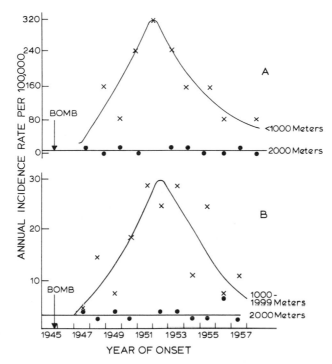

Figure 3–5. Annual incidence rate of leukemia following the atomic bomb explosion among survivors who were residents of Hiroshima city at the time of diagnosis*

* (A) Persons less than 1000 meters from hypocenter compared with persons 2000 or more meters from hypocenter at time of explosion. (B) Persons 1000 to 1999 meters from hypocenter compared with persons 2000 or more meters from hypocenter at time of explosion.

Source: Cobb, Miller, and Wald (7).

lated that the increased use of X-rays during this period, which were known to be leukemogenic, was a possible explanation. This analysis provided the basis for a field investigation of the possible influence of prenatal and postnatal X-rays and other procedures on the occurrence of childhood leukemia (24). Their finding of a connection between intrauterine radiation (mainly X-ray pelvimetry) and childhood leukemia stimulated many others to investigate this relationship (10, 14, 18, 19). Several of these studies suggested that although the entire increase in death rates could not be explained by intrauterine radiation, certainly a portion of the increase could be so explained (10, 14, 19). It must be admitted, however, that

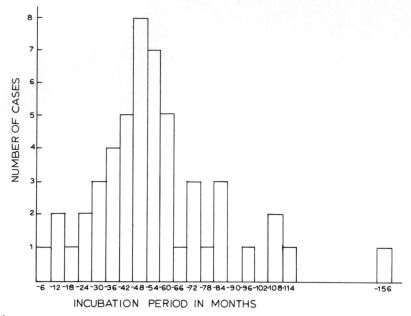

Figure 3–6.   Distribution of incubation periods of leukemia cases following irradiation for ankylosing spondylitis

Source: Cobb, Miller, and Wald (7).

there are still differences of opinion among those who have investigated the problem (18).

More recently, Armenian and Lilienfeld analyzed the incubation periods of certain neoplastic diseases, including several with known etiological factors and specific exposure times such as thyroid adenomas, cancers following childhood exposure to radiation, bronchogenic carcinoma in asbestos workers, and bladder tumors among dyestuff workers (1). Figure 3–8 shows the distribution of incubation periods for 281 cases of bladder tumors that occurred among dyestuff workers.

The shape of the distribution is skewed to the right and was demonstrated to be log-normal with a median incubation period of about seventeen years. It was also observed that the distribution of the age of onset of Burkitt's lymphoma could be described by a log-normal distribution. Since this lymphoma is a childhood disease, it appears that one or more etiological factors may be operating during the prenatal period or perhaps early in infancy.

If, in infectious diseases, the incubation period reflects the multi-

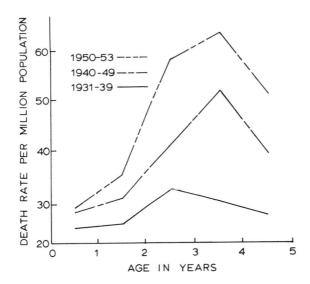

Figure 3–7. Age-specific death rates from leukemia among children under five years of age, England and Wales, 1931–1953

Source: Hewitt (17).

plication of an organism and its interaction with host defenses, it is interesting to speculate on the biological model that underlies the incubation period (or "latency" period as investigators have called it) when exposure to a chemical carcinogenic agent is the etiologic factor. Doll and Pike have each postulated that the neoplastic transformation of a number of individual cells is necessary in order to produce a "nest" of transformed cells which constitute the beginning of a tumor (11, 20). It is also possible that a carcinogenic agent initiates a malignant transformation that requires an additional promoting agent for further growth of the malignancy. Thus, an individual is exposed at a specific point in time to an initiating agent that transforms the cell, and only after an interval of years does exposure to a promoting agent occur, which stimulates growth leading to a malignant tumor (4). Most recently, Polednak proposed the two models presented in Figure 3–9 (21). To these concepts must be added the recent work on the probably important role of immunological factors in the genesis of cancer (9). In cancer, the incubation period may thus result from the interaction between the growth of neoplastic cells and the development of immune responses by the host.

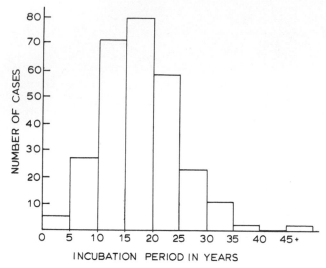

Figure 3–8. Distribution of incubation periods for 281 cases of bladder tumors among dyestuff workers

Source: Case et al. (6).

D. SPECTRUM OF DISEASE

The spectrum of disease may be defined as the sequence of events that occurs in the human organism from the time of exposure to the etiological agent to death, as shown in Figure 3–10. It is composed of two general components, a subclinical one and clinical illness. Whether an individual with the disease progresses through the entire spectrum depends upon the availability and efficacy of preventive and/or therapeutic measures that, if introduced at a particular point of the spectrum, will completely prevent or retard any further development of the disease. In the case of cancer of the cervix, the spectrum might consist of three stages: dysplasia, carcinoma *in situ,* and invasive carcinoma. Similarly, cerebrovascular disease may consist of the following stages: atherosclerotic changes in carotid arteries, transient ischemic attacks, and stroke. The atherosclerotic changes in the carotid arteries are subclinical and require special diagnostic tests for their ascertainment, such as angiograms.

In infectious diseases, this spectrum is usually known as the "gradient of infection," which refers to the sequence of manifestations of illness in the host reflecting his response to the infectious agent.

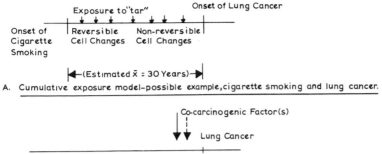

A. Cumulative exposure model–possible example, cigarette smoking and lung cancer.

B. One insult co-carcinogenic model–possible example, pulmonary scars and lung cancer.

Figure 3–9. Two hypothetical models of carcinogenesis

Source: Polednak (21).

This extends from "inapparent infections" at one extreme to death at the other (Fig. 3–11). The frequency with which these different manifestations occur varies with the specific infectious disease. For example, in measles, the vast majority (over 90 percent) of infected persons exhibit clinical illness; in mumps, the proportion is somewhat less, approximately 66 percent; and in poliomyelitis, over 90 percent of the infections are not clinically apparent.

Clinicians and epidemiologists are usually only aware of a small part of the spectrum of a given disease and the gradient of infection, proverbially known as the "tip of the iceberg." However, epidemiologists try to determine the entire range of the spectrum since it may provide a very different picture of a disease than that which clinicians see in fully developed cases. Histoplasmosis is a case in point. From its first description in 1906 until the 1940s, histoplasmosis was regarded as a rare and usually fatal disease. Epidemiologic surveys by the Public Health Service in the 1940s, using the histoplasmosis skin test, completely changed this view. They revealed that most nonepidemic histoplasmosis infections produce no symptoms, or a mild influenzalike disorder, and rarely lead to a progressive systemic disease. In certain areas of the country (parts of Kentucky, Tennessee, Missouri, Indiana, Ohio, Arkansas),

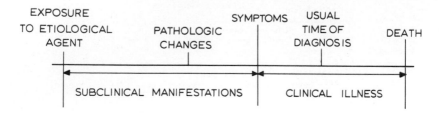

Figure 3–10. Spectrum of disease

the frequency of infections was found to be higher than 80 percent (8). It should be emphasized that one of the major deterrents in elucidating the epidemiology of diseases of unknown etiology is the absence of methods to detect the subclinical state—the bottom of the "iceberg."

Inapparent infections are important because they play a role in the transmission of infectious agents. The spread of poliomyelitis, meningococcal meningitis, and other diseases can only be explained on this basis. It is also necessary to take into account the frequency of these clinically inapparent infected persons by means of tests for antibodies or skin tests for a specific disease, if available, in order to estimate the number of individuals in the population who have become immune to the infectious agent.

Epidemiologists also have to consider the role of latent, as well as inapparent, infections in the study of certain diseases, particularly viral diseases. Latent infection is distinguished from inapparent infection in that the host does not shed the infectious agent, which lies dormant in the host cells. A viral disease may occur early in life in one clinical form, and in later life, the dormant virus may produce a different clinical disease due to some, as yet unknown, mechanism; these are referred to as "slow virus diseases" (13). Recent studies showing a relationship of measles virus to subacute sclerosing panencephalitis and possibly to multiple sclerosis suggest that

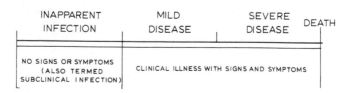

Figure 3–11. Gradient of infection

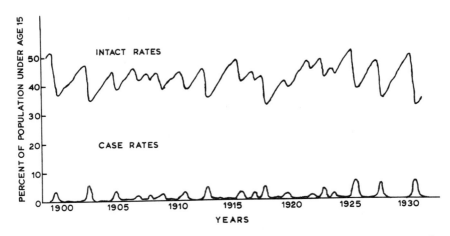

Figure 3–12. Estimated complete monthly attack rates from measles and intact rates (proportions not previously attacked) for the population under fifteen, Old Baltimore, Md., July 1899–December 1931

Source: Hedrich (15).

these latter diseases may represent late manifestations of measles infections and may be slow virus diseases. A similar situation may exist with regard to the relationship of herpes simplex virus to a variety of malignancies.

E. HERD IMMUNITY

Just as individual immunity decreases the probability that an individual will develop a particular disease when exposed to an infectious agent, herd immunity indicates the decreased probability of a group or community developing an epidemic upon the introduction of an infectious agent, although there are a certain number of persons who are individually susceptible to the agent. This concept is helpful in understanding why an epidemic does not occur in a community and in explaining the periodic variation of some infectious diseases, particularly those that are transmitted from one person to another. It is measured in terms of the proportion of immune, or conversely, of susceptible, persons in a social group. Clearly, the presence of a large proportion of immune individuals in a community decreases the chances of contact between infected and susceptible persons. By acting as a barrier between the two, the immune population decreases the rate of spread of the infectious agent. The degree of herd immunity necessary to prevent the development of an epidemic varies with the specific disease. It depends upon such factors as the degree to which an infected individual is capable of transmitting the infection, the length of time during which he is infectious, and the size and social behavior of the community.

The relationship between the proportion of the susceptible individuals in a community and the periodicity of disease is illustrated by the analysis of case rates of measles in Baltimore for the period 1899–1931 (Fig. 3–12) (15). The incidence of measles increases at a time when the number of susceptible persons is highest and herd immunity is lowest. Mathematical models have shown that the smaller the community, the longer is the interval between epidemics (2).

A very practical aspect of this concept of herd immunity is in indicating that an entire population (100 percent) does not have to be immunized to prevent the occurrence of an epidemic (12). This has also been demonstrated by mathematical models. However, in the large metropolises of modern urban society, one must recognize that the socialization and interpersonal contacts necessary for the spread of an infectious agent occur in smaller neighborhood groups and not in the entire metropolis. Consequently, from the viewpoint of public health immunization practice, it is the herd immunity of these smaller groups that must be taken into consideration.

STUDY PROBLEMS

1. A local health officer in a small community received reports from three physicians that they were taking care of persons who had diarrhea, abdominal cramps, vomiting, chills, and fever. From stools collected from several patients, a strain of Salmonella (*S. typhimurium*) was isolated. A total of 119 patients were identified and the times of onset of the disease in this group were tabulated as follows:

January 7		January 8		January 9	
Time	No. of Ill Persons	Time	No. of Ill Persons	Time	No. of Ill Persons
6–7 A.M.	2	12–1 A.M.	5	12–1 A.M.	3
8–9 A.M.	5	2–3 A.M.	3	2–3 A.M.	2
10–11 A.M.	11	4–5 A.M.	3	4–5 A.M.	0
12–1 P.M.	18	6–7 A.M.	3	6–7 A.M.	1
2–3 P M	10	8–9 A.M.	4	8–9 A.M.	0
4–5 P.M.	7	10–11 A.M.	6	10–11 A.M.	1
6–7 P.M.	5	12–1 P.M.	8	12–1 P.M.	0
8–9 P.M.	4	2–3 P.M.	4	2–3 P.M.	0
10–11 P.M.	4	4–5 P.M.	3		
		6–7 P.M.	3		
		8–9 P.M.	2		
		10–11 P.M.	2		

   a) Make a graph of the epidemic curve.
   b) What type of outbreak does this curve resemble? Why?
   c) What are the possible reasons for the bimodality of this epidemic curve?
   d) Describe the investigation that the health officer should conduct.
2. What is the biological basis for the incubation period of a non-infectious disease, such as ischaemic heart disease or chronic obstructive pulmonary disease?
3. Contrast the epidemic curves encountered in a:
   a) common vehicle continuous exposure outbreak
   b) serial transfer propagated epidemic
   c) epidemic resulting from a slow-virus disease.
4. Of what importance is the concept of herd immunity to the public health administrator?

5. Subclinical cases have always posed a problem in investigating the etiology of both infectious and noninfectious diseases. Discuss the reasons for this.
6. One often hears that there is a venereal disease epidemic in the United States today. Into what categories would you classify this epidemic?
7. How would you categorize the epidemics that were investigated by William Budd and John Snow (see Chap. 2)?

REFERENCES

1. Armenian, H.K., and Lilienfeld, A.M. 1974. "The distribution of incubation periods of neoplastic diseases." *Amer. J. Epid.* 99:92–100.
2. Bartlett, M.S. 1957. "Measles periodicity and community size." *J. Roy. Stat. Soc.* 120:48–70.
3. Benenson, A.S., ed. 1970. *Control of Communicable Diseases in Man.* 11th Edition. New York: American Public Health Association.
4. Berenblum, I. 1941. "The mechanism of carcinogenesis. A study of the significance of cocarcinogenic action and related phenomena." *Cancer Res.* 1:807–814.
5. Burnet, M., and White, D.O. 1972. *Natural History of Infectious Disease.* 4th Edition, Cambridge, England: Cambridge University Press.
6. Case, R.A.M., Hosker, M.E., McDonald, D.B., and Pearson, J.T. 1954. "Tumours of the urinary bladder in workmen engaged in the manufacture and use of certain dyestuff intermediates in the British chemical industry. Part 1. The role of aniline, benzidine, alpha-naphthylamine and beta-napthylamine." *Brit. J. Indust. Med.* 11:75–104.
7. Cobb, S., Miller, M., and Wald, N. 1959. "On the estimation of the incubation period in malignant disease." *J. Chron. Dis.* 9:385–393.
8. Comstock, G.W. 1973. "Histoplasmosis." In *Maxcy-Rosenau Preventive Medicine and Public Health.* 10th Edition, E.P. Sartwell, ed. New York: Appleton-Century-Crofts, pp. 399–401.
9. Conference on Immunology of Carcinogenesis. 1972. *National Cancer Institute Monograph No. 35.* Washington, D.C.: United States Department of Health, Education and Welfare.
10. Diamond, E.L., Schmerler, H., and Lilienfeld, A.M. 1973. "The relationship of intrauterine radiation to subsequent mortality and development of leukemia in children: A prospective study." *Amer. J. Epid.* 97:283–313.
11. Doll, R. 1971. "The age distribution of cancer: Implications for models of carcinogenesis." *J. Roy. Stat. Soc.* 134:133–166.
12. Fox, J.P., Elveback, L., Scott, W., Gatewood, L., and Ackerman, E. 1971. "Herd mmunity: Basic concept and relevance to public health immunization practices." *Amer. J. Epid.* 94:179–189.
13. Fucillo, D.A., Kurent, J.E., and Sever, J.L. 1974. "Slow virus diseases." *Ann. Rev. Microbiol.* 28:231–264.

14. Graham, S., Levin, M.L., Lilienfeld, A.M., Schuman, L.M., Gibson, R., Dowd, J.E., and Hempelman, L. 1966. "Preconception, intrauterine, and postnatal irradiation as related to leukemia." In *Epidemiological Approaches to the Study of Cancer and Other Chronic Diseases.* W. Haenszel, ed. Natl. Cancer Inst. Monogr. No. 19. Washington, D.C., United States Government Printing Office.
15. Hedrich, A.W. 1933. "Monthly estimates of the child population 'susceptible' to measles, 1900–1931, Baltimore, Md." *Amer. J. Hyg.* 17:613–636.
16. Hess, A.D., and Holden, P. 1958. "The natural history of the arthropod-borne encephalitides in the United States." *Ann. N.Y. Acad. Sci.* 70:294–311.
17. Hewitt, D. 1955. "Some features of leukemia mortality." *Brit. J. Prev. Soc. Med.* 9:81–88.
18. Kato, H. 1971. "Mortality in children exposed to A-bombs while *in utero,* 1945–1969." *Amer. J. Epid.* 93:435–442.
19. MacMahon, B. 1962. "Prenatal X-ray exposure and childhood cancer." *J. Natl. Cancer Inst.* 28:1173–1191.
20. Pike, M.C. 1966. "A method of analysis of a certain class of experiments in carcinogenesis." *Biometrics* 22:142–161.
21. Polednak, A.P. 1974. "Latency periods in neoplastic diseases." *Amer. J. Epid.* 100:354–356.
22. Sartwell, P.E. 1950. "The distribution of incubation periods of infectious disease." *Amer. J. Hyg.* 51:310–318.
23. ———. 1966. "The incubation period and the dynamics of infectious disease." *Amer. J. Epid.* 83:204–216.
24. Stewart, A., Webb, J., and Hewitt, D. 1958. "A survey of childhood malignancies." *Brit. Med. J.* 1:1495–1508.

4 Mortality Statistics

A. INTRODUCTION

Death certificates were not introduced for epidemiologic studies, but rather as legal documents. Graunt's use of the Bills of Mortality and Farr's adaptation of the Registration System to portray the health and social conditions of the population initiated the broad epidemiologic use of data that were regularly collected. Although this chapter deals with mortality statistics, it should be noted that these are only part of a system of vital records existing today in most industrialized countries. In addition to deaths, such vital events as births, marriages, and divorces are also recorded. Such reporting systems, however, are most highly developed for births and deaths.

In the United States, state laws require the registration of births, deaths, marriages, and divorces as they occur. Local registrars transmit these records to the state registrars, who maintain them for permanent reference; copies are sent to the National Center for Health Statistics for the tabulation of national statistics. In 1902, the collection of copies of death certificates by a permanent Bureau of Census began as an annual procedure in ten states and in several additional cities that had an adequate registration system, thereby creating a Death Registration Area (1). This Area was predominantly urban and included about 40 percent of the U.S. population (2). In 1933, with the admission of Texas, the Death Registration Area covered the entire United States. These developments must be considered when evaluating mortality trends in the United States.

B. CLASSIFICATION OF CAUSE OF DEATH

A standard death certificate, developed by the National Center for Health Statistics, has been adopted, with minor modifications, by most states (Fig. 4–1); there is a separate certificate for fetal deaths. Information is requested on demographic factors such as place of residence, occupation, national origin, age, and sex, as well as cause of death. The latter, as stated on the certificate, must be accepted with caution. Figure 4–1 shows that the immediate cause is entered first, then any intermediate conditions, and finally, the underlying cause. A separate space allows for the inclusion of other significant conditions. In official tabulations, the cause of death is, in fact, the underlying cause, classified according to the International Statistical Classification of Diseases, Injuries, and Causes of Death (ICD), which is revised about every ten years by the World Health Organization in cooperation with several national committees. Since 1900, the United States has adhered to the International List in its classification procedures.

In 1948, the revision in ICD classification radically departed from previous versions by including in a single list the classification of both mortality and morbidity. This was a direct consequence of both an increased interest in morbidity studies and the need for comparability of classification by various health agencies.

Multiple Causes

An important problem develops when the physician enters two or more causes on the death certificate. Before 1949, a *Manual of Joint Causes of Death,* specifying rules for assigning priorities to various causes, was used to assure standardization for selecting the cause of death, based on both the sequence of pathogenetic events accepted at the time and the information required for public health programs. This manual was updated periodically, but coincident with the adoption of the ICD revision in 1949, its use was terminated and the physician became responsible for determining the underlying cause of death. Although a manual is used to correct illogical

FORM APPROVED
BUDGET BUREAU NO. 68-R190)

U.S. GOVERNMENT PRINTING OFFICE : 1967 OF—241-661

(PHYSICIAN)

U.S. STANDARD
CERTIFICATE OF DEATH

STATE FILE NUMBER

TYPE, OR PRINT IN
PERMANENT INK
SEE HANDBOOK FOR
INSTRUCTIONS

LOCAL FILE NUMBER

DECEASED

DECEASED—NAME					
FIRST	MIDDLE	LAST	SEX	DATE OF DEATH (MONTH, DAY, YEAR)	
1.			2.	3.	

AGE—LAST BIRTHDAY (YEARS)	UNDER 1 YEAR		UNDER 1 DAY		DATE OF BIRTH (MONTH, DAY, YEAR)	COUNTY OF DEATH
	MOS.	DAYS	HOURS	MIN.		
5a.	5b.		5c.		6.	7a.

RACE WHITE, NEGRO, AMERICAN INDIAN, ETC. (SPECIFY)
4.

CITY, TOWN, OR LOCATION OF DEATH
7b.

INSIDE CITY LIMITS (SPECIFY YES OR NO)
7c.

HOSPITAL OR OTHER INSTITUTION—NAME (IF NOT IN EITHER, GIVE STREET AND NUMBER)
7d.

STATE OF BIRTH (IF NOT IN U.S.A., NAME COUNTRY)
8.

CITIZEN OF WHAT COUNTRY
9.

MARRIED, NEVER MARRIED, WIDOWED, DIVORCED (SPECIFY)
10.

SURVIVING SPOUSE (IF WIFE, GIVE MAIDEN NAME)
11.

SOCIAL SECURITY NUMBER
13a.

USUAL OCCUPATION (GIVE KIND OF WORK DONE DURING MOST OF WORKING LIFE, EVEN IF RETIRED)
13a.

KIND OF BUSINESS OR INDUSTRY
13b.

USUAL RESIDENCE WHERE DECEASED LIVED. IF DEATH OCCURRED IN INSTITUTION, GIVE RESIDENCE BEFORE ADMISSION.

RESIDENCE—STATE	COUNTY	CITY, TOWN, OR LOCATION	INSIDE CITY LIMITS (SPECIFY YES OR NO)	STREET AND NUMBER
14a.	14b.	14c.	14d.	14e.

PARENTS

FATHER—NAME			MOTHER—MAIDEN NAME		
FIRST	MIDDLE	LAST	FIRST	MIDDLE	LAST
15.			16.		

INFORMANT—NAME	MAILING ADDRESS
	(STREET OR R.F.D. NO., CITY OR TOWN, STATE, ZIP)

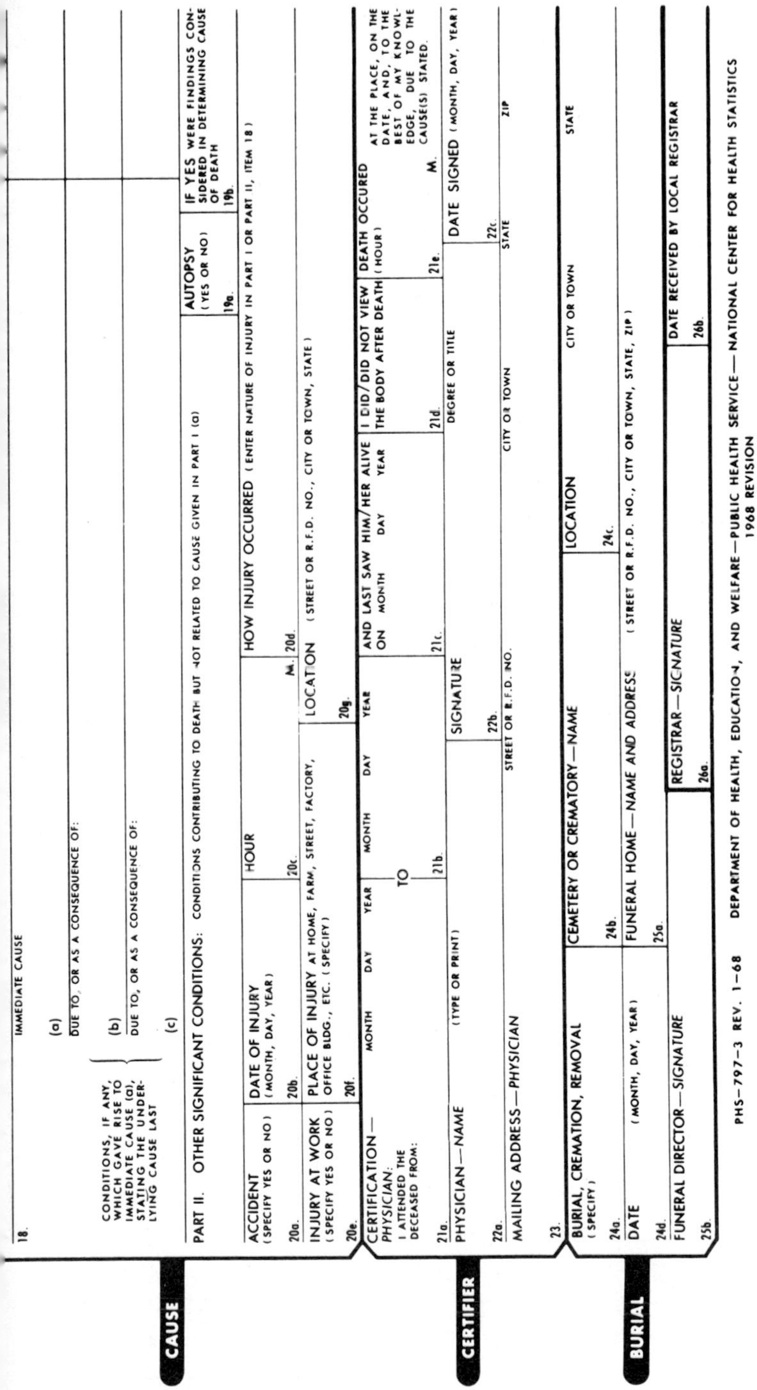

18. | IMMEDIATE CAUSE

(a)

DUE TO, OR AS A CONSEQUENCE OF:

(b)

DUE TO, OR AS A CONSEQUENCE OF:

CONDITIONS, IF ANY, WHICH GAVE RISE TO IMMEDIATE CAUSE (a), STATING THE UNDERLYING CAUSE LAST

(c)

PART II. OTHER SIGNIFICANT CONDITIONS: CONDITIONS CONTRIBUTING TO DEATH BUT NOT RELATED TO CAUSE GIVEN IN PART I (a)

AUTOPSY (YES OR NO) 19a.

IF YES WERE FINDINGS CONSIDERED IN DETERMINING CAUSE OF DEATH 19b.

ACCIDENT (SPECIFY YES OR NO) 20a.

DATE OF INJURY (MONTH, DAY, YEAR) 20b.

HOUR 20c. M.

HOW INJURY OCCURRED (ENTER NATURE OF INJURY IN PART I OR PART II, ITEM 18) 20d.

INJURY AT WORK (SPECIFY YES OR NO) 20e.

PLACE OF INJURY AT HOME, FARM, STREET, FACTORY, OFFICE BLDG., ETC. (SPECIFY) 20f.

LOCATION (STREET OR R.F.D. NO., CITY OR TOWN, STATE) 20g.

CERTIFICATION—PHYSICIAN: I ATTENDED THE DECEASED FROM:
MONTH DAY YEAR TO MONTH DAY YEAR 21b.
AND LAST SAW HIM/HER ALIVE ON MONTH DAY YEAR 21c.
I DID/DID NOT VIEW THE BODY AFTER DEATH 21d.
DEATH OCCURRED (HOUR) M. 21e.
AT THE PLACE, ON THE DATE, AND, TO THE BEST OF MY KNOWLEDGE, DUE TO THE CAUSE(S) STATED.
DATE SIGNED (MONTH, DAY, YEAR) 21f.

PHYSICIAN—NAME (TYPE OR PRINT) 21a.

SIGNATURE 22b.

DEGREE OR TITLE 22c.

MAILING ADDRESS—PHYSICIAN 22a.
STREET OR R.F.D. NO. CITY OR TOWN STATE ZIP

BURIAL, CREMATION, REMOVAL (SPECIFY) 24a.

CEMETERY OR CREMATORY—NAME 24b.

LOCATION 24c.

CITY OR TOWN STATE

DATE (MONTH, DAY, YEAR) 24d.

FUNERAL HOME—NAME AND ADDRESS (STREET OR R.F.D. NO., CITY OR TOWN, STATE, ZIP) 25a.

FUNERAL DIRECTOR—SIGNATURE 25b.

REGISTRAR—SIGNATURE 26a.

DATE RECEIVED BY LOCAL REGISTRAR 26b.

CAUSE

CERTIFIER

BURIAL

PHS-797-3 REV. 1-68   DEPARTMENT OF HEALTH, EDUCATION, AND WELFARE—PUBLIC HEALTH SERVICE—NATIONAL CENTER FOR HEALTH STATISTICS
1968 REVISION

Figure 4–1. Model certificate of death recommended by the National Center for Health Statistics

and confusing reported sequences of events leading to death, it was thought that the physician's statement of the underlying cause of death would be more useful in planning programs for their prevention, since he would be more familiar with them. These changing methods of tabulating causes of death have had marked effects on the pattern of mortality trends of certain diseases, such as diabetes; but for most diseases, these effects have been small. The effects of each ICD revision and its comparability with existing statistics have been studied (3–6). These facts must be kept in mind in the interpretation of mortality trends.

The use of a single or only a primary cause of death for routine statistical tabulations has been criticized as not providing a complete representation of events (9). For deaths in the United States in 1955, special tabulations of the multiple causes were prepared, thereby providing information for evaluating the routine tabulations of death (15). It has been suggested that epidemiologists should really be interested in "those diseases that one dies with as well as from."

Accuracy of Statement of Cause of Death

As the physician completing the death certificate may not have been the attending physician and, therefore, would be unfamiliar with the deceased's medical history, the reliability of statements of causes of death has been questioned. Even if an autopsy is performed, the results may not be available in time to be entered on the death certificate, which by law is also required for burial.

Many studies have been conducted to evaluate the accuracy of the cause of death statements on the certificate (7, 10–13). Moriyama and his colleagues studied certificates from a sample of 1,837 deaths in Pennsylvania during a three-month period in 1956, obtaining supplementary information from the qualifying physician by questionnaire (10). The returns from these physicians were reviewed, together with the original statement of cause of death on the certificates, under the supervision of an internist, who also gave his opinion as to the certainty of the diagnoses. The reviewer's evaluations indicated that the different cause of death statements were fairly variable with respect to the percent of diagnoses he considered to have been solidly established (Table 4–1). For the major cardiovascular-renal diseases, only 32.8 percent of deaths so certified were solidly established as compared to 89.3 percent for malignant neoplasms of the lymphatic and hematopoietic tissues. However, at the other end of the scale, the percent of cause-of-death statements that were considered to be probably wrong varied from 0 to 20.3 percent. For the majority of causes of death, they were 5 percent or less. These results indicate that epidemiologists utilizing death-certificate information in studying a particular disease may have to incorporate validation procedures for the cause of death statements.

C. MEASURES OF MORTALITY

Mortality Rates

Several methods of measuring mortality in a population are described in biostatistics and demography texts. However, it may be worthwhile to present briefly a few measures that are frequently used in epidemiologic studies. The most frequently used measure of mortality is the mortality or death rate, which has three essential elements:

1. A population group exposed to the risk of death.
2. A time period.
3. The number of deaths occurring in that population group during that time period.

The numerator of the rate consists of the number of deaths that occurred in the specified population and the denominator is obtained either from a census, or estimates, of that population:

$$\begin{matrix} \text{Annual death rate} \\ \text{from all causes} \\ \text{(per 1,000} \\ \text{population)} \end{matrix} = \frac{\begin{matrix}\text{Total number of deaths during}\\ \text{a specified twelve-month period}\end{matrix}}{\begin{matrix}\text{Number of persons in the popula-}\\ \text{tion at the middle of the period}\end{matrix}} \times 1,000$$

It is important to note that the numerator and denominator are related to each other in that the numerator represents those individuals who died, and the denominator those who are exposed to the risk or probability of death. For example, in the U.S. there were 1,892,879 deaths in 1978 in a population of 212,946,226; thus:

Table 4–1.   Reviewer's Evaluation of Diagnostic Information in the Deaths Certified by Physicians: Pennsylvania Sample, Three-month Period, 1956*

Cause of Death	Total Number	Percent Distribution				
			Diagnosis of Cause of Death			
		Total	Solidly Estab-lished	Reason-able	In Doubt	Probably Wrong
Tuberculosis, all forms	25	100.0	72.0	12.0	0	4.0
Malignant neoplasms, including neoplasms of lymphatic and hematopoietic tissues†	433	100.0	67.7	14.1	7.4	7.2
Malignant neoplasm of diges-tive organs and peritoneum	185	100.0	65.4	13.0	9.2	8.1
of stomach	47	100.0	44.7	21.3	10.6	19.1
Malignant neoplasm of respi-ratory system†	58	100.0	61.1	21.8	12.4	5.0
of trachea, and of bronchus and lung specified as primary	21	100.0	61.9	23.8	4.8	4.8
of lung and bronchus, un-specified as to whether pri-mary or secondary	33	100.0	57.6	21.2	9.1	6.1
Malignant neoplasm of breast and female genital organs	66	100.0	81.8	9.1	4.5	1.5
Malignant neoplasm of male genital organs	20	100.0	65.0	25.0	5.0	0
Malignant neoplasm of urinary organs	16	100.0	87.5	6.3	6.3	0
Malignant neoplasm of lym-phatic and hematopoietic tissues	28	100.0	89.3	10.7	0	0
Diabetes mellitus	60	100.0	50.0	36.7	6.7	5.0

$$\text{Annual death rate in 1978 (per 1,000 population)} = \frac{1{,}892{,}879 \text{ deaths during 1978}}{212{,}946{,}226 \text{ persons estimated to be present on July 1, 1978}} = 8.89 \text{ per 1,000 population.}$$

This particular death rate is expressed in terms of a single year and a population of 1,000. The unit of time can be selected by the investigator, but it should be specified. Also, the population unit can vary but must be specified. For total deaths, the population unit is usually 1,000. For specific causes of death a unit of 100,000 is usually used because the larger population results in a rate that can be expressed in whole numbers. Thus, in countries the size of

Table 4–1 cont.

Cause of Death	Total Number	Percent Distribution Diagnosis of Cause of Death				
		Total	Solidly Estab-lished	Reason-able	In Doubt	Probably Wrong
Major cardiovascular-renal diseases†	1194	100.0	32.8	46.5	10.3	6.0
Vascular lesions affecting central nervous system†	236	100.0	31.8	53.8	7.2	2.1
Rheumatic fever and rheumatic heart disease	38	100.0	58.0	23.7	7.9	2.6
Arteriosclerotic heart disease so described†	260	100.0	30.0	51.9	9.2	3.5
Heart disease specified as involving coronary arteries†	271	100.0	39.1	45.0	10.7	3.0
Hypertensive diseases†	128	100.0	32.8	40.6	16.4	3.1
Other cardiovascular-renal diseases†	261	100.0	26.4	42.1	11.1	17.2
Influenza and pneumonia, except pneumonia of newborn	30	100.0	20.0	40.0	16.7	16.7
All other	148	100.0	45.9	18.9	12.2	20.3
Total weighted sample†	1,890	100.0	42.7	36.0	9.6	7.5

* Excludes 232 medicolegal cases. Deaths for which no information was reported are included in totals.
† Figures adjusted to represent one-tenth of the deaths for the three-month period, i.e., the number of deaths in the Current Mortality Sample.
Source: Moriyama et al. (10).

the United Kingdom, death rates may be expressed per 1,000,000 population. These rates can be made explicit for a variety of characteristics, such as age and specific causes:

Annual age-specific death rate from all causes for those under 10 yrs of age in 1976 (per 1000 population) $= \dfrac{\text{Number of all deaths under 10 yrs of age in 1976}}{\text{Number of individuals in the population under 10 at July 1, 1976}}$

$$= \frac{62,905}{32,688,000} \times 1,000$$

$$= 1.92 \text{ per } 1,000 \text{ population.}$$

$$\begin{array}{l}\text{Annual death rate} \\ \text{from lung cancer} \\ \text{in 1978 (per} \\ \text{100,000 population)}\end{array} = \dfrac{\begin{array}{l}\text{Number of deaths from} \\ \text{lung cancer in 1978}\end{array}}{\begin{array}{l}\text{Number of persons in} \\ \text{the population at} \\ \text{July 1, 1978}\end{array}} \times 100{,}000$$

$$= \dfrac{82{,}025}{212{,}946{,}226} \times 100{,}000$$

$$= 38.5 \text{ per 100,000 population.}$$

Such rates can also be specified by sex, various socioeconomic characteristics of the population, marital status, and color.

Another type of rate, frequently and confusingly termed a "mortality rate" in the clinical literature, is the "case fatality rate":

$$\begin{array}{l}\text{Case fatality rate} \\ \text{(percent)}\end{array} = \dfrac{\begin{array}{l}\text{Number of individuals dying during} \\ \text{specified period of time after} \\ \text{disease onset or diagnosis}\end{array}}{\begin{array}{l}\text{Number of individuals with the} \\ \text{specified disease}\end{array}} \times 100$$

This rate represents the risk of dying during a definite period of time for those individuals who have the particular disease. Again, the period of time during which the deaths occurred should be specified. Case fatality rates can also be made specific for age, sex, severity of disease, and any other factors of clinical and epidemiologic importance.

The proportionate mortality rate (or ratio), which represents the proportion of total deaths that are due to a specific cause, is also frequently used:

$$\begin{array}{l}\text{Proportionate mortality} \\ \text{rate from cardiovascular} \\ \text{diseases in the U.S. in 1978}\end{array} = \dfrac{\begin{array}{l}\text{Number of deaths from cardiovascular} \\ \text{diseases in the U.S. in 1978}\end{array}}{\text{Total deaths in the U.S. in 1978}}$$

This rate is usually multiplied by one hundred and expressed as a percentage. Since it depends on two variables, both of which may differ, it is of limited value in making comparisons between different population groups or different time periods.

The proportionate mortality rate does not directly measure the risk or probability of a person in a population dying from a specific disease as does a cause-specific mortality rate. To illustrate its limitation in a simple way, let us assume that there are two countries,

A and B, each with a population of one million. Furthermore, Country A had a death rate from all causes of death of thirty per 100,000 population in 1978, representing 300 deaths, and Country B had an all-cause death rate of 10 per 100,000 in 1978, representing 100 deaths. Each country had the same death rate from cardiovascular diseases of 5 per 100,000 representing 50 deaths and a person's risk of dying from cardiovascular disease in each country was therefore the same. The proportionate mortality rates expressed as the percent of all deaths that were from cardiovascular diseases in each country would then be as follows:

Country A: $\frac{50}{300} = 17$ percent

Country B: $\frac{50}{100} = 50$ percent

Clearly, this difference in proportionate mortality rates does not reflect the risk of dying from cardiovascular diseases in these countries—which is the same—but the difference in mortality from other causes of death. However, the proportionate mortality rate is useful in indicating within any population group the relative importance of specific causes of death in the total mortality picture. This rate aids the epidemiologist in selecting areas for further study and the health administrator in determining priorities for planning purposes.

Age Adjustment of Mortality Rates

Among the principal determinants of mortality is, of course, age (Fig. 4–2) (8). Since differences in the age composition of the population will influence the total mortality rates, it is preferable to use age-specific mortality rates in comparing the mortality experiences in different geographical areas, population groups, or time periods. However, it is sometimes convenient to have a summary statistic of such comparisons that takes into account the differences in the age distribution of the population. This is accomplished by a computational process known as "age adjustment" or "age standardization." Of the several such summary statistics that are available, two will be used in presenting illustrative material in this book: The Direct Method of Age Adjustment, and the Standardized Mortality Ratio.

It should be emphasized that the procedure of standardization provides a summary index and is not a substitute for a careful ex-

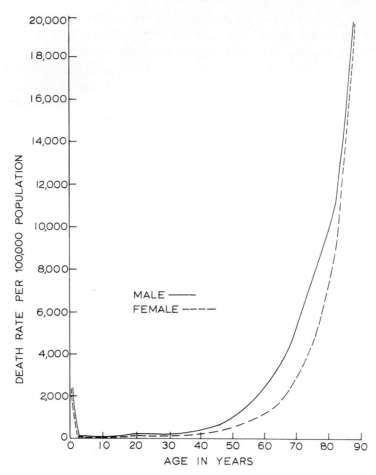

Figure 4–2.   Age-specific death rates by sex, United States, 1969

Source: Klebba, Mauer, and Glass (8).

amination of age-specific rates. It is, however, a generally useful procedure. Although it was originally developed to analyze and present mortality statistics and still is most frequently used for that purpose, it can be applied in the other types of epidemiologic studies discussed in this book. And, the same method of adjustment can be used for taking into account other factors besides age, such as sex, social class, number of cigarettes smoked, or size of family.

DIRECT METHOD OF AGE ADJUSTMENT

A "standard population" is first selected. Then, one applies the age-specific mortality rates of the two groups being compared to

Table 4–2. Calculation of the Age-adjusted Mortality Rates from all Causes by the Direct Method: United States, 1950 and 1960

Age Group (Years)	Mortality from All Causes per 100,000 Population		Standard Population: Total U.S. Enumerated Population per 1,000,000	Expected Number of Deaths that Would Occur in Standard Population at Rates in	
	1950 (1)	1960 (2)	1940 (3)	1950 (4)	1960 (5)
<1	3,299.2	2,696.4	15,343	506.2	413.7
1–4	139.4	109.1	64,718	90.2	70.6
5–14	60.1	46.6	170,355	102.4	79.4
15–24	128.1	106.3	181,677	232.7	193.1
25–34	178.7	146.4	162,066	289.6	237.6
35–44	358.7	299.4	139,237	499.4	416.9
45–54	853.9	756.0	117,811	1,006.0	890.7
55–64	1,901.0	1,735.1	80,294	1,526.4	1,393.2
65–74	4,104.3	3,822.1	48,426	1,987.5	1,850.9
75–84	9,331.1	8,745.2	17,303	1,614.6	1,513.2
85+	20,196.9	19,857.5	2,770	559.5	550.4
Total death rate all ages	963.8	954.7	—	—	—
Total population	—	—	1,000,000	—	—
Total expected number of deaths	—	—	—	8,414.5	7,609.7
Age-adjusted death rate per 100,000	—	—	—	841.45	760.97

Source: Klebba, Mauer, and Glass (8).

the number in the same age groups of that standard population. This gives the number of deaths that can be expected in the standard population if these age-specific rates had prevailed. As an example, in Table 4–2, we are comparing the United States mortality experience for 1950 and 1960 (cols. 1 and 2). In the 1–4 age group (underlined), the 1950 death rate of 139.4 per 100,000 (col. 1) is multiplied by 64,718 (col. 3), the number in that age group of the standard population of 1,000,000. This results in an expected number of 90.2 deaths (col. 4), that is, the number of deaths that would have been expected if that age-specific death rate of 139.4 had prevailed in that age group of the standard population. In 1960, the same age group had a death rate of 109.1 (col. 2), which, when multiplied by 64,718 (col. 3), resulted in 70.6 expected deaths (col. 5). In a similar manner, the age-specific death rates for each year and age group are multiplied by the number in the appropriate age group of the standard population yielding the expected number of deaths for 1950 and 1960, as shown in columns 4 and 5 of Table 4–2. Separately, for 1950 and 1960, the expected number of deaths in each age group are totaled to determine the total number of expected deaths. These are divided by the total standard population of 1,000,000 to yield "age-adjusted" death rates that are expressed in terms of 100,000 population to make them comparable to the original death rates (cols. 4 and 5).

In the example given in Table 4–2, the age-adjusted rate in 1960 is much lower than in 1950, in contrast to the total death rates where the 1960 death rate is only slightly lower. Examination of the age-specific death rates indicates a much larger decline from 1950 to 1960 for most of the age groups (except for the older ones) than is reflected in the total death rates. The difference between the changes in the total and age-adjusted death rates results from the fact that the 1960 population has a larger proportion of people in the older age groups than the 1950 population. The much higher mortality rates in the older age groups have a large effect on the total death rate. The total death rate is affected by both the age specific death rates *and* the age distribution of the population. The age-adjustment procedure is used to remove the influence of the age distribution of the population by the use of a standard population. Thus, the differences in the computed age-adjusted death rates in Table 4–2 more closely reflect the differences in the age-specific death rates. The formulas for the variance and standard error of the age-adjusted death rate are presented in Appendix 1 (p. 353).

STANDARDIZED MORTALITY RATIO

Another type of age-adjustment is the standardized mortality ratio (SMR), which is defined by the Registrar General of England and Wales for studies of occupational mortality as "the number of deaths occurring among men aged 20–64 in a given occupation, expressed as a percentage of the number of deaths that might have been expected to occur if the given occupation had experienced within each age group the same rate as that of a standard population" (14). It has one advantage over the direct method of age-

Table 4–3. Calculation of the Standardized Mortality Ratio for Occupation of Male Farmers and Farm Managers for All Causes of Death: England and Wales, 1951

Age Group	Number of Farmers and Farm Managers (Census, 1951) (1)	Standard Death Rates per 1,000,000 (All Causes of Death) (2)	Expected Number of Deaths for Farmers and Farm Managers per 1,000,000 (3) = (1) × (2)
20–24	7,989	1,383	11
25–34	37,030	1,594	59
35–44	60,838	2,868	174
45–54	68,687	8,212	564
55–64	55,565	22,953	1,275

Total expected deaths per year: 2,083
Total observed deaths per year: 1,464

$$\text{SMR} = \frac{1,464}{2,083} \times 100 = 70.3\%$$

Source: Registrar General's Decennial Supplement (14).

adjustment in that knowledge of the age distribution of deaths in the population subgroup is not necessary for its computation. One need only know the number of persons in each age group in that population segment and age-specific death rates for the entire population.

The Registrar General's Decennial Supplement for 1951, *Occupational Mortality,* provides an example of the computation of the SMR (Table 4–3). Column 1 of this table shows the number of male farmers and farm managers by age group, as enumerated in the 1951 census. During the five-year period 1949–1953, there were 7,320 deaths from all causes in this occupational group, or an average of 1,464 deaths per year. Does this figure indicate a normal, high, or low mortality risk for the group? In order to answer this question, the expected number of deaths according to a selected standard is computed. The standard in this table is the average annual death rate for all causes, at specified ages, for all employed and retired males in England and Wales during 1949–1953 (col. 2). Multiplying, within each age group, the figures in column 1 with those in column 2 and dividing by 1,000,000—since the rates are given per million males—results in the number of deaths in column 3. The sum total is 2,083, which is more than the number of deaths that actually did occur. The SMR is finally obtained by expressing the observed number as a percentage of the expected.

$$\text{SMR} = \frac{\text{Observed number of deaths per year}}{\text{Expected number of deaths per year}} = \frac{1,464}{2,083} \times 100 = 70.3 \text{ percent}$$

This indicates that the mortality experience of farmers and farm managers was only 70.3 percent of the total population rate from all causes of death.

This general computational procedure would be the same if deaths from a specific cause rather than from all causes were considered. Also, the formulas for the variance and standard error of the SMR are presented in Appendix 1 (p. 353).

STUDY PROBLEMS

1. Usually, the epidemiologist prefers to use the direct method of age adjustment, since it results in an estimate of the *average* probability of death. However, sometimes the indirect method (the standardized mortality ratio or SMR) is preferred, even though all the data required for the use of the direct method is available. Under what circumstances would the SMR be preferred?
2. What are the major limitations in the use of "official mortality statistics"?
3. Usually, age-specific mortality rates for disease X can be viewed as the probability of an individual of a given age dying of disease X. How does the epidemiologist view an age-adjusted rate?
4. The age-sex-specific death rates per 1,000,000 persons for diabetes in 1960 (ICD 260) in the United States were as follows:

Age	Male	Female
0–4	8	6
5–14	3	5
15–24	8	10
25–34	27	20
35–44	51	40
45–54	121	121
55–64	319	437
65–74	761	1084
75–84	1446	1785
85+	1706	1887

Three standard populations are:

Age	African	World (Segi)	European
0–4	10,000	12,000	8,000
5–9	10,000	10,000	7,000
10–14	10,000	9,000	7,000
15–19	10,000	9,000	7,000
20–24	10,000	8,000	7,000
25–29	10,000	8,000	7,000
30–34	10,000	6,000	7,000
35–39	10,000	6,000	7,000
40–44	5,000	6,000	7,000
45–49	5,000	6,000	7,000
50–54	3,000	5,000	7,000
55–59	2,000	4,000	6,000
60–64	2,000	4,000	5,000
65–69	1,000	3,000	4,000
70–74	1,000	2,000	3,000
75–79	500	1,000	2,000
80–84	300	500	1,000
85+	200	500	1,000
TOTAL	100,000	100,000	100,000

a) Which standard population might be preferred to calculate age-adjusted death rates for a country whose population is:
   i) young (over 50% of the population is less than 30 years of age)?
   ii) old (over 50% of the population is over 30 years of age)?
   iii) representative of the world as a whole?
b) Calculate the age-adjusted rates for diabetes for males and females using each of the standard populations. Are the age-adjusted rates the same for males? for females? For each of the standard populations, calculate the ratio of the male age-adjusted rate to that for females. Are the ratios the same?
c) What can one conclude about the importance of the standard population selected for determining:
   i) the absolute magnitude of the death rate?
   ii) the relative magnitude of the death rate?
5. What are the alternatives to using the three standard populations presented in Problem 4? For each alternative, discuss the effect on the inferences made.

REFERENCES

1. Cassedy, J.H. 1965. "Registration area and American vital statistics: Development of a health research resource, 1885–1915." *Bull. Hist. Med.* 39: 221–231.
2. Dorn, H.F. 1966. "Mortality." In *Chronic Diseases and Public Health.* A.M. Lilienfeld and A.J. Gifford, eds. Baltimore: The Johns Hopkins Press, pp. 23–54.
3. Dunn, H.L., and Shackley, W. 1945. *Comparison of cause of death assignments by the 1929 and 1938 revisions of the International List: Deaths in the United States, 1940 Vital Statistics—Special Reports 19:153–277, 1944.* Washington, D.C.: United States Department of Commerce, Bureau of the Census.
4. Faust, M.M., and Dolman, A.B. 1963. *Comparability of mortality statistics for the fifth and sixth revisions: United States, 1950.* Vital Statistics—Special Reports, Selected Studies 51: No. 2:133–178. Washington, D.C.: U.S. Government Printing Office, United States Department of Health, Education and Welfare, Public Health Service.
5. ———. 1964. *Comparability ratios based on mortality statistics for the fifth and sixth revisions: United States, 1950.* Vital Statistics—Special Reports, Selected Studies 51: No. 3:181–245. Washington, D.C.: United States Department of Health, Education and Welfare, Public Health Service.
6. ———. 1965. *Comparability of mortality statistics for the sixth and seventh revisions: United States, 1958.* Vital Statistics—Special Reports, Selected Studies 51: No. 4:248–297. Washington, D.C.: United States Department of Health, Education and Welfare, Public Health Service.
7. James, G., Patton, R.E., and Heslin, A.S. 1955. "Accuracy of cause-of-death statements on death certificates." *Pub. Health Reps.* 70:39–51.
8. Klebba, A.J., Mauer, J.D., and Glass, E.J. 1973. *Mortality Trends: Age, Color, and Sex: United States, 1950–69.* National Center for Health Statistics, Vital and Health Statistics Series 20, No. 15. Washington, D.C.: Public Health Service, U.S. Government Printing Office.
9. Krueger, D.E. 1966. "New enumerators for old denominators—Multiple causes of death." In *Epidemiological Approaches to the Study of Cancer and Other Chronic Diseases.* W. Haenszel, ed. Natl. Cancer Inst. Monogr. No. 19, Washington, D.C.: United States Government Printing Office, pp. 431–443.
10. Moriyama, I.M., Baum, W.S., Haenszel, W.M., and Mattison, B.F. 1958. "Inquiry into diagnostic evidence supporting medical certifications of death." *Amer. J. Pub. Health* 48:1376–1387.
11. ———, Dawber, T.R., and Kannel, W.B. 1966. "Evaluation of diagnostic information supporting medical certification of deaths from cardiovascular diseases." In *Epidemiological Approaches to the Study of Cancer and Other Chronic Diseases.* W. Haenszel, ed. Natl. Cancer Inst. Monogr. No. 19, Washington, D.C., United States Government Printing Office, pp. 405–419.
12. Pohlen, K., and Emerson, H. 1942. "Errors in clinical statements of causes of death." *Amer. J. Pub. Health* 32:251–260.
13. ———. 1943. "Errors in clinical statements of causes of death: Second report." *Amer. J. Pub. Health* 33:505–516.
14. Registrar General's Decennial Supplement. 1958. *1951 Occupational Mortality, Part II, Vol. 2.* London: Her Majesty's Stationery Office.

15. Vital Statistics of the United States. 1965. *1955 Supplement: Mortality Data, Multiple Causes of Death.* United States Department of Health, Education and Welfare, Public Health Service, National Center for Health Statistics, Washington, D.C.: United States Government Printing Office.

5 Epidemiologic Studies
of Mortality

> The death rate is a fact; anything beyond this is
> an inference.
>
> WILLIAM FARR, 1874

A. DISTRIBUTION OF MORTALITY IN POPULATIONS

Mortality statistics, reflecting the frequency of occurrence of mortality-producing diseases in the population, are routinely collected in many countries. They provide a readily available indicator of the frequency of disease as it occurs in time, place, and persons and, therefore, are important to the epidemiologist's view of disease.

Time: Trends in Mortality Rates

Figure 5–1 shows the age-adjusted mortality trends from selected sites of cancer among white males in the United States from 1930 to 1976 (1). These trends show considerable differences: lung cancer shows a marked increase; stomach cancer, a marked decrease; and liver cancer, a moderate, but continuous, decline. Slight but consistent increases are noted for pancreatic cancer, leukemia, and esophageal cancer. Colon, rectum, and prostate cancer rates increased slightly until about 1950, after which the rates remained essentially stable.

Epidemiologists constantly search for explanations of such trends. Table 5–1 provides a broad outline for systematically considering possible reasons for changes in mortality trends.

One explanation to be considered immediately is the possibility that the trends may not be real, but rather artifactual—the result of errors in the numerator or denominator of the mortality rates. Im-

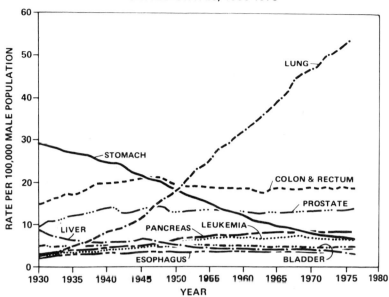

MALE CANCER DEATH RATES* BY SITE
UNITED STATES, 1930-1976

Figure 5–1. Age-adjusted death rates from selected cancer sites among males, United States, 1930–1976

Source: American Cancer Society (1).

provements in medical services over any given period of time are reflected in improved diagnoses of disease and, in turn, in the accuracy of statements of the cause of death on death certificates. For example, the decline in mortality from liver cancer may reflect diagnostic improvements, since we know from clinical experience that many cancers spread to the liver from their primary sites. With improved diagnostic techniques, the original site will be diagnosed more frequently and the certifying physician will designate it as the underlying cause on the death certificate, even if metastases to other organs have occurred. The extent to which this happens and the degree of its influence on mortality trends are difficult to determine. If there is a marked change in a mortality trend, however, knowledge of specific diagnostic improvements in the disease category

Table 5–1.   Outline of Possible Reasons for Changes in Mortality Trends of Disease

---

A. *Artifactual*
1. Errors in the numerator due to
     a)   changes in the recognition of disease
     b)   changes in rules and procedures for classification of causes of death
     c)   changes in the classification code of causes of death
     d)   changes in accuracy of reporting age at death
2. Errors in the denominator due to
     a)   errors in the enumeration of the population
B. *Real*
1. Changes in age distribution of the population
2. Changes in survivorship
3. Changes in incidence of disease: the result of
     a)   genetic factors
     b)   environmental factors

---

usually permits a judgment as to whether they can reasonably be expected to be responsible for the change.

The International Classification of Diseases (ICD) is revised every ten years to improve its efficiency in classifying causes of death (see Chap. 4, p. 67). The revisions entail changes in code numbers and the addition of different disease entities to categories within a specific code. Special studies have been conducted to determine the effect of these changes, if any, on comparability of death rates in different years. When it was noted that the percent increase in the number of reported lung cancer deaths in 1968 was 9.6 percent over 1967—in contrast to an annual percent increase of approximately 5.7 percent between 1963 and 1967, which then fell to 4.1 percent in 1969—a study was conducted to determine whether the eighth ICD revision, which went into effect in 1968, had any influence on cancer mortality rates from all sites (43). The procedure was to code a sample of death certificates where cancer was mentioned, either as an underlying or contributory cause, using both the seventh and eighth revisions of the code. The survey showed that the increases and decreases, listed in Table 5–2, could be attributed to changes in classification for selected groups of cancers. The 17.2 percent decrease in the category of other and unspecified sites suggests an overall improvement in specification of diagnoses. Although these differences attributed to coding changes are not large, they indicate that ICD revisions must be taken into account when evaluating mortality trends.

Table 5–2. Number of Deaths and Percent Change Coded for Each Group of Malignant Neoplasms According to Seventh and Eighth Revisions of International Classification of Diseases (ICD): Special Sample of Death Certificates, 1966–1971

Site	Percent Change in Number of Deaths Coded by Eighth Revision Compared to Seventh Revision
Buccal cavity and pharynx	+5.8*
Digestive system	−0.8
Respiratory system	+1.6
Lung cancer	+2.4
Breast	+0.4
Genitourinary organs	−1.5
Lymphoma	−0.8
Other specified sites†	+1.4
Other and unspecified sites	−17.2
Total malignant neoplasms	−0.4

* Plus sign indicates an increased number in those coded by the eighth revision.
† Includes melanoma, skin, eye, brain and other parts of nervous system, thyroid gland, other endocrine glands, bone, connective tissue, lymph nodes, leukemias.

Source: Percy et al. (43).

Another approach to assessing the accuracy of mortality trends is by a direct numerical estimate of whether an increase in mortality from one cause of death can be explained by a decline in another. For example, Gilliam attempted to determine whether the increase in death rates from lung cancer could be explained by errors in certification of deaths from other pulmonary diseases, such as tuberculosis (15). This hypothesis arose from the observation that, during the period in which lung cancer mortality was increasing, mortality from tuberculosis was decreasing. Perhaps some of the deaths that had been attributed to tuberculosis in the earlier half of the twentieth century were actually due to lung cancer. Gilliam computed the degree of error in the certification of deaths from lung cancer, tuberculosis, and all respiratory diseases that would be necessary to produce the amount of the observed increase in lung cancer mortality from 1914 to 1950. He concluded that only part of the increase in mortality attributed to cancer of the lung since 1941 in the United States among white males and females could be accounted for by erroneous death certification of other respiratory diseases,

Table 5–3. Estimates of the Net Census Undercount of the Population by Broad Age Groups, Color, and Sex in the Census of 1970*

| | | Percent of Expected Population | | | |
| | | White | | Black | |
Age	Total	Male	Female	Male	Female
<5	−3.5	−2.3	−2.0	−10.4	−9.8
5–9	−3.0	−2.4	−2.2	−7.7	−6.9
10–14	−1.3	−1.1	−0.9	−3.5	−2.8
15–19	−1.2	−1.3	−0.5	−4.3	−3.2
20–24	−2.3	−2.5	−1.1	−12.1	−5.2
25–34	−4.3	−4.3	−2.4	−18.5	−6.7
35–44	−3.1	−3.6	−0.5	−17.7	−4.0
45–54	−2.1	−2.7	−0.1	−12.4	−5.3
55–64	−2.6	−2.2	−1.9	−9.2	−7.0
65+	−1.8	−1.2	−2.2	+3.1†	−4.2
All ages	−2.5	−2.5	−1.4	−9.9	−5.5

* These estimates are a composite of analytic methods.
† Plus sign indicates a net overcount.

Source: Siegel (48).

"without unreasonable assumptions of age and sex differences in diagnostic error." The fact that, since 1950, lung cancer mortality has continued to increase at a rate that is substantially greater than the decline in tuberculosis mortality confirms that earlier misdiagnoses could not entirely explain the trend.

Another possibility is that artifacts in mortality trends may result from errors in the population census, taken every ten years in the United States (51). In analyzing trends in mortality rates, one must keep in mind that the denominators for the rates are obtained from the decennial census, and that the degree of error in the census may differ from one decade to another. More important, however, is the observation that the errors in the census vary by age, sex, and color, and undoubtedly other characteristics. This is illustrated in Table 5–3, which shows the estimated net census undercount by broad age groups, color, and sex for the 1970 census.

Of special interest is the fact that there is a substantial undercount in estimates of the nonwhite population, the 18.5 percent undercount among males in the 25–34 age group representing the largest error. Obviously, mortality rates among nonwhite males in this age group, assuming nearly complete death registration in the

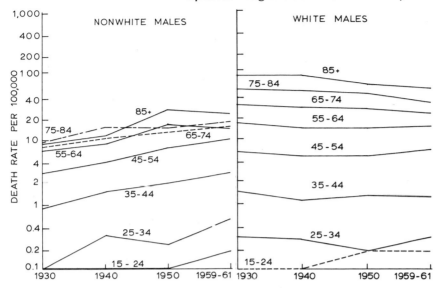

Figure 5–2. Age-specific death rates from malignant neoplasms of buccal cavity and pharynx (ISC 140–148) among males by color, United States, 1930 to 1959–1961

Source: Lilienfeld, Levin, and Kessler (34). Copyright © 1972, The President and Fellows of Harvard College.

group, would be significantly overestimated. If the degree of under-count changes in the different census years with no change in the quality of death certification, artifactual trends of mortality will result. This possibility must be considered, for example, in evaluating the observed increase in mortality trends from cancer of the buccal cavity, pharynx, and esophagus among nonwhite in contrast to white males (Figs. 5–2 and 5–3) (18, 34).

Other methods are available to evaluate trends. One can, for example, determine whether the increases or decreases in mortality agree with the analyses of trends based on autopsies (11), or whether there is consistency between the sexes, or between the trend of a specific cause of death and that of the organ system in which it is classified.

If a mortality trend is real, it may be a result of changes in the age distribution of the population. It is preferable to make this assessment by analyzing the trends of age-specific death rates and then summarizing them by age adjustment.

A decline in mortality might indicate an increase in survivorship, reflecting improvements in the treatment of a disease. However,

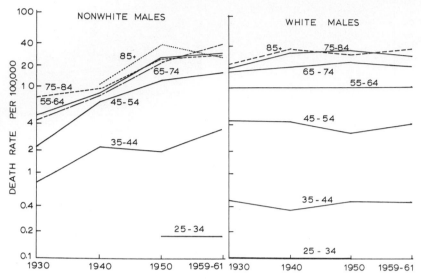

Figure 5–3.   Age-specific death rates from malignant neoplasm of esophagus (ISC 150) among males by color, United States, 1930 to 1959–1961

Source: Lilienfeld, Levin, and Kessler (34). Copyright © 1972, The President and Fellows of Harvard College.

the decline in mortality from gastric cancer shown in Figure 5–1 cannot be attributed to improvements in survivorship since the five-year survivorship rate from gastric cancer has remained at approximately nine to ten percent (5).

Once these possibilities of artifactual error are eliminated, two broad explanatory hypotheses for the trends must be considered in the search for the etiology of disease, namely, genetic and environmental causes. Environmental causes may include changes in personal living habits (e.g. smoking, diet), occupation, air and water pollution, and increased use of drugs.

Ordinarily, genetic factors, per se, do not produce marked mortality changes over a short period of time, unless a specific genetic factor present in the population interacts with a newly introduced agent in the environment. Thus, large increases or decreases in mortality trends usually indicate that a new environmental agent has been introduced into or removed from the population in question. The relationship of asthma mortality to the use of pressurized aerosols is a recent example. Between 1959 and 1966, mortality attributed to asthma steadily increased in England and Wales, after remaining stable for a century (49). In the 5–34 age group, the mortality rate trebled, and in the 10–14 age group, the increase was

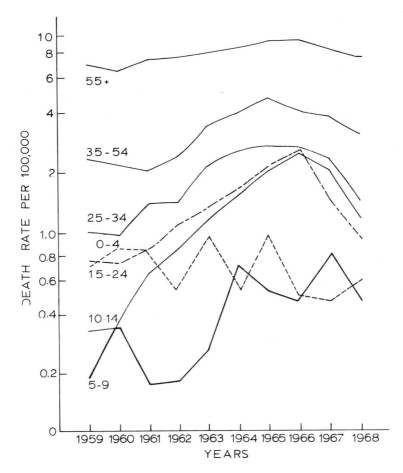

Figure 5–4. Age-specific death rates from asthma (ICD 241), England and Wales, 1959–1968

Source: Inman and Adelstein (22).

sevenfold (Fig. 5–4) (22, 49). A detailed analysis led to the conclusion that the increase was not artifactual and that the mortality trend most likely resulted from new methods of treating asthma, including corticosteroids and pressurized aerosols (49). A study of about 180 deaths attributed to asthma in persons 5–34 years of age during 1966–1967 indicated that in 84 percent of the cases, pressurized aerosol bronchodilators were known to have been used, and probably in excess, whereas only about 66 percent had received corticosteroids (50). The period of introduction of these bronchodilators, particularly isoprenaline, coincided with the increase in asthma mortality. These analyses confirmed prior clinical reports of several patients who had died suddenly following excessive use of aerosol inhalers (19, 20, 40). In June 1967, the Committee on Safety of Drugs issued a warning to all physicians in the United Kingdom, and in 1968 aerosols were made available by prescription only. Both deaths from asthma and aerosol sales declined and by 1969 asthma mortality had almost reached its earlier level (22). A further analysis of mortality rates from asthma in different countries, some showing a rise in asthma mortality and others not, strongly suggested a relationship between increased asthma mortality and high sales volumes of a highly concentrated form of isoprenaline (isoproterenol) in pressurized aerosol nebulizers. The countries that did not show an increase in asthma mortality were those that had not licensed the concentrated nebulizers (52). Subsequent pharmacologic studies provided information on the possible mechanisms by which high concentrations of isoprenaline could result in asthma deaths (10).

Mortality trends also provide a means of evaluating hypotheses developed from other types of studies. A variety of epidemiologic studies, for example, showed a relationship between cigarette smoking and lung cancer (see Chaps. 8 and 9). In light of the evidence indicating a marked increase in the consumption of cigarettes among males since 1920, one would expect to see a corresponding increase in lung cancer mortality. The absence of an observed increase would have been inconsistent with the hypothesis that cigarette smoking was a causal factor in lung cancer.

Place

The distribution of mortality by place will be discussed first in terms of international comparisons and then in terms of regional comparisons within a country.

INTERNATIONAL COMPARISONS OF MORTALITY

Mortality statistics for many countries are available for international comparisons in the compilations of national statistics that appear regularly in the World Health Organization Epidemiological and Vital Statistics Reports. Segi and Kurihara have collated some extremely useful tables and graphs, such as the one in Figure 5–5, comparing the age-adjusted rates for female breast cancer in several countries for the period 1958–1959 (46). Most striking is the very low mortality rate for female breast cancer in Japan. In an

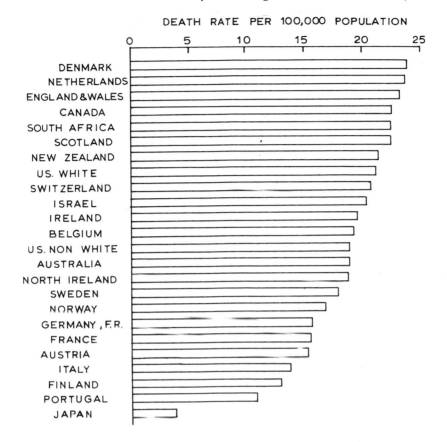

Figure 5–5. Age-adjusted death rates from malignant neoplasm of breast among females in selected countries, 1958–1959

Source: Segi and Kurihara (46).

attempt to explain this, several investigators noted that Japanese children were breast-fed for longer periods of time (one to two years) than was the practice in Western countries. This was consistent with the hypothesis that lactation protects against the development of breast cancer and several studies explored this hypothesis (32). An international collaborative study that reevaluated this hypothesis in populations at low, intermediate, and high risk of breast cancer concluded that lactation had little, if any, protective effect (37). The possibility that endocrine factors could explain the international differences was a natural hypothesis in view of the influence of hormones on the breast. The international differences

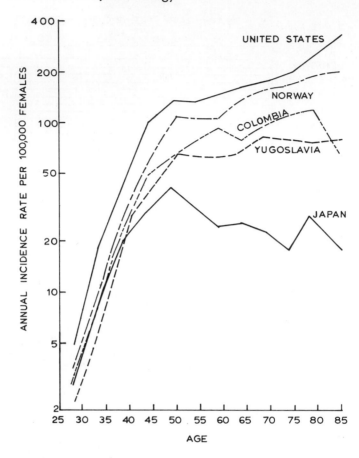

Figure 5–6. Annual age-specific incidence rates of malignant neoplasm of breast among females in selected countries around 1965*

* Colombia (Cali), 1962–1966; Japan (averages of Miyogi Prefecture, 1962–1964, and Okayama Prefecture, 1966); Norway, 1964–1966; United States, 1966–1968; Yugoslavia (Slovenia), 1961–1965.

Source: Seidman (47).

led to studies of Japanese and Caucasian women, which showed different estrogenic profiles, although they were not sufficiently large to explain the mortality differences (35, 36). DeWaard subsequently pointed out that the international differences in mortality and incidence were essentially limited to the postmenopausal period, hypothesizing that there may be two etiologically different types of breast cancer, and that, in addition to endocrine factors, differences in environmental factors in these countries could be

Table 5–4. Coronary Heart Disease and All-cause Death Rates per 100,000 Population, Age-adjusted within Ten-year Age Groups among Males Aged 35–64 in Selected Countries: 1965

Country	Death Rates	
	Coronary Heart Disease	All Causes
Greece	78	712
Japan	79	986
Yugoslavia	116	950
Italy	187	985
Netherlands	243	831
United States	461	1,286
Finland	534	1,432

Source: Keys (24). Reprinted by permission of The American Heart Association, Inc.

etiologically important (Fig. 5–6). He further suggested that the environmental factors might affect endocrine regulation (13).

In evaluating the reported international differences in mortality, one can follow the same sequence of reasoning that was applied in evaluating mortality trends (Table 5–1), substituting only the word "differences" for "changes." However, greater care must be exercised in determining whether the differences are artifactual, that is, due to errors in the numerators and denominators of the mortality rates. International differences in the availability of medical services, diagnostic practices of physicians, and classification procedures must be carefully considered. Some countries do not conduct population censuses; also, it may be necessary to assess carefully the completeness of those which have been done, particularly in developing countries.

Special surveys in individual countries must often be conducted in order to determine definitively whether mortality differences actually reflect differences in disease frequency. Reports of marked mortality differences from arteriosclerotic heart disease (ASHD) in selected countries prompted Keys to organize an international cooperative study of coronary heart disease using samples of men aged 40–59 (Table 5–4) (24). A total of 12,770 men were included in the study, with eleven samples in Europe, two in Japan, and a large group of United States railroad employees. In addition to obtaining information on the frequency of cardiovascular diseases at the initial examination, the plan was to follow and reexamine these men for ten or more years.

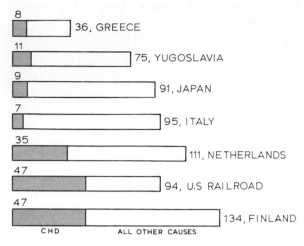

Figure 5–7. Average annual age-standardized death rates from coronary heart disease (CHD) and all causes among males, 40–59 years of age, in five years of follow-up in study countries

Source: Keys (24). Reprinted by permission of The American Heart Association, Inc.

The mortality experience and the major changes in health status as reported by local physicians and health workers were periodically (1–4 times yearly) checked by physicians of the research teams responsible for each of the samples in Europe and in Japan. Detailed examinations approximately five years after entry were carried out on survivors in all samples. Figure 5–7 presents the death rates based on the five-year follow-up of the selected samples.

The pattern of differences in coronary heart-disease mortality between the different groups observed in the follow-up study was generally consistent with the officially reported mortality statistics. Additional analysis of the development of illness from coronary heart disease showed an even greater degree of consistency with the officially reported mortality statistics. Keys also investigated the possible influence on cardiovascular morbidity of various environmental factors, such as diet, obesity, serum cholesterol levels, and smoking habits. The investigators found that cigarette smoking, physical inactivity, and obesity did not explain the differences in morbidity from coronary heart disease. However, elevated blood pressure, higher serum cholesterol levels, and increased percentage of diet calories provided by saturated fatty acids were found to be related to an increased frequency of coronary heart disease.

MIGRANT STUDIES

If one can reasonably eliminate the possibility that mortality differences are artifactual and assume that they do reflect actual differences in disease frequency, it then becomes essential to resolve the issue of whether they are due to different environmental factors in the countries studied or to different genetic compositions of the populations. Migrant studies are being used more and more frequently for this purpose.

These studies take advantage of migration to one country by people from other countries with different mortality experiences from many diseases (12, 21). Comparisons are made between the mortality experience of the migrant groups with that of their country of origin and of their current country of residence.

The rationale for these comparisons and the inferences derived from them can be stated in the following simplified form, where CO = country of origin, M = migrants, and CA = natives of the country of adoption:

1. If the change in environment is the explanation for an observed difference in death rates, one would expect that,
   a) CO rates would differ from M rates and
   b) M rates would approximate CA rates.
2. On the other hand, if genetic factors are of prime importance, one would expect that,
   a) CO rates would equal M rates and
   b) CO and M rates will differ from CA rates.

Other factors that may influence these differences in mortality rates must also be taken into consideration:

1. *Premigration Environment.* If the premigration environment in the country of origin is of primary etiological importance, the pattern of mortality differences would be erroneously interpreted as being genetically determined, according to the reasoning outlined above.
2. *Age at the Time of Migration.* This may be significant since exposure to an etiological factor in the environment may occur at a certain age or period of life. Such information would assist in further determining whether genetic, premigration, or postmigration environmental factors are operating.

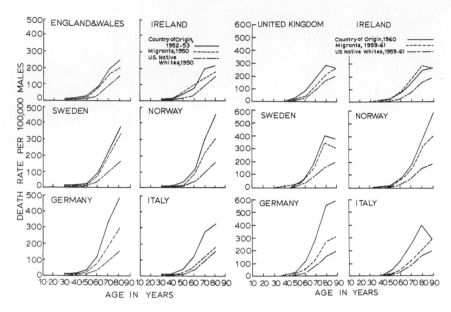

Figure 5–8. Age-specific death rates from malignant neoplasm of stomach (ISC 151) among males, for United States native whites, for migrants to the United States from selected countries, and for residents of these countries of origin, 1950–1953, 1960, and 1959–1961

Source: Lilienfeld, Levin, and Kessler (34). Copyright © 1972, The President and Fellows of Harvard College.

3. *Selective Factors.* Individuals who migrate may differ in ways that influence the occurrence of disease in contrast to those who remain in the country of origin. For example, the healthier and more physically fit would tend to migrate more often than those who are ill. Immigration laws of some countries may require potential migrants to pass a physical and mental examination.

Figure 5–8 presents death rates from malignant neoplasms of the stomach for United States native whites, migrants to the United States from selected countries, and for residents of these countries of origin for 1950–1953, 1960, and 1959–1961 (34). One notes that, in general, the migrant death rates tend to approximate those of the country of adoption, which suggests that changes in the environment and/or living habits are of etiological importance. Figure 5–9 presents the same type of data for female breast cancer,

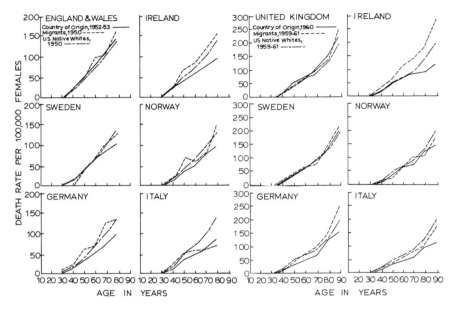

Figure 5–9. Age-specific death rates from malignant neoplasm of the breast (ISC 170) among females, for United States native whites, for migrants to the United States from selected countries, and for residents of these countries of origin, 1950–1953, 1960, and 1959–1961

Source: Lilienfeld, Levin, and Kessler (34). Copyright © 1972, The President and Fellows of Harvard College.

where the differences are not as large as those found in cancer of the stomach. In fact, for some countries (England, Wales, and Sweden, for example), no differences are observed between the various groups, which indicates that possible etiological factors in the environment of these countries and the United States are similar and that the genetic characteristics of these populations are either similar or play no etiological role.

This kind of analysis provides a basis for further study of specific environmental factors to which migrants have been exposed or of changes in their personal living habits that may be of etiological importance. Field epidemiologic studies of these population groups then become necessary.

A study of this type was carried out to investigate the frequency of coronary heart disease and stroke in Japanese men living in Japan, Hawaii, and California (23). It was conducted because of previously observed differences in reported mortality from heart dis-

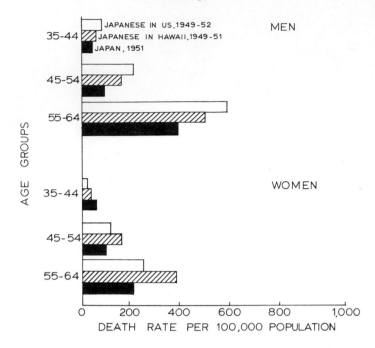

Figure 5–10. Age-specific death rates from diseases of the heart among adult Japanese in continental United States, Hawaii, and Japan by sex, 1949–1952

Source: Gordon (17).

ease and stroke in these groups (17). The Japanese in Hawaii, particularly men, had heart disease mortality rates that were intermediate between Japanese in the United States, who had higher rates, and males in Japan, who had lower rates (Fig. 5–10). Japanese of both sexes in the United States had lower rates from heart disease than the United States white population (Fig. 5–11).

Since the Japanese in Hawaii and the United States are migrants, these data suggest that environmental changes, including living habits, may be etiologically important in heart disease. Many epidemiologic studies have provided evidence to indicate that elevated blood lipid and blood pressure levels, and heavy cigarette smoking, termed "risk factors," increase a person's risk of developing coronary heart disease (45).

A major objective of the previously mentioned study of Japanese men in Japan, Hawaii, and the United States was to determine if the observed differences in mortality among the native and migrant

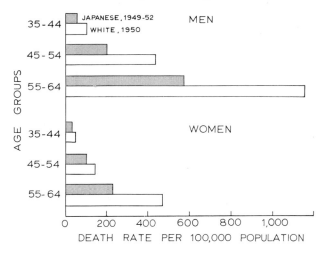

Figure 5–11. Age-specific death rates from diseases of the heart among adult Japanese and whites in continental United States by sex, 1949–1952

Source: Gordon (17).

populations were consistent with the frequency of some risk factors. The first report's findings showed consistency for selected risk factors but not for others. Figure 5–12 shows that the serum cholesterol levels in these groups are consistent with mortality differences; in contrast, blood pressure levels are not (Fig. 5–13 and 5–14). Japanese in Hawaii and in Japan have similar blood pressure levels, but those in California are the highest. Differences in diet, adiposity, and uric acid levels were found to be consistent with the mortality differences, but pulmonary function as measured by "vital capacity" and glucose tolerance were equivocal.

Migrant studies can be further refined to differentiate genetic and environmental reasons for international differences in mortality by comparing the characteristics of migrants with their non-migrant siblings who remained in the country of origin. Each of these groups would also be compared with those of population samples of the native-born in both the countries of origin and of adoption. Since siblings are more similar genetically than nonsiblings, studying certain personal characteristics may provide information on the relative importance of genetic and environmental factors. However, similarities in morbidity, mortality, or personal characteristics in siblings may reflect similarities in the familial en-

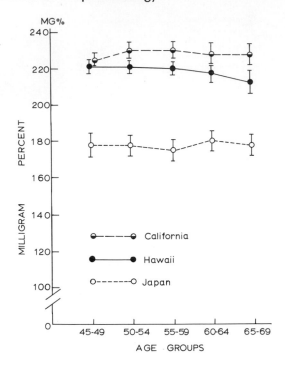

Figure 5–12. Mean values (±2 standard errors) of serum cholesterol for Japanese males in Japan, Hawaii, and California by age

Source: Kagan et al. (23).

vironment, as well as genetic factors. Possible factors influencing the migration of some siblings and not others must also be considered.

This approach is demonstrated by the Ireland–Boston Heart Study, which attempted to explain the reported higher mortality from arteriosclerotic heart disease for males aged 45–64 in the United States than in Ireland (7). In this study, Irish-born men in the Boston area, 30–65 years of age, who had a brother still living in Ireland and who volunteered to cooperate, were enrolled. Because of the urban-rural differences between these groups, two urban groups and one rural male group were also recruited in Ireland. As most of the brothers in Boston were over 20 years of age when they had migrated, they would have been affected by environmental factors in both Ireland and Boston. Consequently, a sample of comparable men in Boston who had been born in the United States, both of whose parents had been born in Ireland,

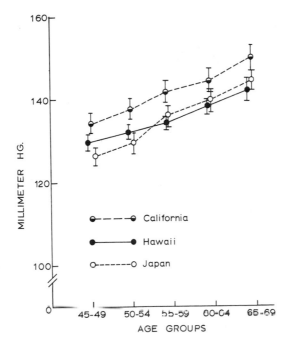

Figure 5–13. Mean values (±2 standard errors) of systolic blood pressure for Japanese males in Japan, Hawaii, and California by age

Source: Kagan et al. (23).

were also recruited. A total of 1994 men in these six groups were enrolled. The investigators studied the intake of calories, complex carbohydrates, magnesium and fluorides, the proportion of calories derived from both saturated and unsaturated fats, serum cholesterol and blood pressure levels, cigarette smoking, weight, skinfold thickness, and electrocardiograms. They concluded that greater physical activity appeared to be an important factor in the lower risk of coronary heart disease in Ireland.

REGIONAL DIFFERENCES WITHIN A COUNTRY

There are geographical differences in mortality from many diseases in the United States and other countries, such as multiple sclerosis, coronary heart and cerebrovascular disease, anencephaly, and cancer of the esophagus (16, 26, 34, 41, 44, 55). In fact, for some diseases, these regional differences are greater than those between countries. Such a regional difference is illustrated by the reported mortality from

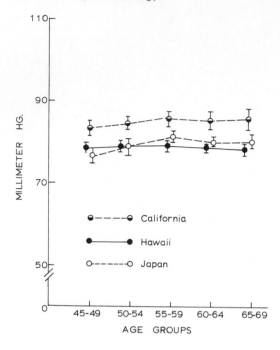

Figure 5–14.   Mean values (±2 standard errors) of diastolic blood pressure for Japanese males in Japan, Hawaii, and California by age

Source: Kagan et al. (23).

cerebrovascular diseases for white males in the United States (Fig. 5–15) (41). A generally similar pattern is found for white females and nonwhites of both sexes. For white males, ages 35–74, the age-adjusted death rates vary from 50–59 (per 100,000) in parts of Colorado to 240–249 (per 100,000) in areas of South Carolina (30). The possible reasons for these differences are similar to those outlined in the previous discussion of changes in mortality trends:

1. Artifactual
   a) resulting from errors in the numerator (such as diagnostic differences, methods of certification) or
   b) errors in the denominator (i.e., in the population census);
2. Real
   a) differences in survivorship, i.e., in case fatality rates due to differences in medical services and facilities or

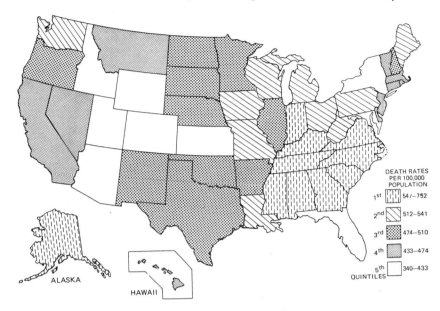

Figure 5–15. Average annual state death rates from cerebrovascular diseases among white males, ages 65–74, by quintile rank, United States, 1959–1961

Source: Moriyama, Krueger, and Stamler (41). Copyright © 1971, The President and Fellows of Harvard College.

b) differences in the actual incidence of the disease in these areas, probably the result of differences in environment. The likelihood that genetic factors are responsible for these differences in the United States would appear small.

In the case of cerebrovascular diseases, possible errors in the numerator must be seriously considered because cerebrovascular disease is frequently listed on the death certificate as a contributory condition rather than an underlying cause of death. This was found in the study of multiple causes of death shown in Table 5–5 (56). Although cerebrovascular disease is frequently mentioned on the death certificate, it is stated as an underlying cause of death in only 57.1 percent of the cases. (The reader will recall that reported causes of death are derived from the underlying causes as stated on the death certificate.) Table 5–5 also indicates a variation in the percentages reported for the various subgroups of cerebrovascular

Table 5–5. Estimated Number of Cerebrovascular Disease Deaths Coded on Death Certificates, Total Coded Conditions, and Those Coded as Underlying Cause: United States, 1955

Cause of Death	(ICD Code)	Total Coded Conditions	Coded as Underlying Cause	
			Number	Per cent of Total
Cerebrovascular diseases (Vascular lesions of the nervous system)	(330-334)	304,004	173,541	57.1
Subarachnoid hemorrhage	(330)	7,458	5,216	69.9
Cerebral hemorrhage	(331)	162,435	109,076	67.2
Cerebral embolism and thrombosis	(332)	67,308	41,326	61.4
Spasm of cerebral arteries	(333)	91	11	12.1
Other and ill-defined vascular lesions of the nervous system	(334)	66,712	17,912	26.8

Source: Vital Statistics of the United States (56).

disease (12.1–69.9 percent). If there are differences in the percentages of cerebrovascular diseases reported as an underlying cause of death in different parts of the country, they could explain in whole, or in part, the regional differences in reported mortality (Fig. 5–15). Another possible source of artifactual distortion is error in the population census; however, this is unlikely for white males in the United States.

The epidemiologic approach to such differences is well illustrated by a series of studies conducted to explore these geographical differences in reported mortality from cerebrovascular diseases. A nationwide study of cerebrovascular disease mortality was conducted to ascertain whether the regional differences in the United States were artifactual or real (30). Because the methods used in this validation study are generally applicable, they are worth reporting.

To validate the differences in cerebrovascular disease mortality, nine areas of the country were selected—three with reported high rates, three with intermediate rates, and three with low rates. In each area, a sample of death certificates for white males and females, ages 45–69, who died during 1965, was reviewed. These death certificates were categorized into five strata based on the underlying cause of death. A systematic sample of certificates was selected from each strata (Table 5–6). Other causes of death were included because of their possible relationship to cerebrovascular disease.

Table 5-6. Number of Death Certificates Selected from Each Stratum of Underlying Causes of Death for White Males and Females 45–69 Years of Age: United States, 1965

Underlying Cause of Death (ICD Code)	Number of Death Certificates Selected in	
	Each Area	All Nine Areas
Cerebrovascular disease (330–334)	Up to 200	1,232
Arteriosclerotic heart disease (420–422)	Up to 200	1,979
Hypertension (440–447)	All certificates	466
Diabetes, other cardiac diseases, other neurologic diseases, senility and ill-defined causes (260, 340–369, 250–256, 753, 754, 780, 795)	All certificates	855
Remaining causes, except trauma	Up to 200	1,782
Total	—	6,314

Source: Kuller et al. (30).

Information on the death certificates was compared with clinical data obtained from hospital records, physicians' reports, and medical examiners' or coroners' records. If such information was not available, the family was contacted to ascertain the circumstances surrounding the death and the previous medical history of the dead person. Information was obtained for over 95 percent of the death certificates in the study.

Approximately 90 percent of the stroke diagnoses on the death certificates, stated as either an underlying or contributory cause of death, were validated by either an autopsy examination of the brain, arteriography, hemorrhagic spinal fluid, or the presence of hemiplegia or coma on hospital admission. Differences in certification, coding practices, or clinical diagnosis did not account for the differences in the reports of the underlying cause of death.

In Table 5–7, the nine study areas are combined into three groups—low, intermediate, and high—and reported death rates are compared with death rates that have been corrected for all stroke diagnoses stated on the death certificates. The differences in cerebrovascular disease mortality among these areas do not appear to be artifactual, although the validation procedure indicates that the differences in the corrected rates are not as large as in the reported rates; the ratio of high-to-low reported rates is 2.6, in contrast to 2.1 for corrected rates. Also, the differences between low and inter-

Table 5–7. Age-adjusted Death Rates from Cerebrovascular Disease, White Males, 35–74 Years of Age, Corrected to Include All Stroke Diagnoses Listed on Death Certificates and Clinical Stroke Diagnoses: Selected Areas, United States, 1965

Area	Age-adjusted Rates Based on		
	Underlying Cause of Death	All Stroke Diagnoses on Death Certificates	All Stroke Diagnoses on Death Certificates and Clinical Stroke Diagnoses not on Death Certificates
Low (Dade County, Florida; Denver, and selected economic area in Kansas)	84	134	202
Intermediate (Alameda County, California; King County, Washington; Erie County, New York)	117	176	263
High (Selected census-designated state economic areas in Georgia; North and South Carolina)	218	305	427

Source: Kuller et al. (30).

mediate corrected rates are not as great as those observed in the reported rates.

It is still possible, however, that the differences might be due to differences in either the case fatality rates or the frequency of the disease in these areas. The case fatality rates could be higher in the high-death-rate areas and the frequency of the disease the same in all areas. Conversely, the frequency of the disease could be higher in the high-death-rate areas and the case fatality rates the same in all areas.

Ideally, the next step would be to select samples of the population in each area and follow them to determine how frequently stroke occurs. But, because of the relatively low frequency of stroke, this approach would necessitate a difficult and expensive study of large groups of people. The alternative of implementing a reporting system for cerebrovascular diseases in both hospitals and among physicians would also be a difficult and time-consuming venture. To provide a reasonable initial estimate of differences in disease frequency, the investigators decided to limit their study to hospi-

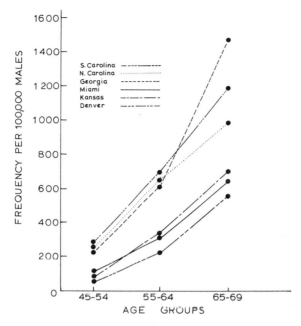

Figure 5–16. Frequency of hospitalized stroke cases among males in six areas of the United States by age, 1965

Source: Kuller et al. (29).

talized stroke cases and evaluate admission policies and case fatality rates (29). Over 90 percent of the hospital records were reviewed in six of the areas, the three low and three high areas, and the frequency of cerebrovascular disease in white males and females was compared (Figs. 5–16 and 5–17). Figure 5–16 indicates a consistency of differences in the frequency of hospitalized rates with those of death rates in the high and low areas for white males; Figure 5–17 shows that for white females these differences are limited to the older age group, 65–69. This sequence of studies thus indicates that regional differences in the frequency of cerebrovascular diseases in the United States are real and paves the way for the investigation of etiological factors.

Persons

The third general category that may influence the distribution of mortality consists of the characteristics of persons. In mortality data, the number of personal characteristics that can be analyzed is limited by the information available on death certificates. They in-

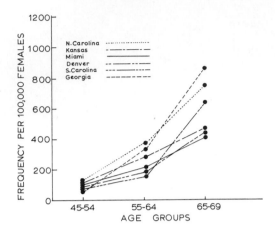

Figure 5–17.   Frequency of hospitalized stroke cases among females in six areas of the United States by age, 1965

Source: Kuller et al. (29).

clude age, sex, color, occupation (from which one can infer socioeconomic status), marital status, and birth cohort (people born during specific years).

AGE

The general increase in mortality with increasing age (see Fig. 4–2) has been attributed to a variety of biological factors:

1. Cumulative exposure of an individual during his lifetime to environmental insults through diet, smoking, occupation, and other factors.
2. Decrease, with age, in immunological defenses of the human organism.
3. Increase in frequency of somatic mutations or chromosomal abnormalities with age, which may result from either cumulative effects of the environment or decreased efficiency of such biological mechanisms as mitosis.
4. Hormonal changes throughout a lifetime.
5. Exposure to an agent, early in life, that may impair the immunological status of the aging person.
6. A nonspecific, genetically determined "wearing out" of the human organism (8). To determine whether this occurs, it is necessary to develop methods to measure "biological age" in contrast to "chronological age" (6, 9, 53).

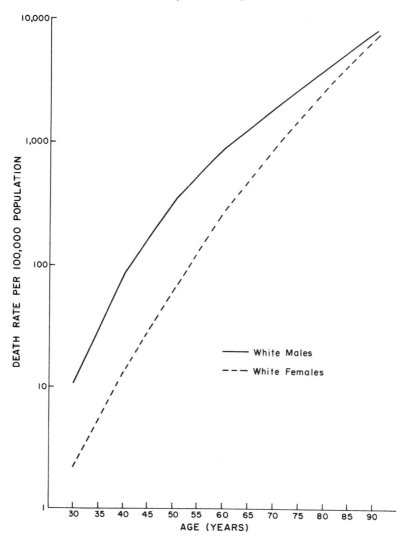

Figure 5–18. Average annual age-specific death rates from arteriosclerotic heart disease, including coronary artery disease (ISC 420, 422), among whites by sex, United States, 1959–1961

Source: Moriyama, Krueger, and Stamler (41). Copyright © 1971, The President and Fellows of Harvard College.

Age patterns differ in different diseases. Figure 5–18 provides an example in the average annual age-specific mortality rates from arteriosclerotic heart disease for white males and females in the United States. The death rates for both males and females increase with age, but the difference between the higher rates for males and the lower ones for females decreases with age, beginning at 45–50

Table 5–8.   Ratio of Male to Female Age-adjusted Cancer Death Rates by Primary Site for Whites: United States, 1959–1961

Primary Site (ICD Code)	Male/Female Ratios
	Ratios 3 or More
Larynx (161)	10.50
Bronchus and lung specified as primary and unspecified (162.1, 163)	6.79
Esophagus (150)	4.13
Tongue (141)	4.00*
Buccal cavity and pharynx (140–148)	4.00
Nasopharynx (146)	3.00
Parotid gland (142.0)	3.00
	Ratios 2–2.99
Bladder and other urinary organs (181)	2.89
Mediastinum (164)	2.84
Other malignant neoplasm of skin (191)	2.20
Lymphatic leukemia (204.0)	2.11
Bone (196)	2.00
	Ratios 1–1.99
Stomach (151)	1.97
Kidney (180)	1.94
Liver, primary (155.0)	1.83
Hodgkin's disease (201)	1.77
Pancreas (157)	1.68
Other and unspecified leukemia (204.4)	1.60
Rectum (154)	1.56
Lymphosarcoma and reticulosarcoma (200)	1.54
Leukemia and aleukemia (204)	1.54
Other endocrine glands (195)	1.50
Liver (primary, secondary, and unspecified) (155.0, 156)	1.50
Nose, nasal cavities, middle ear, and accessory sinuses (160)	1.50
Brain and other parts of nervous system (193)	1.50
Other forms of lymphoma and mycosis fungoides (202, 205)	1.50
Multiple myeloma (203)	1.45
Acute leukemia (204.3)	1.45
Myeloid leukemia (240.1)	1.44
Small intestine including duodenum (152)	1.33
Melanoma of skin (190)	1.27
Monocytic leukemia (204.2)	1.20
	Ratios Less Than 1
Large intestine, except rectum (153)	0.98
Thyroid gland (194)	0.67
Gall bladder and extrahepatic gall ducts including ampulla of Vater (155.1)	0.56
Breast (170)	0.01

* Based on crude death rates

Source: Lilienfeld, Kessler, and Levin (34). Copyright © 1972, The President and Fellows of Harvard College.

and continuing to decline until the male and female rates approximate each other. In view of the hormonal changes in women that occur during this age period, one might infer that hormonal factors are important in the development of arteriosclerotic heart disease. It is also possible that these male/female differences reflect the different environmental exposure of males and females, including occupational and social factors.

SEX

Males and females experience differences in mortality from many diseases, as is clearly shown by the marked sex differences in various forms of cancer mortality (Table 5–8). For only three cancer sites—gall bladder, thyroid gland, and breast—is the mortality higher among females than males. For many sites, those with male/female ratios of the order 1–1.99 the degree of difference is not very large, but for six sites these ratios exceed three. The lowest male/female ratios in cancer rates occur in the thyroid and breast—the former, an endocrine gland, and the latter, strongly influenced by the endocrine system. Thus, hormonal factors may play a role in the genesis of these cancers.

In contrast, the six cancer sites with male/female ratios of three or more are all in the respiratory tract, an area of the body exposed to the environment. One environmental factor that is known to be of etiological importance in cancer at several of these sites is cigarette smoking, a habit more common among males than females. In addition, environmental factors to which men are occupationally exposed (as in the asbestos, uranium mining, and arsenical industries) have been incriminated in the etiology of cancer of the upper respiratory tract.

ETHNIC CHARACTERISTICS

Color is the main ethnic characteristic on death certificates available for epidemiologic study. Table 5–9 shows the white/nonwhite ratios for the average annual age-adjusted cancer death rates by primary site and sex in the United States for 1959–1961 (34). For a number of sites, there is a higher mortality among nonwhites. This may be partially artifactual because of the underestimation of the nonwhite male population in the census (Table 5–3). It could, however, indicate a lower survival rate among nonwhites due to inadequate medical care. Or it might actually represent a higher frequency of cancer

Table 5–9. Ratio of Nonwhite to White Age-adjusted Cancer Death Rates, by Primary Site and Sex: United States, 1959–1961

Primary Site (ICD Code)	Nonwhite/White Ratios	
	Males	Females
Penis (179.0)	4.00	. . .
Cervix uteri (171)	. . .*	2.53
Esophagus (150)	2.52	2.50
Liver, primary (155.0)	2.18	1.17
Uterus, unspecified (174)	. . .	2.06
Nasopharynx (146)	2.00	1.00
Uterus, except cervix (172, 173, 174)	. . .	1.85
Stomach (151)	1.76	1.52
Prostate (177)	1.69	. . .
Nose, nasal cavities, middle ear, and accessory sinuses (160)	1.67	1.50
Peritoneum and unspecified digestive organs (155.8, 158, 159)	1.50	1.57
Connective tissue, lymph nodes, secondary and unspecified and other unspecified sites (197, 198, 199)	1.27	1.54
Liver, secondary and unspecified (156)	1.50	1.44
Larynx (161)	1.14	1.50
Breast (170)	1.50	0.91
Multiple myeloma (203)	1.44	1.45
Bladder and other urinary organs (181)	0.81	1.44
Corpus uteri (172)	. . .	1.36
Bone (196)	1.00	1.33
Digestive organs and peritoneum (150–159)	1.27	1.08
Oral mesopharynx (145)	1.25	—
Buccal cavity and pharynx (140–148)	1.02	1.25
Female genital organs except ovary and uterus (175.1, 175.8, 175.9, 176)	. . .	1.25
Thyroid gland (194)	0.75	1.17
Pancreas (157)	1.14	1.15
Respiratory system (160–165)	1.00	1.09
Male genital organs, except prostate (178, 179)	1.09	. . .
Bronchus and lung, specified as primary and unspecified (162.1, 163)	0.98	1.06
Bronchus and trachea and lung specified as primary (162)	1.01	1.00
Small intestine, including duodenum (152)	1.00	1.00
Tongue (141)	0.92	1.00
Other and unspecified leukemia (204.4)	0.88	1.00
Rectum (154)	0.79	1.00
Other forms of lymphoma and mycosis fungoides (202, 205)	1.00	0.75
Parotid gland (142.0)	0.67	1.00
Other malignant neoplasm of skin (191)	0.64	1.00

Table 5–9 cont.

Primary Site (ICD Code)	Nonwhite/White Ratios	
	Males	Females
Hypopharynx (147)	1.00	—
Mediastinum (164)	1.00	—
Lymphatic and hematopoietic tissues, excluding leukemia (lymphomas) (200–203, 205)	0.88	0.79
Large intestine, except rectum (153)	0.75	0.83
Myeloid leukemia (204.1)	0.69	0.78
Lymphatic leukemia (204.0)	0.68	0.78
Ovary (175.0)	. . .	0.78
Kidney (180)	0.70	0.76
Brain and other parts of nervous system, malignant, benign and unspecified (193, 223, 237)	0.70	0.76
Leukemia and aleukemia (204)	0.64	0.74
Lymphosarcoma and reticulosarcoma (200)	0.73	0.58
Gall bladder and extrahepatic gall ducts, including ampulla of Vater (155.1)	0.71	0.60
Hodgkin's disease (201)	0.70	0.62
Monocytic leukemia (204.2)	0.67	0.00
Other endocrine glands (195)	0.67	0.50
Acute leukemia (204.3)	0.53	0.64
Brain and other parts of nervous system (193)	0.52	0.54
Eye (192)	—	0.50
Testis (178)	0.33	. . .
Melanoma of skin (190)	0.29	0.27

* . . . = category not applicable; — = quantity zero.

Source: Lilienfeld, Kessler, and Levin (34). Copyright © 1972, The President and Fellows of Harvard College.

in several of these sites among nonwhites, perhaps from increased exposure to etiological factors in the environment.

SOCIOECONOMIC STATUS

This has been receiving a great deal of attention, particularly in the analysis of rates for noninfectious diseases. This does not imply that socioeconomic status has no influence on the occurrence of infectious diseases, since those who live in crowded quarters are more vulnerable to the transmission of infectious agents. In assessing socioeconomic status, one must recognize its broad nature and the variety of elements that it includes. Table 5–10 illustrates the sequence of possible components within a social class that lead to disease or death.

Table 5–10. Possible Relationship between Selected Population Variables and Specific Components Influenced by Social Class

	Population Variable	Components	Physiological or Cellular	End Result
Social Class	Medical care Diet Working conditions Psychosocial stress Other	Specific therapy Occupational exposures Other components	Biochemical mechanism	Specific disease or Cause of death

A study of mortality from cirrhosis of the liver provides an example of the use of mortality data analyzed by socioeconomic status in two countries to determine their consistency with a specific hypothesis (54). Table 5–11 presents the standardized mortality ratios from

Table 5–11. Standardized Mortality Ratios for Cirrhosis of the Liver among Men 20–64 Years of Age, by Occupation Levels: United States, 1950

Occupational Level	Standardized Mortality Ratio Total
I. Professional workers	90
II. Technical, administrative, and managerial workers, except farm	88
III. Clerical, sales, and skilled workers	105
IV. Semiskilled workers	118
V. Laborers, except farm	148
Agricultural workers	51

Source: Terris (54).

cirrhosis of the liver for men, aged 24–64 years, by the socioeconomic classification of occupations in the United States for 1950. An inverse relationship between cirrhosis mortality and occupational level is demonstrated, which is consistent with similar findings in Buffalo, New York, and in California (33, 42). The fact that lower social classes have higher cirrhosis mortality rates than the upper classes might be interpreted as indicating that occupational

Table 5–12. Standardized Mortality Ratios for Cirrhosis of the Liver among Men 20–64 Years of Age, by Social Class: England and Wales, 1949–1953

Social Class	Standardized Mortality Ratio
I. Professional occupations	207
II. Intermediate occupations	152
III. Skilled occupations	84
IV. Partly skilled occupations	70
V. Unskilled occupations	96

Source: Terris (54).

factors are of etiological importance in this disease. On the other hand, a different pattern was found in a similar analysis in England and Wales (Table 5–12). There, the upper social classes have a higher mortality from cirrhosis than the lower, and the mortality risk decreases as one descends the scale of social class. More detailed analyses of several occupational groups in the United States revealed that the three groups with the highest mortality were workers in eating and drinking facilities, hotels and lodging places, and entertainment and recreational services who are more "exposed" to alcoholic beverages.

Terris postulated that the very high taxes on alcohol in England and Wales have put alcoholic beverages out of the reaches of the lower classes, "where only the well-to-do can really afford the luxury of dying from cirrhosis of the liver" (54). This would be consistent both with the hypothesis developed from clinical and animal studies that alcohol consumption is a major etiological factor in hepatic cirrhosis and with the correlation between cirrhosis mortality trends and estimated alcohol consumption in various countries.

BIRTH COHORTS

A personal characteristic that has proved very useful in the analysis of mortality statistics is the year of birth or "generation period." An analysis of age-specific death rates in a specific calendar year does not account for the fact that persons in particular age groups in that year were at younger ages in past calendar years. For example, those persons in the 40–45-year age group in 1975 were five years younger in 1970 and, thus, in the 35–39-year age group. Therefore, any environmental events occurring in a given calendar year may have different effects on each age group, depending upon that group's past experience (3). For example, if an epidemic oc-

Table 5–13. Age-specific Death Rates per 100,000 from Tuberculosis (All Forms) among Males, with Rates for Cohort of 1880 Indicated: Massachusetts, 1880–1930

			Year			
Age	1880	1890	1900	1910	1920	1930
0–4	760	578	309	209	108	41
5–9	43	49	31	21	24	11
10–19	126	115	90	63	49	21
20–29	444	361	288	207	149	81
30–39	378	368	296	253	164	115
40–49	364	336	253	253	175	118
50–59	366	325	267	252	171	127
60–69	475	346	304	246	172	95
70+	672	396	343	163	127	95

Source: Frost (14).

curred many years ago and conferred immunity on persons living at that time, they may later remain unaffected by the recurrence of an epidemic of the same disease. (Recall the measles epidemic in the Faroe Islands, Chap. 2, p. 40.)

Cohort analysis of mortality statistics first described by Farr in 1870, was used by Andvord in an attempt to explain the changing age distribution of tuberculosis (2). The technique was elaborated by Frost, who appreciated its biological implications (14). Utilizing age-specific tuberculosis mortality rates among males at ten-year intervals in Massachusetts, Frost noted that:

1. at every age mortality is lowest in the latest calendar year (1930);
2. in each year, mortality is higher in infancy, declining in childhood, and increasing during adolescence to a higher level in adult life, and
3. in the latest year (1930), the highest rate of mortality among males occurred in the 50–59-year age group, while in 1880 it occurred in the 0–4 age group (Table 5–13).

The 1930 age-specific death rates suggest that an individual encounters his greatest risk of death from tuberculosis between 50 and 60 years of age. But Frost pointed out that this was not really so; in 1930, the people in the 50–59 age group had, in earlier life, passed

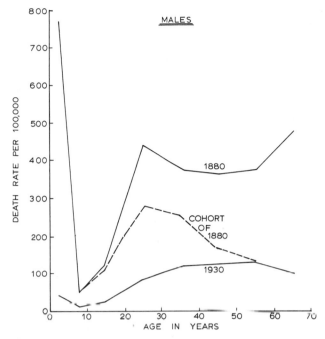

Figure 5–19. Age-specific death rates from tuberculosis (all forms) among males in 1880 and 1930 and for the birth cohort of 1880, Massachusetts

Source: Frost (14).

through greater risks of mortality. This is shown in Table 5–13 and illustrated in Figure 5–19 for the age-specific male death rates in 1880 and 1930 and also the "cohort of 1880," consisting of those born during 1871–1880. Those who were 50–59 years of age in 1930 had passed through greater risks of mortality in two earlier age periods, 0–9 and 20–29. This *analysis by cohort* indicates that the pattern of the age distribution of the risk of dying from tuberculosis had remained relatively the same, although mortality rates had been at increasingly lower levels (Fig. 5–20).

These analyses led Frost to infer that:

1. constancy of the relative mortality at successive ages in successive cohorts suggests constancy in physiological changes in resistance with age;
2. if the frequency and extent of exposure to infection in early life have progressively decreased over time, the lack of oppor-

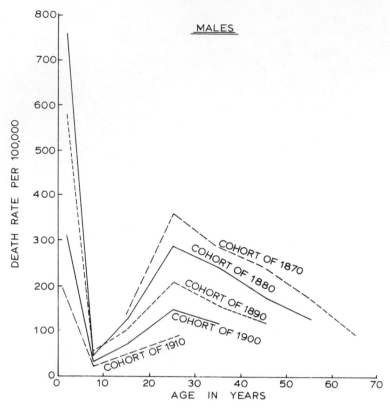

Figure 5–20. Age-specific death rates from tuberculosis (all forms) among males in successive ten-year birth cohorts, Massachusetts

Source: Frost (14).

tunity to acquire immunity in childhood was probably not the reason for the increased mortality in adult life;

3. the mortality peak later in life—in 1930—does not represent the postponement of maximum risk, but suggests that the high rates in old age are the residuals of higher rates in earlier life. The latter inference indicates that tuberculosis mortality (and morbidity) in adults is probably the result of reactivation of an infection acquired early in life and not a newly acquired infection or reinfection.

Cohort analysis has also been applied to the study of lung cancer mortality (Fig. 5–21). Age-specific death rates by calendar year (the solid lines in Fig. 5–21) increase to 60–69 years of age and then

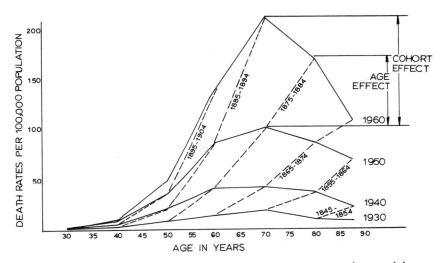

Figure 5–21. Age-specific death rates from malignant neoplasm of lung among white males by calendar year (solid lines) and birth cohorts (broken lines), United States, 1930–1960

Source: Levin (31).

decline in ages over 70. This could be explained by different hypotheses:

1. that exposure to the etiological agent decreases after a certain age during the calendar period considered here;
2. that there was no cumulative effect of the hypothesized etiological agent;
3. that a physiological change related to age influences the individual's reaction to an environmental agent.

However, if the mortality is analyzed in terms of birth cohorts (broken lines in Fig. 5–21), it becomes clear that each birth cohort has an increasing rate of mortality with increasing age, although each also has a higher mortality rate at all ages than cohorts born earlier. Therefore, in 1960, the lower death rates for those over eighty years of age are not explained by a decline in mortality risk with age, but by the fact that persons over eighty years of age are members of an earlier birth cohort, which, in earlier life, had a lower exposure to the etiological agent—cigarette smoking—than later cohorts. The contribution of these two different factors—birth cohort and age—to the curve of age-specific mortality from lung cancer is shown in Figure 5–21 (31).

B. LIMITATIONS OF OFFICIAL MORTALITY STATISTICS

The epidemiologic value of mortality statistics depends on how closely they estimate the real frequency of disease in the population. The most important consideration is not whether mortality rates tend to underestimate the actual disease frequency, but whether the differences in mortality by various population characteristics such as age, sex, color, and occupation tend to reflect similar differences in the frequency of disease. In Chapter 4, mention was made of the various factors that might distort the degree to which mortality statistics actually reflect disease frequencies, such as accuracy of cause of death certification, case fatality rates, methods of classification of causes of death, and the statement of multiple causes of death. Additional limitations are imposed by the small number of items of information on the death certificate by which deaths can be classified. Also, there are diseases with low case fatality rates such as arthritis, for which mortality statistics are inadequate for epidemiologic study.

Despite these limitations, the analysis of mortality statistics provides for many purposes an inexpensive and convenient means of obtaining clues to etiological hypotheses, determining consistency between hypotheses and serving as an index of the frequency of certain diseases in the population. The degree of usefulness of mortality statistics quite naturally will depend upon the extent of knowledge of the disease in question. If little is known about the disease, an analysis of the mortality statistics represents an initial step in an epidemiologic study. If epidemiologic data on the disease is extensive and specific etiological hypotheses need to be assessed, the contribution of mortality statistics may be quite limited.

C. STUDIES OF AUTOPSY SERIES

A different aspect of mortality studies is the use of autopsy series as a source of data. It has the great advantage of providing diagnostic accuracy, within the limits of the training and skill of the patholo-

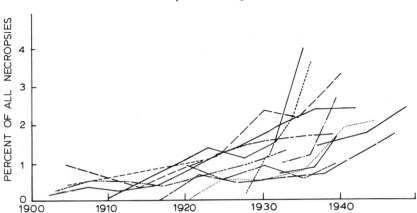

Figure 5–22. Percent of carcinomas of the lung found at autopsy in thirteen series

Source: Cornfield et al. (11).

gist. However, it must be recognized that autopsy series represent a biased and selected sample of hospital admissions (38, 39, 57).

In studying the characteristics of one autopsy series, McMahan made the following interesting observations:

1. The average age at death for autopsied cases was higher for males than for females.
2. Not only were dead males more likely to be autopsied than dead females, but this tendency prevailed in practically all five-year age groups.
3. Among those who died under the age of forty, persons dying in the early "teens" were apparently least likely to be autopsied.
4. Of all the age groups, older persons (those aged seventy-five and over) who die are least likely to be autopsied (39).

In view of such bias in selection, it is practically impossible to refer the usual autopsy series to any well-defined population at risk, and therefore, impossible to use such data for estimating the frequency of a disease. However, if systematic postmortem examinations are performed in a well defined population, as has been done in a part of the city of Prague, Czechoslovakia, and in a few other places, the biases mentioned above will be eliminated, and one can obtain a good estimate of disease frequency in the population.

Table 5–14. Distribution of Subjects According to Percent of Sections of Bronchial Epithelium with Lesions Composed Entirely of Atypical Cells and with Cilia Absent (Carcinoma *in Situ*)

Percent of Sections with Carcinoma *in Situ*	Deaths Not Due to Lung Cancer					Deaths Due to Lung Cancer
	Never Smoked Regularly	Smoked <½ Pack Daily	Smoked ½–1 Pack Daily	Smoked 1–2 Packs Daily	Smoked 2+ Packs Daily	
0	65	32	44	74	9	11
1–4	—	4	13	31	11	8
5–9	—	—	1	18	3	13
10–14	—	—	1	6	—	8
15–19	—	—	—	4	5	8
20–24	—	—	—	4	3	2
25–29	—	—	—	5	2	4
30–34	—	—	—	1	—	4
35–39	—	—	—	—	1	1
40–49	—	—	—	—	1	2
50–59	—	—	—	—	—	1
60+	—	—	—	—	1	1
Number of subjects	65	36	59	143	36	63
Mean percent	0	0.3	0.8	4.2	11.0	14.4
Standard deviation of mean	0	0.14	0.25	0.60	2.41	1.99
Number of sections	3,324	1,824	3,016	7,062	1,787	2,784
Number with carcinoma *in situ*	0	5	24	307	203	417
Percent with carcinoma *in situ*	0	0.3	0.8	4.3	11.4	15.0

Source: Auerbach et al. (4). Reprinted by permission of *The New England Journal of Medicine,* 265:253–267, 1961.

Despite the limitations of autopsy series for determining the frequency of a disease in a population, inferences made from an analysis of autopsy series may provide useful leads for more refined epidemiologic studies. For example, the observation that the relative proportion of lung cancer in different series of autopsies was increasing with time, and that the ratio of squamous cell carcinoma to adenocarcinoma was also increasing (while the proportion of adenocarcinoma remained fairly constant) led to the hypothesis that the total increase of lung cancer might, in fact, be limited to squamous cell carcinoma (Fig. 5–22) (11, 27, 28). Subsequent mortality and morbidity studies confirmed this.

In cancer studies, autopsy series are of value in providing information about the relationship between a possible etiological factor and a form of cancer by determining if a similar relationship also exists between that factor and precancerous lesions (4). By examining serial sections of bronchi in deceased smokers and nonsmokers, for example, Auerbach et al. were able to show changes in smokers which could be interpreted as potentially precancerous lesions (Table 5–14) (4). Such a finding considerably strengthens the inference that there is a relationship between lung cancer and cigarette smoking.

STUDY PROBLEMS

1. The following table presents the time trends of age-adjusted* mortality rates (per 100,000) from gastric cancer in Norway from 1930 to 1965 by sex.

Sex	1930	1935	1940	1945	1950	1955	1960	1965
Male	90	92	80	70	70	50	45	42
Female	65	60	55	45	45	35	30	30

* Adjusted to Norweigan population on January 1, 1956.

Discuss the possible general reasons for these trends.

2. In 1965, the death rate in Greece from athcrosclcrotic heart disease among 35–64 year old males was 78 per 100,000 and in the Netherlands it was 243 per 100,000. List four possible reasons for this difference.

3. During 1959–61, the age-adjusted annual death rates from breast cancer in the United States by marital status were as follows:

Marital Status	Rate (per 100,000 women)
Single	39.9
Married	28.2
Widowed	28.9
Divorced	32.0

Outline the possible reasons for these differences.

4. In 1956, the National Office of Vital Statistics published comprehensive statistical data on mortality by marital status, age, color, and sex based upon the 1950 U.S. census and all deaths from 1949–1951 in the continental United States. A brief review of these data appeared in the *Statistical Bulletin of the Metropolitan Life Insurance Company*. Some points noted in the review were:

    a) married people generally experienced a lower mortality rate than did single, widowed, and divorced people;

    b) the relative excess mortality (1.5 times) in the not-married categories was consistently greater in males than females; and

    c) there was a very large relative excess in mortality (5 or 6 times) among the young widowed group, compared to the young married group.

    1) Discuss possible reasons for these observations, particularly (c);

    2) What are the implications of these reasons for the epidemiologist?

5. Age-sex-specific mortality rates from disease X in a Standard Metropolitan Statistical Area for 1930, 1940, and 1950 are presented in the following table. Describe a study designed to determine whether the change is real or artifactual.

Age	Male			Female		
	1930	1940	1950	1930	1940	1950
0–14	0.1	0.0	0.0	0.0	0.0	0.0
15–24	0.2	0.2	0.1	0.2	0.2	0.1
25–34	1.6	1.1	0.7	1.5	1.0	0.7
35–44	8.8	6.2	3.9	7.5	4.3	2.6
45–54	34.2	26.0	16.0	23.1	14.1	8.5
55–64	99.3	78.1	54.2	61.8	41.1	25.6
65–74	213.8	174.3	126.6	155.5	105.2	64.8
75–84	308.0	288.0	227.7	256.4	199.5	139.5
80+	290.1	287.2	271.8	266.8	233.0	187.3

6. The data on page 127 are taken from an actual human experience, which occurred during a short period of time around 1910 in a completely isolated population. What can you infer, from the information provided, about the nature of the experience, the cause or causes of death and the attendant circumstances?

Mortality by sex, socioeconomic status, and age

Socio-economic status	Adult males			Adult females			Children both sexes			All		
	No. in pop.	Deaths no.	%	No. in pop.	Deaths no.	%	No. in pop.	Deaths no.	%	No. in pop.	Deaths no.	%
High	183	125	68.3	144	5	3.5	5	0	–	332	130	39.2
Medium	160	147	91.9	93	15	16.1	24	0	–	277	162	58.5
Low	454	399	87.9	179	81	45.3	76	53	69.7	709	533	75.2
Unknown	865	676	78.2	23	2	8.7	0	–	–	888	678	76.2
Total	1662	1347	81.0	439	103	23.5	105	53	50.5	2206	1503	68.1

7. Population cause-specific mortality statistics are usually based on the cause of death stated on death certificates. For the most part, the cause-of-death is based upon the physician's diagnosis of the patient's condition before death. Thus, an opportunity to examine the diagnostic accuracy of the physician is welcome. In 1970–71, Britton examined 400 deaths in the Medical Department of Serafimer-lasarettet, a university hospital in Stockholm, Sweden; of the 400 deaths, 383 were autopsied. The following table presents a comparison between the findings on autopsy and the premortem clinical diagnoses for those cases in whom diagnoses had been made.

Disease group (main groups, ICD)	Clinical diagnosis*		Changes after autopsy (major errors)†		Total no. of final diagnoses
	Total errors	Errors— all degrees† (% of total)	Cases removed	Cases added	
Neoplastic, II	50	16	2	11	59
Infective, endocrine, blood, mental, nervous system, I, III–VI	17	41	7	3	13
Circulatory, VII	228	38	10	9	227
Respiratory, VIII	8	29	3	1	6
Digestive, IX	14		2	2	14
Genitourinary, X	7		1	2	8
All others, XI–XVII	9	—	3	0	6
Total	333*	34	28	28	333

* 50 cases had no premortem diagnosis.
† Errors were classified as: 1. *major,* if the final diagnosis belonged to a different main group (I–XVII) of diseases; 2. *intermediate,* if the final diagnosis was in a different subgroup within the same main group; and 3. *minor,* all other errors.

   a) What do these data indicate about the accuracy of cause of death statements on death certificates?

   b) Why are such data important to the epidemiologist? The physician? The public health administrator?

REFERENCES

1. American Cancer Society, 1977. *1978 Cancer Facts and Figures.* New York: American Cancer Society.
2. Andvord, K.F. 1930. "What can we learn by studying tuberculosis by generations?" *Norsk Magizen for Laegevidenskaben* 91:642–660.
3. Armstrong, B., and Doll, R. 1974. "Bladder cancer mortality in England and Wales in relation to cigarette smoking and saccharin consumption." *Brit. J. Prev. Soc. Med.* 28:233–240.
4. Auerbach, O., Stout, A.P., Hammond, E.C., and Garfinkel, L. 1961. "Changes in bronchial epithelium in relation to cigarette smoking and in relation to lung cancer." *N. Eng. J. Med.* 265:253–267.
5. Axtell, L.M., Breslow, L., and Eisenberg, H. 1961. "Trends in survival rates of cancer patients: Connecticut and California." In *End Results and Mortality Trends in Cancer.* Part I. End Results in Cancer. S.J. Cutler and F. Ederer, eds. Natl. Cancer Inst. Monogr. No. 6, United States Department of Health, Education and Welfare, Public Health Service, Washington, D.C.: United States Government Printing Office. pp. 49–67.
6. Bourliere, F. 1970. *The Assessment of Biological Age in Man.* Public Health Papers 37. Geneva: World Health Organization.
7. Brown, J., Bourke, G.J., Gearty, G.F., Finnegan, A., Hill, M., Heffernan-Fox, F.C., Fitzgerald, D.F., Kennedy, J., Childers, R.W., Jessop, W.J.E., Trulson, M.F., Latham, M.D., Cronin, S., McCann, M.B., Clancy, R.E., Gore, I., Stoudt, H.W., Hegsted, D.M., and Stare, F.J. 1970. "Nutritional and epidemiological factors related to heart disease." *World Rev. Nutr. Diet.* 12:1–42.
8. Cohen, B. 1964. "Family patterns of mortality and life span." *Q. Rev. Biol.* 39:130–181.
9. Comfort, A. 1969. "Test battery to measure ageing-rate in man." *Lancet* 2:1411–1415.
10. Conolly, M.E., Davies, D.S., Dollery, C.T., and George, C.F. 1971. "Resistance to B Adrenoceptor stimulants (a possible explanation for the rise in asthma deaths)." *Brit. J. Pharmacol.* 43:389–402.
11. Cornfield, J., Haenszel, W., Hammond, E.C., Lilienfeld, A.M., Shimkin, M.B., and Wynder, E.L. 1959. "Smoking and lung cancer: Recent evidence and a discussion of some questions." *J. Natl. Cancer Inst.* 22:173–203.
12. Davies, A.M., and Sacks, M. Eds. 1971. "Symposium on cancer and other chronic diseases in migrants to Israel." *Israel J. Med. Sci.* 7:1333–1596.
13. DeWaard, F. 1973. "Nurture and nature in cancer of the breast and endometrium." In *Host Environment Interactions in the Etiology of Cancer in Man:* R. Doll and I. Vodopija, eds. Lyon: International Agency for Research in Cancer, pp. 121–129.
14. Frost, W.H. 1939. "The age selection of mortality from tuberculosis in successive decades." *Amer. J. Hyg.* 30:31–96.
15. Gilliam, A.G. 1955. "Trends of mortality attributed to carcinoma of the lung: Possible effects of faulty certification of death to other respiratory diseases." *Cancer* 8:1130–1136.
16. Gordon, P.C. 1966. "The epidemiology of cerebral vascular disease in Canada: An analysis of mortality data." *Can. Med. Assoc. J.* 95:1004–1011.
17. Gordon, T. 1957. "Mortality experience among the Japanese in the United States, Hawaii, and Japan." *Pub. Health Reps.* 72:543–553.

18. ———, Crittenden, M., and Haenszel, W. 1961. "Part II Cancer mortality trends in the United States, 1930–55." In *End Results and Mortality Trends in Cancer*, Natl. Cancer Inst. Monogr. No. 6, United States Department of Health, Education and Welfare, Public Health Service.

19. Greenberg, M.J. 1965. "Isoprenaline in myocardial failure" (letter). *Lancet* 2:442–443.

20. ———, and Pines, A. 1967. "Pressurized aerosols in asthma" (letter). *Brit. Med. J.* 1:563.

21. Haenszel, W., ed. 1970. "Symposium on cancer in migratory populations." *J. Chron. Dis.* 23:289–448.

22. Inman, W.H.W., and Adelstein, A.M. 1969. "Rise and fall of asthma mortality in England and Wales in relation to use of pressurized aerosols." *Lancet* 2:279–285.

23. Kagan, A., Harris, B.R., Winkelstein, W., Jr., Johnson, K.G., Kato, H., Syme, S.L., Rhoads, G.G., Gay, M.L., Nichaman, M.Z., Hamilton, H.B., and Tillotson, J. 1974. "Epidemiologic studies of coronary heart disease and stroke in Japanese men living in Japan, Hawaii, and California: Demographic, physical, dietary, and biochemical characteristics." *J. Chron. Dis.* 27:345–364.

24. Keys, A., ed. 1970. *Coronary Heart Disease in Seven Countries.* Amer. Heart Assoc. Monogr. No. 29. New York: The American Heart Association.

25. Klebba, A.J. 1966. *Mortality from Diseases Associated with Smoking. United States, 1950–64.* National Center for Health Statistics, Series 20, No. 4. Washington, D.C.: United States Department of Health, Education and Welfare, Public Health Service.

26. Kmet, J., and Mahboubi, E. 1972. "Esophageal cancer in the Caspian Littoral of Iran: Initial studies." *Science* 175:846–853.

27. Kreyberg, L. 1954. "The significance of histological typing in the study of the epidemiology of primary epithelial lung tumours: A study of 466 cases." *Brit. J. Cancer* 8:199–208.

28. ———. 1962. *Histological Lung Cancer Types: A Morphological and Biological Correlation.* Oslo, Norway: Norwegian Universities Press.

29. Kuller, L., Anderson, H., Peterson, D., Cassel, J., Spiers, P., Curry, H., Paegel, B., Saslaw, M., Sisk, C., Wilber, J., Millward, D., Winkelstein, W., Jr., Lilienfeld, A.M., and Seltser, R. 1970. "Nationwide cerebrovascular disease morbidity study." *Stroke* 1:86–99.

30. ———, Bolker, A., Saslaw, M.S., Paegel, B.L., Sisk, C., Borhani, N., Wray, J.A., Anderson, H., Peterson, D., Winkelstein, W., Jr., Cassel, J., Spiers, P., Robinson, A.G., Curry, H., Lilienfeld, A.M., and Seltser, R. 1969. "Nationwide cerebrovascular disease mortality study: I. Methods and analysis of death certificates; II. Comparison of clinical records and death certificates; III. Accuracy of the clinical diagnosis of cerebrovascular disease; IV. Comparison of the different clinical types of cerebrovascular disease." *Amer. J. Epid.* 90:536–578.

31. Levin, M.L., 1953. "The occurrence of lung cancer in man." *Acta Unio. Internationalis Contra Cancrum* 9:531–541.

32. Lilienfeld, A.M. 1963. "The epidemiology of breast cancer." *Cancer Res.* 23:1503–1513.

33. ———, and Korns, R.F. 1950. "Some epidemiological aspects of cirrhosis of the liver: A study of mortality statistics." *Amer. J. Hyg.* 52:65–81.

34. ———, Levin, M.L., and Kessler, I.I. 1972. *Cancer in the United States.* Cambridge, Massachusetts: Harvard University Press.

35. MacMahon, B. 1973. "Oestrogens and the etiology of breast cancer: Utilization of demographic differences to test a hypothesis." In *Host Environment Interactions in the Etiology of Cancer in Man*. R. Doll, I. Vodopija, and W. Davis, eds. Lyon: International Agency for Research on Cancer, pp. 163–167.

36. ———, Cole, P., Brown, J.B., Aoki, K., Lin, T.M., Morgan, R.W., and Woo, N-C. 1971. "Oestrogen profiles of Asian and North American Women." *Lancet* 2:900–902.

37. ———, Lin, T.M., Lowe, C.R., Mirra, A.P., Ravnihar, B., Salber, E.J., Trichopoulos, D., Valaoras, V.G., and Yuasa, S. 1970. "Lactation and cancer of the breast. A summary of an international study." *Bull. WHO* 42: 185–194.

38. Mainland, D. 1953. "Risk of fallacious conclusions from autopsy data on incidence of diseases with applications to heart disease." *Amer. Heart J.* 45:644–654.

39. McMahan, C.A. 1962. "Age-sex distribution of selected groups of autopsied cases." *Arch. Path.* 73:40–47.

40. McManis, A.G. 1964. "Adrenaline and isoprenaline: A warning." *Med. J. Aust.* 2:76.

41. Moriyama, I.M., Krueger, D.E., and Stamler, J. 1971. *Cardiovascular Diseases in the United States*. Cambridge, Massachusetts: Harvard University Press.

42. Pearl, A., Buechley, R., and Lipscomb, W.R. 1962. "Cirrhosis mortality in three large cities: Implications of alcoholism and intercity comparisons." In *Society, Culture and Drinking Patterns*. D.J. Pittman, and C.R. Snyder, eds. Carbondale, Illinois: Southern Illinois University Press, pp. 345–352.

43. Percy, C., Garfinkel, L., Krueger, D.E., and Dolman, A.B. 1974. "Apparent changes in cancer mortality, 1968." *Pub. Health Reps.* 89:418–428.

44. Renwick, J.H. 1972. "Hypothesis: Anencephaly and spina bifida are usually preventable by avoidance of a specific but unidentified substance present in certain potato tubers." *Brit. J. Prev. Soc. Med.* 26:67–88.

45. Report of Inter-Society Commission for Heart Disease Resources. 1970. "Primary prevention of the atherosclerotic diseases." Atherosclerosis Study Group, J. Stamler, Chairman. Epidemiology Study Group. A.M. Lilienfeld, Chairman. *Circulation* 42:A55–A95.

46. Segi, M., and Kurihara, M. 1962. *Cancer Mortality for Selected Sites in 24 Countries, No. 2 (1958–1959)*. Sendai, Japan: Department of Public Health. Tohoku University School of Medicine.

47. Seidman, H. 1972. *Cancer of the Breast: Statistical and Epidemiological Data*. New York: American Cancer Society.

48. Siegel, J.S. 1974. "Estimates of coverage of the population by sex, race, and age in the 1970 census." *Demography* 11:1–23.

49. Speizer, F.E., Doll, R., and Heaf, P. 1968. "Observations on recent increase in mortality from asthma." *Brit. Med. J.* 1:335–339.

50. ———, and Strang, L.B. 1968. "Investigation into use of drugs preceding death from asthma." *Brit. Med. J.* 1:339–343.

51. Spiegelman, M. 1968. *Introduction to Demography*. Rev. edit., Cambridge, Massachusetts: Harvard University Press.

52. Stolley, P.D., and Schinnar, R. 1978. "Association between asthma mortality and isoproternol aerosols: A Review." *Prev. Med.* 7:519–538.

53. Strehler, B.L. 1977. *Time, Cells, and Aging*. 2nd ed. New York and London: Academic Press.

54. Terris, M. 1967. "Epidemiology of cirrhosis of the liver: National mortality data." *Amer. J. Pub. Health* 57:2076–2088.
55. Tuyns, A.J. 1970. "Cancer of the oesophagus: Further evidence of the relation to drinking habits in France." *Int. J. Cancer* 5:152–156.
56. *Vital Statistics of the United States. 1965. 1955 Supplement: Mortality Data, Multiple Causes of Death.* United States Department of Health, Education and Welfare, Public Health Service, National Center for Health Statistics, Washington, D.C.: U.S. Government Printing Office.
57. Waife, S.O., Lucchesi, P.F., and Sigmond, B. 1952. "Significance of mortality statistics in medical research: Analysis of 1,000 deaths at Philadelphia General Hospital." *Ann. Intern. Med.* 37:332–337.

6 Morbidity Statistics

> We cannot hope for its (epidemiology) uniform
> development until accurate and complete statistics
> of disease incidence in different population groups
> and under varying conditions of environment are
> collected currently and in . . . detail.
>
> EDGAR SYDENSTRICKER, 1920

A. SOURCES

The limitations of mortality statistics and the need to obtain information on various aspects of illness in the population stimulated the collection of morbidity statistics. Morbidity statistics are essential to health agencies attempting to control disease, especially communicable diseases. Various tax-financed public assistance programs and medical-care plans require knowledge of morbidity of the population groups they serve for planning and evaluation purposes. Industry is concerned with the effect of morbidity on its employees, particularly as it affects absenteeism and productivity. The planning and evaluation of public-health activities and health facilities require knowledge of the extent of morbidity in the population. Morbidity statistics are also the by-products of societal activities such as conscription for the armed services and retirement plans.

In recent years, increased reliance has been placed on a variety of morbidity statistics in order to maintain surveillance of the quality of medical care and the degree of utilization of health facilities. These activities will probably provide an incentive for developing additional methods of collecting morbidity statistics.

Table 6–1 presents a list of sources of morbidity statistics which, although incomplete, does provide an overview. Detailed consideration of many of these can be found in books on demography or vital statistics (30).

In assessing the utility of any of these sources for epidemiologic

Table 6–1.   Various Sources of Morbidity Statistics

  I. Disease Control Programs
        Disease reporting—communicable diseases; case registers of tuberculosis, cancer, and other diseases
        Case-finding programs in selected population groups
  II. Tax-financed Public-assistance Programs
        Public assistance, aid to the blind, aid to the disabled
        State or federal medical-care plans
        Armed forces, including preinduction records
        Veterans Administration
  III. Records of Industrial and School Absenteeism and Preemployment and Periodic Physical Examinations in Industry and Schools
  IV. Data Accumulated as a By-product of Insurance, Prepaid Medical Care Plans, and Other Health-related Activities
        Group health and accident insurance
        Prepaid medical care plans
        State disability insurance plans
        Life insurance companies
        Hospital insurance plans—Blue Cross
        Railroad retirement board
        Selected Service records
        Clinics and hospitals
  V. Biomedical Research Programs
  VI. Morbidity Surveys on Population Samples for Illness in General and for Specific Diseases

---

studies, one must be aware of two factors: 1) the variety of definitions of illness used; and 2) the composition of the population that has served as the source of information. The definition of illness used in a particular instance is influenced by the nature of the program or activity for which the data were collected (Table 6–1). These data serve many different administrative purposes. Statistics derived from disability programs, for example, will vary according to the program's content and purpose (13). Some programs are concerned with specific forms of disability such as blindness, whereas others consider a disabled person in terms of his physical or mental ability to support himself. Thus, disability may be defined with regard to specific types and/or according to a range from temporary and limited to permanent and total.

Determining whether a morbid condition or illness is present in an individual often depends upon the type and method of examination used. In a community case-finding program, for example, a single test such as an X-ray examination may be used to detect individuals with a high probability of having a specific disease, a process known as "screening." Additional examinations would be necessary to determine if they had a specific disease. Statistics derived from such programs provide information on presumptive diagnoses, whereas those obtained from hospitals and clinics usually represent the results of detailed examinations. Illness can also be determined by interview, i.e., by asking a person whether he feels ill or whether he has or has had a specific disease. Thus, the various methods of determining the presence of illness will result in different definitions that must be considered in assessing the usefulness of such data for epidemiologic purposes.

Most sources of morbidity statistics, particularly items II to V in Table 6–1, only provide information on special population groups, i.e., the group covered by a particular health insurance plan or retirement program. In many instances, the population served by a facility, such as a hospital, is not even defined. Studies in the past have shown underreporting of communicable diseases by physicians. This, too, must be considered in evaluating the usefulness of such data (27, 29). Underreporting of a variety of obstetrical conditions and congenital malformations on birth certificates has also been found (17, 20). Case-finding programs have a similar limitation, and it has been particularly difficult to obtain even a 90 percent response to surveys for such conditions as diabetes (18). Those who do respond to case-finding surveys may differ in important ways from those who do not. This may result in biased estimates of the frequency of the disease in the population.

An approach that has proved extremely valuable both in many states of the United States and in a number of other countries is the population-based permanent or long-term registration system for a specific disease, such as cancer or one of the other chronic diseases (4, 9, 11, 21, 36). If these registries are well planned and operated, they can furnish a great deal of information on the frequency of a disease and serve as a base for epidemiologic studies. An attempt is made through these registries to collect as much information as is practical on all newly recognized cases of the disease in a specified population. To achieve the desired degree of completeness, it is necessary to collect information from many sources, including hospitals, pathology laboratories, practicing physicians, and official death certificates.

Some registries require compulsory notification of cases by physicians; others depend on voluntary cooperation. In many instances, the reporting is limited to hospitalized cases (21). If the registry is for a disease such as cancer where a vast majority, if not all cases, are hospitalized, registration is considered as being virtually complete.

The development of a case register is costly. It is, therefore, essential to compare the cost-benefit ratio to that of other methods of obtaining similar information, such as periodic population surveys. After its initiation, the survival of either a voluntary or compulsory case register depends on maintaining the interest of cooperating physicians and hospitals. Interest in a register can generally be sustained if the data collected are actually used as a basis for providing health and social services for patients or for research purposes.

B. MORBIDITY SURVEYS

The limitations of some of the sources of morbidity data mentioned, in particular their restriction to certain population groups, and the desire to obtain information on illness in the general population on a periodic or continuing basis have been responsible for the development of morbidity surveys. This method was initiated on a large scale in continuous studies of all illnesses in a community by the United States Public Health Service in Hagerstown, Maryland, in 1921–1924 (31).

In general, community-wide morbidity surveys have collected information on population samples in two ways, by interview and/or examination. Information obtained by interview can be elicited directly from the respondent about himself or from a member of the household on illnesses among all household members for a specified period of time. Information can be obtained by a complete physical examination or by examination of certain organ systems, e.g., cardiovascular, in a sample of the entire population or selected groups of the population, depending upon the purposes of the survey. Morbidity surveys can be carried out by a single visit to the household, a single examination of a person, or by periodic visits or examinations.

Soon after the Hagerstown surveys, other national morbidity surveys were conducted for different purposes, but generally, they were

Table 6–2. Annual Reported Incidence Rates (per 100 population) of Fractures and Dislocations, Sprains to the Musculoskeletal System,* United States, July 1975–June 1976, by Age

Age (in years)	Percentage Incidence		
	Fractures and Dislocations	Sprains and Strains	Total
< 6	1.3	1.0	2.3
6–16	4.3	7.2	11.5
17–44	2.8	9.9	12.7
≥45	2.9	4.1	7.0
All ages	3.0	6.8	9.8

* Episodes associated with receipt of medical care or with limitation of activity.

Source: Kelsey et al. (12). From National Center for Health Statistics (for numerators); U.S. Bureau of the Census (for denominators). These data are based on information obtained in the Health Interview Survey of the U.S. National Health Survey, and are most likely underestimates.

grossly inadequate. It was not until 1956 that a continuing program of surveying the health status of the United States was begun by the passage of the necessary legislation; this was the United States National Health Survey, which is currently conducted by the National Center for Health Statistics (22).

Essentially, the National Health Survey includes three general programs of survey activities: the Health Interview Survey, the Health Examination Survey, and the Health Record Survey. The Health Interview Survey is based on a sample of the noninstitutionalized population of the United States. It is conducted continuously by interviewing a sample of households each week and combining these findings to provide estimates of illness for longer periods of time.

The Health Examination Survey consists of examinations and a variety of physiological and psychological tests for specific diseases, carried out over a period of two or three years for a selected age group. The first group examined covered the broad range of 18–79 years of age; the second was restricted to children 6–11 years of age, and the third to youths aged 12–17. The sample is selected by methods similar to those of the Health Interview Survey, but it is much smaller. The Health Records Survey involves a sampling of institutions or facilities providing health or medical care services, either on a continuous or periodic basis.

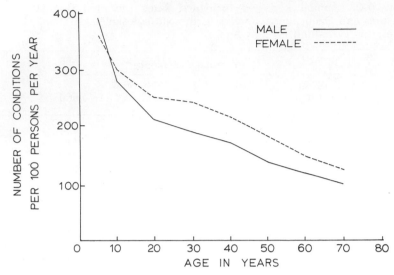

Figure 6–1. Age-specific incidence of acute conditions by sex, National Health Survey, United States, July 1971–June 1972

Source: Wilder (38).

More recently, the scope of these activities was broadened to include a national surveillance of the nutritional status of the population in an attempt to monitor changes in this status (23). In addition to these surveys, there is an ongoing program of data evaluation and methodological research as well as a program of analytical studies of epidemiologic and statistical problems. Table 6–2 and Figures 6–1 and 6–2 show some examples of the types of information provided by the National Health Survey Program (23, 28, 38).

Various types of national health survey systems have been developed by European countries. These systems, their problems and variety of uses were reviewed at a conference in 1975 (3).

C. MEASUREMENT OF MORBIDITY

To express morbidity, two general types of rates are available: incidence and prevalence rates. They are defined as follows:

$$
\text{Incidence rate per 1,000} = \frac{\substack{\text{Number of new cases of a disease}\\\text{occurring in the population}\\\text{during a specified period of time}}}{\substack{\text{Number of persons exposed to}\\\text{risk of developing the disease}\\\text{during that period of time}}} \times 1,000
$$

$$\text{Prevalence rate per 1,000} = \frac{\begin{array}{l}\text{Number of cases of disease}\\\text{present in the population at}\\\text{a specified time}\end{array}}{\begin{array}{l}\text{Number of persons in the}\\\text{population at that specified time}\end{array}} \times 1{,}000$$

The incidence rate is a direct estimate of the probability, or risk, of developing a disease during a specified period of time. This contrasts with the prevalence rate, which measures the number of cases that are present at, or during, a specified period of time. The prevalence rate equals the incidence rate times the average duration of the disease. For example, if the average duration of a disease is three years and its incidence rate is 10 per 1,000, the prevalence rate would be 30 per 1,000. The duration of disease is usually measured from the time of diagnosis to death. Although it would be highly desirable to measure the duration from the time of onset of a disease, it is usually difficult, if not impossible, to ascertain this for most diseases.

The two types of prevalence rates that are used by investigators are point prevalence and period prevalence. *Point prevalence* refers to the number of cases present at a specified moment of time; *period prevalence* refers to the number of cases that occur during a specified period of time—for example, a year. Period prevalence consists of the point prevalence at the beginning of a specified period of time plus all new cases that occur during that period. The distinction between these measures of prevalence (Fig. 6–3) developed from practical considerations since it usually takes a *period of time* to conduct a survey and to ascertain all of the cases. Even if a survey does require some time for its execution, however, it is generally possible to estimate point prevalence.

The cases of disease that would be counted in an incidence rate during the annual period in Figure 6–3 would include case numbers 3, 4, 5, and 8. For measuring point prevalence as of January 1, case numbers 1, 2, and 7 would be included, and for point prevalence on December 31, one would include case numbers 1, 3, 5, and 8. Period prevalence from January 1 to December 31, 1975, would include case numbers 1, 2, 3, 4, 5, 7, and 8.

Clearly, the rates can vary depending upon the measure of morbidity that is used. In evaluating published data, it is important to keep in mind the measure used by the investigator since these terms are often erroneously used in published reports. The term "incidence" has been applied to data when prevalence is actually being

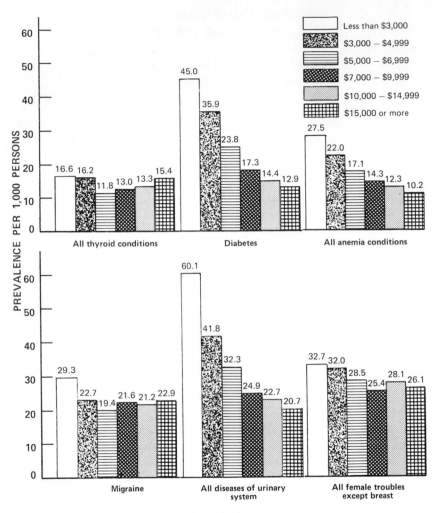

Figure 6–2. Prevalence of selected chronic conditions per 1,000 persons by family income, National Health Survey, 1973

Source: Scott (28).

measured. This creates some difficulties when rates from two different reports are compared.

When an epidemiologist compares the development of disease in different population groups or attempts to determine if a relationship exists between a possible etiological factor and a disease, he generally prefers to use incidence rates. This is because the incidence rate directly estimates the probability of developing a disease during a specified period of time. It permits the epidemiologist to

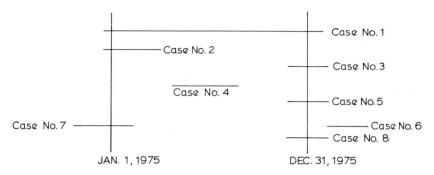

Figure 6–3. Number of cases of disease beginning, developing, and ending during a period of time, January 1–December 31, 1975

determine whether the probability of developing a disease differs in different populations or time periods or in relationship to suspected etiological factors.

All forms of morbidity rates, including incidence, attack, and prevalence rates can be made specific for age, sex, and/or any other personal characteristics. They also can be standardized in the same manner as mortality rates. It is important to distinguish between incidence and prevalence rates in comparing different population groups or different time periods. The incidence rate of a disease may be the same in these comparisons, but the prevalence rates may vary with the availability of medical services that influence duration of the disease. Thus, a higher prevalence rate does not necessarily reflect an increased probability of developing a disease.

Prevalence rates of disease are useful to the health service administrator in planning medical care services. In the absence of incidence rates, differences in prevalence rates between populations have also been useful in stimulating further epidemiologic studies. In some instances, they may be the only rates that are available for studying a particular disease.

A special form of incidence or attack rate, initially developed by C.V. Chapin to measure the spread of infection within a family or household following exposure to the first or primary case in the family, is the *secondary attack rate* (10). It is defined as follows:

$$\begin{matrix}\text{Secondary} \\ \text{attack rate} \\ \text{(percent)}\end{matrix} = \frac{\begin{matrix}\text{Number of exposed persons de-} \\ \text{veloping the disease within the} \\ \text{range of the incubation period}\end{matrix}}{\begin{matrix}\text{Total number of persons exposed} \\ \text{to the primary case}\end{matrix}} \times 100.$$

This rate attempts to measure the degree of spread of an infection within a group that has been exposed to an infectious agent by contact with a case. The numerator can be expressed in terms of clinical disease or any measurable component of the gradient of infection, providing the technical means are available to measure this component. The denominator consists of all persons who are exposed to the case. This can be more specifically defined to include those who are *susceptible* to the specific infectious agent (if means are available to distinguish the immune from the susceptible persons). If the incubation period of a specific disease is unknown, the numerator can be expressed in terms of a specified time period. The primary case is excluded from both the numerator and denominator.

The secondary attack rate is usually applied to biological or social groups such as families, households, friends, or classmates, but it can be used with any closed aggregate of persons who have had contact with a case of disease. Meyer, for example, studied the occurrence of mumps in 170 families, each of which had at least two cases of the disease (19). Table 6–3, taken from this study, presents the distribution of intervals between the day of onset of the first case in the family (designated as day "0") and that of one or more subsequent cases. The secondary cases are those occurring during the interval between 7–8 days and 29–30 days, which would approximate the range of the incubation period and, therefore, represent those cases developing the disease as a result of contact with the first case. The cases that occur after this period are usually called "tertiary" cases and, for the most part, result from contact with secondary cases. They may also be produced by contact with cases outside the family. When the number of secondary cases has been determined and the total number of persons in the household is established, a secondary attack rate can be computed.

The secondary attack rate serves many purposes in addition to reflecting the degree of infectivity of the agent; for instance, in evaluating the efficacy of a prophylactic agent. A study of an outbreak of infectious hepatitis among households in a municipal housing project illustrates this application (15). In this outbreak, some household members had received gamma globulin for prophylaxis at the city hospital nearby, and some had not. The gamma globulin was not administered to the household members in a systematic manner, but varied with the hospital staff member on duty. From the available data, it was possible to compute secondary attack rates for the

Table 6–3. Distribution of Time Intervals between Onset of Initial and Subsequent Cases of Mumps in 170 Families with Two or More Cases

Days Since Initial Case	Number of Subsequent Cases
0	4*
1–2	3
3–4	2
5–6	1
7–8	3
9–10	1
11–12	3
13–14	23
15–16	65
17–18	65
19–20	46
21–22	27
23–24	9
25–26	4
27–28	2
29–30	3
31–32	1
33–34	6
35–36	3
37–38	2
39–40	3
41–42	1
43–44	1
45–56	1
47+	0
Total	279

* Where two cases had onset on day "0," one was arbitrarily designated as a primary, and one as a "subsequent" case. Thus, there were actually 174 cases on day "0."

Source: Meyer (19).

household contacts of the primary case, according to whether or not they had received gamma globulin. Table 6–4 shows that the attack rates were lower among those contacts who had received gamma globulin than among those who had not.

Secondary attack rates are also used to determine whether a disease of unknown etiology is communicable and thus to indicate the possible etiological role of an infectious agent. For example, they have been used to determine whether a transmissible agent may be involved in the etiology of Hodgkin's disease (35). In one study of schools where a case of Hodgkin's disease had initially occurred, secondary attack rates were observed to be higher among both

Table 6–4. Age-specific Secondary Attack Rates of Infectious Hepatitis among Total Number of Persons Exposed to a Case in a Household and among those Receiving or Not Receiving Gamma Globulin

Age	Number of Persons Exposed to a Case	Cases of Hepatitis	
		Number	Percent
0–4	59	3	5.1
5–9	66	5	7.6
10–14	45	6	13.3
15–19	29	3	10.3
20+	100	4	4.0
All Ages	299	21	7.0
Did Not Receive Gamma Globulin			
0–4	42	2	4.8
5–9	45	5	11.1
10–14	32	6	18.8
15–19	26	3	11.5
20+	83	4	4.8
All Ages	228	20	8.8
Received Gamma Globulin			
0–4	17	1	6.0
5–9	21	0	0
10–14	13	0	0
15–19	3	0	0
20+	17	0	0
All Ages	71	1	1.4

Source: Lilienfeld, Bross, and Sartwell (15).

teachers and students than would have been expected from the reported annual incidence rate of Hodgkin's disease. Among the students, the number of secondary cases were about two and one-half times higher than would have been expected from the usual incidence, and among teachers, about seven times higher. This type of aggregation supports the idea that a transmissible agent may be involved in the development of Hodgkin's disease, but further investigations obviously are necessary before reaching any conclusions on its communicability.

D. MORBIDITY SURVEYS—SOME ISSUES AND PROBLEMS

Although there are several advantages in obtaining information on illnesses from a specific population either by interview or examination, inaccuracy and variability of the information presents problems. These difficulties must be considered in assessing the findings from morbidity surveys, for they influence the methods used by epidemiologists in obtaining data and the inferences they derive from the data.

Validity of Interview Surveys

Several studies have addressed the issue of the validity or accuracy of the information on the presence of illness or on other characteristics obtained by interview; these have been summarized recently (6–8, 26, 32, 33). One was conducted in 1958 by the National Health Survey (NHS) in cooperation with the Health Insurance Plan of Greater New York (HIP). Medical records were compared with information obtained by interview from approximately 1400 families, who were a sample of the subscribers and dependents enrolled in HIP. The study was limited to chronic conditions and the sample was divided into two groups: a) families in which one or more members had had contact with a physician in one of the HIP groups within about a year of the interview, and b) families in which no person received such services in the stated period. At the time of physician contact, an HIP Physician Visit Report Form (Med 10) was completed by the physician, indicating the conditions he considered present in the patient. At the time of study, a family member was questioned by an NHS interviewer, using the NHS forms and procedures. The conditions recorded on interview were then compared with the conditions stated on the Med 10 form. Table 6–5 summarizes the general findings on the percentage of possible chronic conditions listed on the Med 10s that were reported during the household interview (33). The table shows that about 32 percent of one or more conditions considered present by the physician were reported on interview. This percentage was somewhat higher for those reporting for themselves (35.6 percent) than for those who responded for their household relatives (28.5 percent). It is clear that there was considerable underreporting of chronic conditions.

A similar study in the Eastern and Midwestern parts of the United States was carried out by the NHS to determine whether a history of hospitalization was accurately reported (32). A sample of 1,505 persons who had been hospitalized during the previous year was interviewed. The respondent was asked to report hospitalizations for the year prior to the Sunday night of the week of the inter-

Table 6–5. Percentage of Possible Chronic Conditions Listed on Med 10 Forms Reported on Household Interview by Number of Conditions and Type of Respondent

Number of Possible Chronic Conditions Inferred from Med 10's in Study Year and Respondent Status	Number of Persons	Number of Conditions Inferred from Med 10's	Percentage of Conditions Correspondingly Reported on Household Interview
All Persons			
Conditions			
One or more	2,934	4,645	31.9
1	1,818	1,818	31.1
2	734	1,468	31.4
3	237	711	33.8
4	97	388	33.8
5+	48	260	31.5
Self-respondents			
Conditions			
One or more	1,260	2,222	35.6
1	674	674	32.6
2	356	712	37.1
3	133	399	37.3
4	64	256	38.3
5+	33	181	33.1
Relatives of Respondents			
Conditions			
One or more	1,659	2,406	28.5
1	1,130	1,130	30.4
2	378	756	26.1
3	103	309	29.4
4	33	132	25.0
5+	15	79	27.8

Source: United States National Health Survey (33).

view. The degree of underreporting of hospitalization is shown in Figure 6–4. It varied with the length of time between hospitalization and interview; the longer the interval, the greater the degree of underreporting, ranging from 10 percent at about six months after hospitalization to about 35–45 percent at one year. It was also found that underreporting varied with the length of stay in the hospital, the reason for hospitalization (whether for a delivery or a surgical or nonsurgical procedure), and other factors.

Another method of validating interview surveys is to compare the information obtained by interview with that obtained by physical

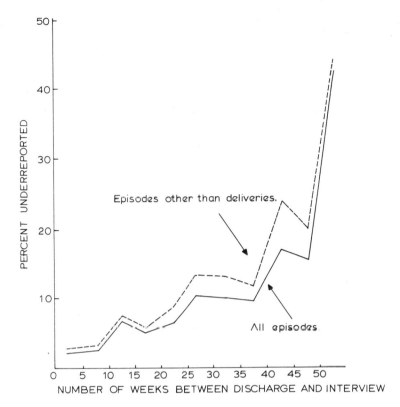

Figure 6–4.   Percent of hospital episodes underreported by the number of weeks between the hospital discharge and interview, including and excluding deliveries

Source: United States National Health Survey (32).

examination. Such comparisons were made in studies conducted by the Commission on Chronic Illness in a rural and an urban area (7, 8).

The study in the rural area was conducted during 1951–1955 in Hunterdon County, New Jersey, which had a population of 42,736. A sample of 13,113 persons in 4,246 households was interviewed with a response rate of 91 percent. Of these, 1,202 persons were categorized into different strata, according to conditions reported on interview, and were invited to a medical center for a complete physical examination, including any indicated laboratory or diagnostic procedures. Seventy-two percent of those who were invited accepted. The conditions reported on interview and on examina-

Table 6–6. Proportions of Match between Interview-reported Conditions and Clinically Evaluated Conditions Which Were Judged to Have Been Present during Year Covered by Family Interview by Disease Classification and Whether or Not Conditions Were Disabling

Disease Classification	Weighted Percent Matching Interview-reported Conditions	
	Disabling	Nondisabling
All conditions present during interview year	24	18
Infective; parasitic	22	8
Neoplasms, benign and malignant	15	7
Allergic	57	12
Diabetes mellitus	63	100
Obesity; endocrine, metabolic, nutritional	6	2
Anemias; other blood conditions	52	0
Mental, psychoneurotic, personality disorders	21	30
Nervous system	39	26
Eye	22	14
Ear	57	54
Heart	38	54
Circulatory, other than heart	26	27
Respiratory	28	54
Dental; buccal cavity and esophageal	15	2
Digestive, other than buccal cavity and esophageal	23	64
Genitourinary	7	16
Skin; cellular tissue	36	3
Arthritis; bone, organs of movement	31	25
Injuries; poisonings	22	46
Impairments (except injuries)	11	9
Symptoms; senility; other ill-defined conditions	15	2

Source: Commission on Chronic Illness (8). © 1959, The Commonwealth Fund.

tion were compared after statistical weighting to adjust for the stratification procedures and different response rates for each stratum. The proportions of match between interview reported and clinically evaluated conditions are shown in Table 6–6 for both disabling and nondisabling conditions. The interview method clearly resulted in underreporting of clinically evaluated conditions. The degree of underreporting varied with the condition and was quite substantial for several disorders. On the other hand, many important conditions reported on interview were validated by clinical evaluation; for example, 80 percent of the reports of a heart condition and 85 percent of reported diabetes were validated. However, for some conditions, such as gastrointestinal disorders, only 48 percent of the reports were clinically confirmed. It was of interest that sex and age did not influence the degree of difference. Strangely enough, those with little education and low family incomes had a higher proportion of validated reports than those in the higher educational and income group.

To illustrate the influence of differences between information obtained by interview and by clinical evaluation, Table 6–7 compares the age-specific annual prevalence rates of selected chronic diseases based on information obtained by interview with that obtained by clinical evaluation (7). Even though there are differences between interview-determined and clinically evaluated conditions in absolute levels for each age group, the age-specific pattern is little affected; either method of determining prevalence shows an increase with age for these conditions.

It can be seen that there are grounds for skepticism as to the accuracy of information obtained by interview (26). This issue is especially relevant in epidemiology, as the search for etiological factors often requires information concerning events that occurred many years in the past. The attempt to determine whether a relationship exists between alcohol consumption and esophageal cancer, for example, may involve interviewing esophageal cancer patients and controls who are mostly over 40–45 years of age. They will be asked about their alcohol consumption over a period of years. It is, therefore, quite reasonable to question the validity of the information that is obtained. All this points to the need to validate information obtained by interview with past medical or other types of records, when conducting epidemiologic studies.

Accuracy and Reproducibility of Examinations, Including Screening and Diagnostic Tests

The uncertainty of information obtained by interview has stimulated a desire to use more objective methods of examination, laboratory tests, or skin tests in measuring morbidity, whenever possible. The procedure selected depends on the component of the disease spectrum (see Chap. 3) which the investigator is studying. Two aspects of these "objective" tests are important in epidemiology: a) accuracy or validity, and b) variability, reproducibility, or precision.

Table 6–7. Comparison of Age-specific Prevalence Rates of Selected Chronic Diseases as Measured by Household Interview and Clinical Evaluation

Age	Annual Prevalence Rate for General Population (per 1,000) from		Ratio Evaluation Rate/Interview Rate
	Interviews	Evaluation	
*All Heart Disease**			
All Ages	24.7	96.4	3.9
<15	7.6	16.4	2.2
15–34	8.6	18.3	2.1
35–64	29.3	122.0	4.2
65+	122.9	574.7	4.7
Hypertension and Hypertensive Heart Disease			
All Ages	36.2	116.6	3.2
<15	0.3	—	—
15–34	10.6	23.3	2.2
35–64	60.2	214.1	3.6
65+	141.3	406.4	2.9
All Arthritis†			
All Ages	47.0	75.2	1.6
<15	—	—	—
15–34	13.7	5.2	0.4
35–64	70.4	98.6	1.4
65+	223.0	514.9	2.3
All Neoplasms			
All Ages	7.5	54.9	7.3
<15	0.9	5.4	6.0
15–34	7.4	49.6	6.7
35–64	11.7	91.1	7.8
65+	9.1	70.3	7.7

* For interview data, incuudes rheumatic fever.
† For interview data, includes "rheumatism."

Source: Commission on Chronic Illness (7). © 1957, The Commonwealth Fund.

ASSESSMENT OF ACCURACY OR VALIDITY

Two indices are used to evaluate the accuracy of a test—those of sensitivity and specificity. These indices are usually determined by administering the test to one group of persons who have the disease

Table 6–8.   Indices to Evaluate the Accuracy of a Test or Diagnostic Examination: Sensitivity and Specificity

Test or Examination	Disease Present	Disease Absent
Positive (Indicating disease is probably present)	A (true positives)	B (false positives)
Negative (Indicating disease is probably absent)	C (false negatives)	D (true negatives)
Totals	A + C	B + D

Sensitivity is defined as the percent of those who have the disease, and are so indicated by the test. Thus,

$$\text{Sensitivity (in percent)} = \frac{A}{A+C} \times 100$$

Specificity is defined as the percent of those who do *not* have the disease and are so indicated by the test. Thus,

$$\text{Specificity (in percent)} = \frac{D}{B+D} \times 100$$

and to another group who do not, and then comparing the results. As indicated in Table 6–8, those testing positive who have the disease are called "true positives"; those testing positive who do not have the disease are called "false positives"; those testing negative who have the disease are called "false negatives"; and those testing negative who do not have the disease are called "true negatives." Using this terminology:

$$\text{Sensitivity} = \frac{\text{True positives}}{\text{True positives plus false negatives}} = \frac{\text{True positives}}{\text{All those with the disease}}$$

$$\text{Specificity} = \frac{\text{True negatives}}{\text{True negatives plus false positives}} = \frac{\text{True negatives}}{\text{All those without the disease}}$$

Sensitivity and specificity are not absolute values. The results of many laboratory tests are not sharply categorized but form a continuous spectrum. Figure 6–5, for example, shows the hypothetical overlap between a normal and diabetic population, in the distribution of blood glucose levels. Table 6–9 presents data obtained from a two-hour postprandial blood test for glucose in a group of 70 **true**

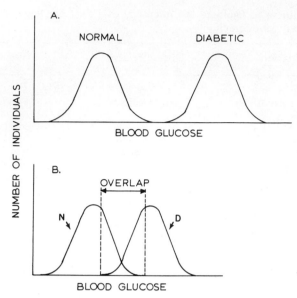

Figure 6–5. Hypothetical distribution of blood glucose values in (A) normal and diabetic population without any overlap and in (B) normal and diabetic populations with overlapping values

Table 6–9. Sensitivity and Specificity of a Two-hour Postprandial Blood Test for Glucose for 70 True Diabetics and 510 True Nondiabetics at Different Levels of Blood Glucose

Blood Glucose Level (mg/100 ml)	Sensitivity (Percent Diabetics So Identified)	Specificity (Percent Nondiabetics So Identified)
80	100.0	1.2
90	98.6	7.3
100	97.1	25.3
110	92.9	48.4
120	88.6	68.2
130	81.4	82.4
140	74.3	91.2
150	64.3	96.1
160	55.7	98.6
170	52.9	99.6
180	50.0	99.8
190	44.3	99.8
200	37.1	100.0

Source: United States Public Health Service (34).

diabetics and 510 true nondiabetics (34). The percentage of diabetics so identified (sensitivity) and the percentage of nondiabetics so identified (specificity) are shown for varying levels of blood glucose. An investigator who decides to use a blood sugar level of 110 mg as a division point for diabetes, for example, would identify

Table 6–10. Sensitivity and Specificity of a Blood Glucose Level of 110 mg/100 ml for Presumptive Determination of Diabetes Status

Blood Glucose Level (mg/100 ml)	Diabetics (Percent)	Nondiabetics (Percent)
All those with level over 110 mg/100 ml are classified as diabetics	92.9 (true positives)	51.6 (false positives)
All those with level under 110 mg/100 ml are classified as nondiabetics	7.1 (false negatives)	48.4 (true negatives)
	100.0	100.0

92.9 percent of the true diabetics and 48.4 percent of the true nondiabetics. Classifying these data into the four categories of Table 6–8 results in Table 6–10. These results are diagrammatically presented in Figure 6–6, which also illustrates the effects of setting different upper limits of normal on blood glucose levels. If the limit is set low, the blood glucose levels become a very sensitive test, i.e., all diabetics have positive tests. However, this is done at the expense of mistakenly identifying many normal subjects as diabetic. If the limit is set high, the blood glucose becomes a highly specific test for diabetes. However, many diabetics are erroneously diagnosed as nondiabetics. The intermediate choice minimizes both types of error— false positive and false negative.

In setting a test level at the point desired to identify those with a specific disease and to omit those without it, one must judge the relative costs of classifying persons as false negatives and false positives. The prevalence of the disease in the community, the cost of additional examinations that may be necessary, and the purpose for applying the test must also be considered (5).

ASSESSMENT OF VARIABILITY OR PRECISION

The problem of variability was initially brought into focus by

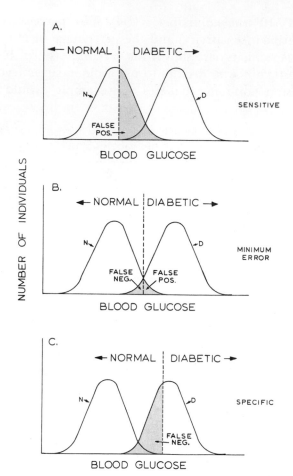

Figure 6–6.   The effect of setting different blood glucose levels on false positives and false negatives: (A) a low limit results in a more sensitive test; (B) intermediate limit results in minimum total error; (C) a high limit results in a more specific test

Yerushalmy in his studies of the interpretation of chest X-ray films in the diagnosis of tuberculosis (39). He found two types of variability in interpretation:

1. Interindividual—representing inconsistency of interpretation among different readers of the X-ray films.
2. Intraindividual—reflecting the failure of a reader to be consistent with himself in independent interpretations of the same set of films.

Table 6–11. Comparison of Independent Interpretations of Chest X-ray Films by Two Different Radiologists A and B: Underlined Numbers Indicate Those Interpretations Where Both Radiologists Agreed

Chest X-ray Interpretation by Radiologist A*	Chest X-ray Interpretation by Radiologist B (Number of Individuals)*						
	SN	OSPA	CV	NSA	NEG	TU	Total
SN	61†	16	1	9	8		95
OSPA	70	1,320	63	861	367	33	2,714
CV	19	151	1,322	369	1,880	62	3,803
NSA	25	407	43	1,716	1,656	40	3,887
NEG	28	157	91	680	8,475	50	9,481
TU		2		4	47		53
Total	203	2,053	1,520	3,639	12,433	185	20,033

* SN—suspect neoplasm; OSPA—other significant pulmonary abnormality; CV—cardiovascular abnormality; NSA—nonsignificant abnormality; NEG—negative; TU—technically unsatisfactory X-ray films.

$$\text{† Percent agreement} = \frac{\text{Total of numbers in diagonals (underlined)}}{\text{Total number of satisfactory films}}$$

$$= \frac{61 + 1,320 + 1,322 + 1,716 + 8,475}{20,033 - (185 + 53)} = \frac{12,894}{19,795} = 65.1$$

Source: Lilienfeld and Kordan (16).

Both types of variability are illustrated by drawing on the results of a study that was designed to evaluate the efficacy of periodic sputum cytologic and X-ray examinations in the early detection of lung cancer (2, 14, 16). This was a cooperative study conducted by the American Cancer Society and the Veterans Administration (VA), which attempted to obtain sputum and chest X-rays about every six months from 14,607 residents of VA domiciles, a group that essentially consisted of veterans receiving pensions. All chest X-ray films were initially read at the VA domiciles. They were then mailed to a radiology center, together with all previous screening films of the individual made during the study. At the radiology center, two of a total of nine qualified radiologists independently read and interpreted each set of films without knowledge of the clinical history or age of the subject. X-ray films for about 97 percent of the study group were obtained.

A comparison between the interpretations of one of the pairs of

Table 6–12. Summary of Percent Agreement of Independent Interpretations of Chest X-ray Films by Two Radiologists

Comparisons	Number of Pairs of Films	Percent Agreement between Radiologists	
		Five Categories	Two Categories
One Reader versus Other Reader*	6,135	67.0	85.1
A versus B	19,795	65.1	89.4
A versus I	29	58.6	82.8
A versus C	1,295	62.2	85.1
A versus D	558	59.5	86.9
A versus E	8,183	59.0	89.2
A versus F	310	31.6	87.1
A versus G	1,438	55.2	90.5
A versus H	521	55.9	89.4
B versus I	213	76.1	89.2
B versus C	388	60.3	80.9
G versus H	256	68.8	91.8

* During early part of study, individual radiologists were not identified.

Source: Lilienfeld and Kordan (16).

radiologists indicated a 65.1 percent agreement when the radiologists placed the films into one of five categories: suspect neoplasm (SN), other significant pulmonary abnormality (OSPA), cardiovascular abnormality (CV), nonsignificant abnormality (NSA), and negative (Neg.) (Table 6–11). If these are combined into two categories—for example, if SN and OSPA are combined and CV, NSA, and Neg. are combined, which would represent a natural combination for this study—the agreement between the two readers increased to 89.4 percent. This has been observed in other studies of variability: the fewer the categories, the greater the degree of agreement between readers.

The agreement between the interpretations of all the different pairs of radiologists from the total group of nine who read the films is presented in Table 6–12. The range of agreement varied from 31.6 to 76.1 percent for five categories and from 80.9 to 91.8 percent for two categories. In this same study, it was also possible to obtain an estimate of the degree of intraindividual variability. By chance, a few films were unknowingly read twice by the same radiologist at different times, with the results shown in Table 6–13.

Table 6–13. Percent Agreement of Independent Interpretations of Chest X-ray Films by the Same Radiologist at Different Times

Comparisons	Number of Pairs of Films	Percent Agreement	
		Five Categories	Two Categories
A versus A	69	55.1	91.3
B versus B	26	46.2	80.8

Source: Lilienfeld and Kordan (16).

Archer and colleagues (2) also investigated the extent of variability in classifying the sputum cytology slides into four categories: positive for lung cancer, suspect, ambiguous cells, and negative. A set of one hundred slides was sent at two different times to the cytologists participating in the study. The extent of intraindividual variability between two of these cytologists is shown in Table 6–14.

Table 6–14. Comparison of First and Second Independent Interpretations for Lung Cancer by Cytologists A and D: Underlined Numbers Indicate Those Interpretations in Which Each Cytologist Agreed with Himself

First Interpretation	Second Interpretation					
	Unsatisfactory	Negative	Ambiguous Cells	Suspect	Positive	Total
Cytologist A						
Unsatisfactory	<u>2</u>	1	1	0	0	4
Negative	7	<u>26</u>	19	1	0	53
Ambiguous cells	4	2	<u>11</u>	5	3	25
Suspect	0	0	1	<u>6</u>	6	13
Positive	1	0	0	0	<u>4</u>	5
Total	14	29	32	12	13	100
Cytologist D						
Unsatisfactory	<u>0</u>	0	0	1	0	1
Negative	1	<u>60</u>	7	2	0	70
Ambiguous cells	0	2	<u>1</u>	0	1	4
Suspect	1	3	0	<u>5</u>	3	12
Positive	0	0	1	4	<u>8</u>	13
Total	2	65	9	12	12	100

Source: Archer et al. (2).

If one eliminates the technically unsatisfactory readings, the degree of agreement for cytologist *A* is about 56 percent and for cytologist *D*, about 76 percent.

It is desirable to determine whether variability in classifying X-ray films and sputum cytology slides have any influence on the accuracy or validity of these tests. In contrast to previous studies, it was possible to answer this question by following the persons tested to ascertain their cause of death—particularly from lung cancer—within the three-year period during which the original tests were administered.

Table 6–15. Percentage of Screened Veterans Administration Domiciliary Members Who Died from All Causes and Types of Cancer by Chest X-ray Interpretation That Was Most Suspicious of Lung Cancer during a Three-year Study Period

Chest X-ray Screening Interpretation Most Suspicious for Lung Cancer*	Number of Screened Members	Percentage of Screened Members Who Died from All Causes or Types of Cancer					
		All Causes	Primary Lung Cancer	Secondary Lung Cancer	Cancer of Upper Respiratory Tract	Cancer of Other Sites	No Cancer Present
SN	535	25.4	10.8	1.5		2.6	10.5
OSPA	3,913	13.4	1.2	0.4	0.3	1.3	10.2
CV, NSA NEG, none	10,159	11.4	0.4	0.3	0.2	1.7	9.1
All screened members	14,607	12.4	1.0	0.4	0.2	1.4	9.4

* SN—suspect neoplasm; OSPA—other significant pulmonary abnormality; CV—cardiovascular abnormality; NSA—nonsignificant abnormality; NEG—negative. The screened member was classified by the X-ray screening interpretation that was most suspicious of lung cancer during the three-year study period.

Source: Lilienfeld et al. (14).

Table 6–15 shows that 10.8 percent of those who had a chest X-ray film interpretation that was suspicious of lung cancer had died from primary lung cancer in contrast to 0.4 percent of those who did not have any, or no significant pulmonary abnormalities. Table 6–16 shows that 30 percent of those who had sputum cytology findings that were positive for cancer cells died from lung cancer,

Table 6–16. Percentage of Screened Veterans Administration Domiciliary Members Who Died from All Causes and Types of Cancer by Sputum Cytology Finding That Was Most Positive for Cancer Cells during Three-year Study Period

Sputum Cytology Screening Finding for Lung Cancer*	Number of Screened Members	Percentage of Screened Members Who Died from All Cancer or Types of Cancer					
		All Causes	Primary Lung Cancer	Secondary Lung Cancer	Cancer of Upper Respiratory Tract	Cancer of Other Sites	No Cancer Present
Positive	50	40.0	30.0	2.0	2.0	2.0	4.0
Suspect	139	13.7	5.0			2.2	6.5
Ambiguous cells	377	11.1	2.4	0.8	1.2	0.3	6.6
Negative	12,162	11.3	0.8	0.4	0.2	1.3	8.6
None	1,879	19.4	1.2	0.4	0.4	2.0	15.1
All screened members	14,607	12.4	1.0	0.4	0.2	1.4	9.4

* The screened member was classified by the sputum cytology finding that was most positive for cancer cells during the three-year study period.

Source: Lilienfeld et al. (14).

and 5.0 percent of those who had suspicious cytology findings in contrast to 0.8 percent of those whose sputum cytology findings were negative. It is clear that the positive and suspect results of these tests are related to subsequent mortality from lung cancer despite variability in their interpretation, although the accuracy of these tests would, no doubt, be enhanced by reducing the variability of interpretation.

E. RECORD LINKAGE

Information on the characteristics of individuals from birth to death exists in the records of many institutions and agencies, private as well as governmental. At birth, a birth certificate is filled out and, when one is hospitalized, a medical record of the hospitalization is initiated and usually maintained. A record in the Social Security system is filed at the beginning of employment; personnel records are maintained at the place of employment; school records are kept, including health as well as scholastic information; and at the time of death, a death certificate is completed. In many epidemiologic studies, some of these records are combined on an ad hoc basis. A good example is the combination of birth and infant mortality certificates to investigate prenatal and perinatal factors that influence infant mortality.

Since the advent of the computer, it has become feasible to develop a systematic method of integrating all these records. This could be useful not only for epidemiologic research but also for genetic studies, the planning of medical care facilities and determining the pattern of patient referral in a community. A pioneering effort in record linkage was made by Newcombe in British Columbia (Canada) for both population and genetic studies. He suggested that such a system could be valuable in the study of environmental carcinogenesis (24, 25).

In 1962, a study was initiated in Oxford, England, to determine the feasibility, cost, and methods of medical record linkage for an entire community. Acheson's report of the results of this pilot study noted that such a system permitted the linking of morbidity and mortality information for the population. This system would provide the necessary knowledge for planning the allocation of various types of medical facilities as well as for facilitating clinical and epidemiologic studies (1). It would also be possible to use the system for a variety of inquiries into the etiology and natural history of different diseases.

Despite the potential value of a system of record linkage, the ethical issue of confidentiality of the information recorded has to be considered. This has been the subject of current public debate, which must be resolved before any attempt is made to establish such a system in the United States (37).

STUDY PROBLEMS

1. Draw a graph of the data presented in Table 6–3 and compute the median incubation period for both the secondary and tertiary cases.
2. A new test has been developed for diagnosing rheumatoid arthritis. The test was evaluated in four communities with the following results:

Community A:

Rheumatoid Arthritis

		Present	Absent	Total
	Positive	887	888	1775
Test Result	Negative	99	7989	8088
	Total	986	8877	9863

Community B:

Rheumatoid Arthritis

		Present	Absent	Total
	Positive	1485	385	1870
Test Result	Negative	165	3465	3630
	Total	1650	3850	5500

Community C:

Rheumatoid Arthritis

		Present	Absent	Total
	Positive	3634	269	3903
Test Result	Negative	404	2423	2827
	Total	4038	2692	6730

Community D:

Rheumatoid Arthritis

		Present	Absent	Total
	Positive	2866	56	2922
Test Result	Negative	318	506	824
	Total	3184	562	3746

a) Calculate the prevalence of arthritis in each of these communities.

b) Calculate the sensitivity and specificity of the test for each community. Graph the sensitivity percentages against the prevalence for the communities. Do the same for the specificity percentages.

c) In addition to sensitivity and specificity, another commonly used criterion for the effectiveness of a diagnostic procedure is the "predictive value":

$$\text{predictive value} = \frac{\text{true positives}}{\text{all who tested positive}} \times 100\%.$$

Calculate the predictive values for each community. Graph the predictive value against the prevalence for the community. What problems might one have in applying the predictive value if, as is usually done, a test is first evaluated in a hospital population and then used in the community?

3. The secondary attack rate was originally developed as a measure of the extent of familial aggregation of infectious diseases. Name at least four explanations for the observation of familial aggregation in a disease of unknown etiology.

4. Under what circumstances would it be desirable to minimize the percentage of individuals with false negative results on a test? Or with false positive results?

5. a) Discuss the advantages and disadvantages of continuous reporting and registering of specific illnesses in a community.

   b) Compare the advantages and disadvantages of maintaining a continuous register for a specific disease with that of periodic ad hoc surveys.

6. What are the advantages and disadvantages in using sensitivity rather than specificity to evaluate a test?

7. In what situations does one find only interindividual variability? Only intraindividual variability? Both?

8. Of what value is the prevalence rate to the epidemiologist for an infectious disease? For a noninfectious disease?

9. a) Outline a study to determine the prevalence rate for an infectious disease, and another, for a noninfectious disease. How would these studies differ from ones attempting to determine the incidence rate for an infectious disease and for a noninfectious disease?

   b) Suppose an investigator reports that the prevalence rate for a disease is 5 percent. How might one validate such a statistic?

REFERENCES

1. Acheson, E.D. 1967. *Medical Record Linkage,* London: Oxford University Press.
2. Archer, P.G., Koprowska, I., McDonald, J.R., Naylor, B., Papanicolaou, G.N., and Umiker, W.O. 1966. "A study of variability in the interpretation of sputum cytology slides." *Cancer Res.* 26:2122–2144.

3. Armitage, P., ed. 1977. *National Health Survey Systems in the European Economic Community*. Luxembourg: Commission of the European Communities.

4. Bahn, A.K., Gorwitz, K., Klee, G.D., Kramer, M., and Tuerk, I. 1965. "Services received by Maryland residents in facilities directed by a psychiatrist." *Pub. Health Reps.* 80:405–416.

5. Blumberg, M.S. 1957. "Evaluating health screening procedures." *Operations Res.* 5:351–360.

6. Cannell, C.F. and Marquis, K.H. 1976. *A Summary of Research Studies of Interviewing Methodology, 1959–1970*. Vital and Health Statistics: Series 2, Data evaluation and methods research; No. 69; DHEW publication No. (HRA) 77-1343, Washington, D.C.: U.S. Government Printing Office.

7. Commission on Chronic Illness. 1957. *Chronic Illness in the United States Vol. IV, Chronic Illness in a Large City: The Baltimore Study*. Cambridge, Massachusetts: Harvard University Press.

8. ———. 1959. *Chronic Illness in the United States Vol. III, Chronic Illness in a Rural Area: The Hunterdon Study*. Reported by R.E. Trussell and J. Elinson. Cambridge: Massachusetts, Harvard University Press.

9. Doll, R., Payne, P., and Waterhouse, J., eds. 1966. *Cancer Incidence in Five Continents: A technical report. Un. Int. Contre Cancer*. Berlin and New York: Springer-Verlag.

10. Frost, W.H. 1941. "The familial aggregation of infectious diseases." In *Papers of Wade Hampton Frost*, K.F. Maxcy, ed. New York: The Commonwealth Fund, pp. 543–552.

11. Gordis, L., Lilienfeld, A.M., and Rodriguez, R. 1969. "An evaluation of the Maryland Rheumatic Fever Registry." *Pub. Health Reps.* 84:333–339.

12. Kelsey, J.L., Pastides, H., and Bisbee, G., Jr. 1978. *Musculo-Skeletal Disorders. Their Frequency of Occurrence and Their Impact on the Population of the United States*. New York: Prodist.

13. Lerner, P.R. 1974. *Social Security Disability Applicant Statistics, 1970*. United States Department of Health, Education and Welfare, Social Security Administration, Office of Research and Statistics Pub. No. (SSA)75-11911, Washington, D.C.: United States Government Printing Office.

14. Lilienfeld, A.M. (Chairman), Archer, P.G., Burnett, C.H., Chamberlain, E.W., Chazin, B.J., Davies, D., Davis, R.L., Haber, P.A., Hodges, F.J., Koprowska, I., Kordan, B., Lane, J.T., Lawton, A.H., Lee, L., Jr., MacCallum, D.B., McDonald, J.R., Milder, J.W., Naylor, B., Papanicolaou, G.N., Slutzker, B., Smith, R.T., Swepston, E.R., and Umiker, W.O. 1966. "An evaluation of radiologic and cytologic screening for the early detection of lung cancer: A cooperative pilot study of the American Cancer Society and the Veterans Administration." *Cancer Res.* 26:2083–2121.

15. Lilienfeld, A.M., Bross, I.D.J., and Sartwell, P.E. 1953. "Observations on an outbreak of infectious hepatitis in Baltimore during 1951." *Amer. J. Pub. Health* 43:1085–1096.

16. ———, and Kordan, B. 1966. "A study of variability in the interpretation of chest X-rays in the detection of lung cancer." *Cancer Res.* 26:2145–2147.

17. ———, Parkhurst, E., Patton, R., and Schlesinger, E.R. 1951. "Accuracy of supplemental medical information on birth certificates." *Pub. Health Reps.* 66:191–198.

18. McDonald, G.W., Fisher, G.F., and Pentz, P.C. 1966. "Diabetes screening activities, July 1958 to June 1963." In *Chronic Diseases and Public Health*, A.M. Lilienfeld and A.J. Gifford, eds. Baltimore: The Johns Hopkins Press, pp. 652–662.

19. Meyer, M. (unpublished data).

20. Milham, S., Jr. 1963. "Underreporting of incidence of cleft lip and palate." *Amer. J. Dis. Child.* 106:185–188.

21. Most, A.S., and Peterson, D.R. 1969. "Myocardial infarction surveillance in a metropolitan community." *JAMA* 208:2433–2438.

22. National Center for Health Statistics. 1963. *Origin, Program, and Operation of the U.S. National Health Survey.* PHS Pub. No. 1000, Series 1, No. 1, United States Department of Health, Education and Welfare, Washington, D.C.: United States Government Printing Office.

23. ———. 1974. *Preliminary Findings of the First Health and Nutrition Examination Survey, United States, 1971–1972, Dietary Intake and Biochemical Findings.* Department of Health, Education and Welfare Pub. No. (HRA) 74–1219–1, Washington, D.C.: United States Government Printing Office.

24. Newcombe, H.B. 1969. "The use of medical record linkage for population and genetic studies." *Methods Inf. Med.* 8:7–11.

25. ———. 1974. "Record linkage for studies of environmental carcinogenesis." In *Proceedings Tenth Canadian Cancer Conference, 1973,* Toronto: University of Toronto Press.

26. Sanders, B.S. 1962. "Have morbidity surveys been oversold?" *Amer. J. Pub. Health* 52:1648–1659.

27. Schaffner, W., Scoot, H.D., Rosenstein, B.J., and Byrne, E.B. 1971. "Innovative communicable disease reporting." *HSMHA Health Reps.* 86:431–436.

28. Scott, G. 1977. *Prevalence of Chronic Conditions of the Genitourinary, Nervous, Endocrine, Metabolic, and Blood and Blood-forming Systems and of Other Selected Chronic Conditions, United States, 1973.* Vital and Health Statistics: Series 10, Data from the National Health Survey; No. 109, DHEW publication No. (HRA) 77-1536, Washington, D.C.: U.S. Government Printing Office.

29. Sherman, I.L., and Langmuir, A.D. 1952. "Usefulness of communicable disease reports." *Pub. Health Reps.* 67:1249–1257.

30. Spiegelman, M. 1968. *Introduction to Demography.* Rev. ed. Cambridge, Massachusetts: Harvard University Press.

31. Sydenstricker, E. 1974. "Statistics of morbidity." In *The Challenge of Facts, Selected Public Health Papers of Edgar Sydenstricker,* R.V. Kasius, ed. New York: Milbank Memorial Fund, Prodist. pp. 228–245.

32. United States National Health Survey. 1961. *Reporting of Hospitalization in the Health Interview Survey. Health Statistics Series D, No. 4,* United States Department of Health, Education and Welfare, Washington, D.C.: Public Health Service.

33. ———. 1961. *Health Interview Responses Compared with Medical Records. Health Statistics Series D, No. 5,* United States Department of Health, Education and Welfare, Washington, D.C.: Public Health Service.

34. United States Public Health Service. 1960. *Diabetes Program Guide, Division of Special Health Services. PHS Pub. No. 506,* Washington, D.C.: United States Government Printing Office.

35. Vianna, N.J., and Polan, A.K. 1973. "Epidemiologic evidence for transmission of Hodgkin's disease." *N. Engl. J. Med.* 289:499–502.

36. Waterhouse, J., Muir, C., Correa, P., and Powell, J., eds. 1976. *Cancer Incidence in Five Continents.* Vol. III. Lyon, France: Int. Agency for Research on Cancer.

37. Westin, A.F. 1967. *Privacy and Freedom*. New York: Atheneum.
38. Wilder, C.S. 1974. *Acute Conditions: Incidence and Associated Disability, United States, July 1971–June 1972*. National Center for Health Statistics Series 10, No. 88, Department of Health, Education and Welfare, Pub. No. (HRA) 74–1515, Washington, D.C.: United States Government Printing Office.
39. Yerushalmy, J. 1947. "Statistical problems in assessing methods of medical diagnosis, with special reference to X-ray techniques." *Pub. Health Reps.* 62:1432–1449.

7 Epidemiologic Studies of Morbidity

> In the conduct of . . . inquiries . . . keep the great object of prevention constantly in view . . . because (it) is the ultimate aim of all investigations of this sort [and] . . . preventive measures may be made a test of the truth of theory itself.
>
> WILLIAM BUDD, "Investigation of Epidemic and Epizotic Diseases," 1864

As with mortality, epidemiologists are interested in the occurrence of morbidity by time, place, and persons. The reasoning processes used in interpreting morbidity data are similar to those discussed for mortality statistics, but such data are not bound by the limited information usually available on death certificates. One can, therefore, use more personal characteristics for analysis. In addition, epidemiologists often conduct their own morbidity studies in selected communities and thus obtain information that is particularly relevant to the etiological hypotheses for the specific disease under consideration.

A. TIME

One aspect of the distribution of an illness in time was considered in the discussion of incubation periods in Chapter 3; basically, these periods represent the temporal distribution of the onset of disease after exposure to an etiological agent. Much of the discussion of temporal trends of mortality in Chapter 5 applies equally well to trends in the incidence of disease.

An aspect of time distribution that has not been discussed previously is the seasonal trend of disease. Many diseases, particularly the infectious ones occur more frequently at particular times of the year. In some instances, there are clear-cut explanations for the

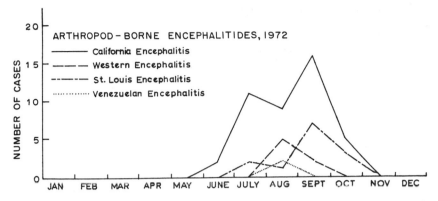

Figure 7–1. Number of reported cases of arthropod-borne encephalitides by etiology and month, United States, 1972

Source: Center for Disease Control (7).

seasonality; the arthropod-borne encephalitides occur more frequently during the summer months since the arthropod vectors of the disease are then present (Fig. 7–1) (7). The seasonal distribution of mumps is quite different, showing an increase in the fall and reaching its highest levels in the winter months (Fig. 7–2) (7). Mumps is a disease that spreads by personal contact, and it is quite possible that the increased crowding within families or other aggre-

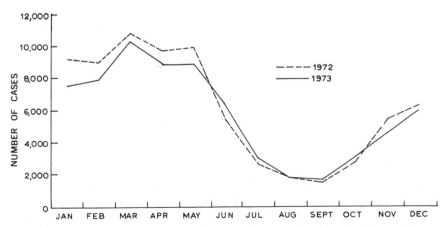

Figure 7–2. Number of reported cases of mumps by month, United States, 1972 and 1973

Source: Center for Disease Control (7).

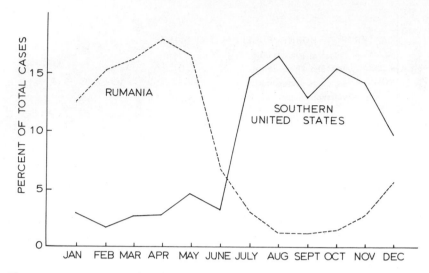

Figure 7–3. Percent distribution of cases of endemic typhus fever by month, Southern United States (Alabama and Savannah, Ga.), 1922–1925 and epidemic typhus fever in Rumania, 1922–1924

Source: Maxcy (22).

gates of the population—such as schools—during certain periods of the year may be responsible for its seasonal pattern.

The seasonal occurrence of a disease has been used to differentiate between diseases. In his classic study of endemic typhus fever conducted at a time when many investigators thought that endemic typhus in the United States was identical to epidemic typhus fever in Europe, Maxcy noted that the two diseases differed in their seasonal distribution (Fig. 7–3). Together with other epidemiologic evidence (to be discussed below), this observation indicated that these were different diseases with different modes of transmission (22).

There is current interest in the possible seasonal variation in human leukemia because of an hypothesized viral etiology, but available data are not consistent (18). In the nutritional deficiency disease pellagra, an increased incidence during the spring months was consistently observed. This was so striking in Italy that the disease was known as *mal del sole* and was attributed to sunstroke (29). No definitive explanation exists for the seasonal distribution.

B. PLACE

The same issues that have been considered in interpreting the occurrence of mortality by place also apply to morbidity. Morbidity data, however, make it possible to analyze disease distribution in smaller geographic areas than do mortality data. Therefore, one can consider very specific factors that influence such distributions from which more specific and definitive etiological hypotheses can be developed.

A classic example of the use of place in deriving etiological inferences is the above-mentioned study of endemic typhus fever (22). At the time of that study, it was known that Old World (epidemic) typhus fever was transmitted from man to man by the louse. From clinical, serological, and experimental evidence, many investigators considered the two diseases to be similar and therefore inferred that endemic typhus was also louse-borne.

Maxcy observed the focal distribution of the disease in certain areas, among them Montgomery, Alabama. Using what is known as a "spot map," he analyzed the distribution of cases of disease by place of residence (Fig. 7–4) and found no distinct localization of cases. Considering the question of contact, however, he felt that an employed person would be exposed to an even greater number of contacts at his place of occupation than at home and, therefore, he distributed the cases according to place of employment (Fig. 7–5). This suggested a focal center of the disease in the heart of the business district. A more detailed analysis of the places of employment indicated a high attack rate among those working at food depots, groceries, feed stores, and restaurants. This led Maxcy to suggest a rodent reservoir of the disease—rats or mice—and fleas, mites, or ticks as possible insect vectors. He summarized the evidence against louse transmission in terms of the differences in the cases' seasonal distribution (Fig. 7–3), their distribution by place of employment and residence (Figs. 7–4 and 7–5), and the lack of evidence of communicability from person to person. His inferences were subsequently shown to be correct in an investigation by Dyer that incriminated the rat as the reservoir and the rat flea as the insect vector of Rickettsia Mooseri (*R. Typhi*) (22, 33).

A more recent example of the use of place in epidemiologic investigations is found in studies of Burkitt's lymphoma, a disease of children 2–14 years of age first described in 1958 (2). Burkitt first

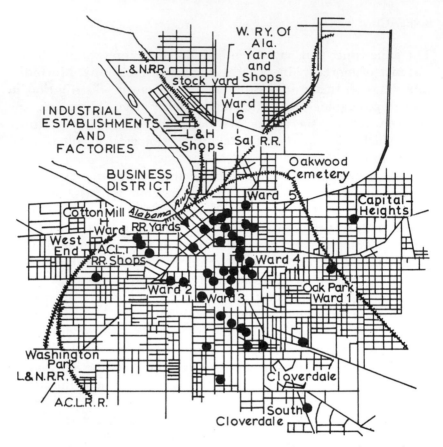

Figure 7–4. Distribution of cases of endemic typhus fever by residence, Montgomery, Alabama, 1922–1925

Source: Maxcy (22).

observed the disease in Uganda and then mapped its geographical distribution from published reports and by visiting hospitals in Africa in a "tumor safari" that covered over 10,000 miles (Fig. 7–6) (4). He noted the absence of the disease in areas over 5000 feet above sea level, where the annual rainfall was below 30 inches and the mean temperature was below 60° F (Fig. 7–7) (3), which suggested an insect vector of a viral or other infectious etiological agent. The areas of disease occurrence in Africa overlapped with those of other infectious diseases, such as malaria and yellow fever.

This led to virological studies that resulted in the identification of the Epstein-Barr (EB) virus, and indicated that it was a likely

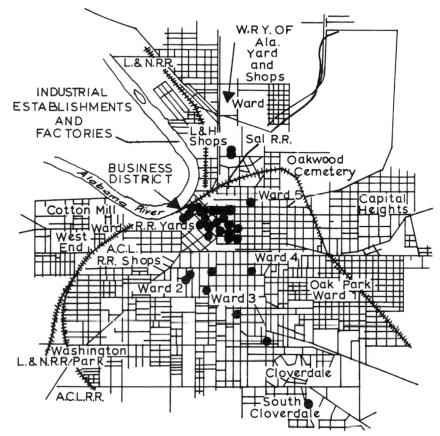

Figure 7–5. Distribution of cases of endemic typhus fever by place of employment, or, if unemployed, by place of residence, Montgomery, Alabama, 1922–1925

Source: Maxcy (22).

etiological agent (12, 13, 16). Reviews of previously collected histological material, however, indicated that the disease was also present in nontropical countries, such as the United States and France, although it was relatively rare in these countries (5). It was also observed that the disease, although rarely, can occur in moist tropical areas (1). The EB virus is not normally transmitted by an insect and was found to be equally prevalent in areas of both high and low incidence of Burkitt's lymphoma. This led to a reconsideration of an earlier suggestion that malarial infection, which has the same geographical distribution as the tumor, might be influential in its

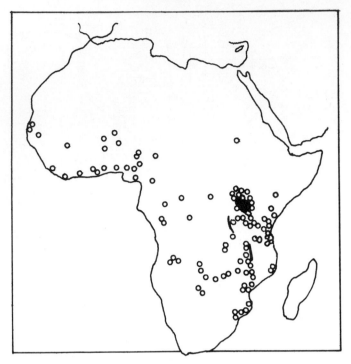

Figure 7–6.   Distribution of known cases of Burkitt's lymphoma, including those obtained on tumor safari, Africa, 1962

Source: Burkitt (4).

etiology (9, 16). This hypothesis was supported by findings of other characteristics of chronic malaria and a reduced frequency of sickle cell hemoglobin in patients with Burkitt's lymphoma (27). Previous observations had indicated that sickle cell hemoglobin protected against malarial infection. Meanwhile, the EB virus had been shown to be etiologically related to infectious mononucleosis. Experimental work also showed a relationship between virus-induced lymphoma and murine malarial infection in mice (31). Furthermore, it has been shown that this virus causes fatal, malignant reticulo-proliferative disease upon inoculation into South American subhuman primates. Thus, one current hypothesis (Fig. 7–8) suggests that when the EB virus acts on normal tissue, it is usually nonpathogenic or, occasionally, causes infectious mononucleosis and rarely causes malignant lymphoma. However, when acting on lymphoid cells that are immunologically altered by chronic ma-

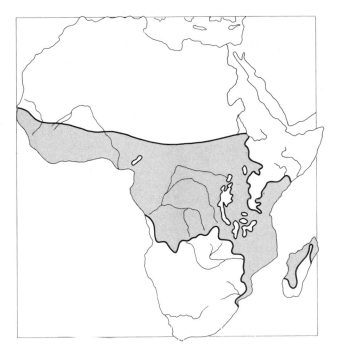

Figure 7–7. Map of Africa where shaded areas indicate those less than 5000 feet above sea level and mean temperature is above 60° F and mean annual rainfall is above 30 inches

Source: Burkitt (3). Copyright © 1961, *East African Medical Journal.*

larial infection, the virus would more likely produce malignant lymphoma although it might, occasionally, result in infectious mononucleosis (6, 12, 16). This concept is still speculative and viral causation of the disease has not been proven; nevertheless, the hypothesis is consistent with present epidemiologic and experimental evidence.

The direct influence of place on the occurrence of a disease is illustrated by coccidioidomycosis, a disease that is caused by a fungus, *coccidioides immitis,* whose spores lie dormant in the dust and soil of arid regions in the southwestern part of the United States, which are almost dry and without much rainfall. The spores are inhaled with the dust, producing a respiratory disease. This was recently illustrated when college students from the east on an archaeological exploration of Indian mounds on the West Coast developed the disease (32). The localization of this disease to the south-

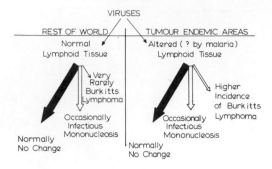

western United States is based on a study of positive reactors to a coccidioidin skin testing program of young adults in various parts of the United States (Fig. 7–9) (11).

These examples of studies illustrate the various ways in which place influences the occurrence of disease. In one instance, endemic typhus, the important place was that of employment in which a dis-

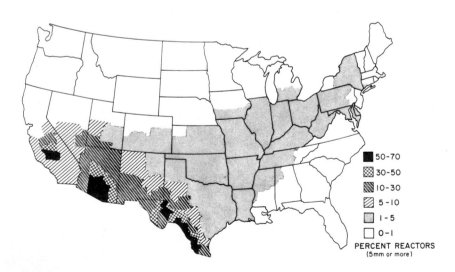

Figure 7–9. Percent reactors to coccidioidin skin test among white men and women, 17–21 years of age, by county of residence, United States, 1945–1951

Source: Edwards and Palmer (11).

ease reservoir was present. In another, Burkitt's lymphoma, current speculation suggests that a different disease, malaria, in a specific geographical place may influence the immunological characteristics of persons to increase their susceptibility to a viral agent. In, the last example, coccidioidomycosis, the place represents the climatic conditions necessary for the continued maintenance of the etiological agent.

C. TIME AND SPACE CLUSTERS

A term that has been increasingly used in recent years to describe the distribution of disease in time or place, or both, is "a cluster." A clustering of cases in time might indicate that certain etiological factors were introduced into the environment at that time, for example, an infectious agent or drug. The food-poisoning outbreak discussed in Chapter 1 was a clustering of cases of gastroenteritis due to exposure to contaminated food. The increase in asthmatic mortality discussed in Chapter 5 also represents a temporal clustering that resulted from the introduction of a particular "therapeutic" agent. In these instances, it was possible to compute either attack rates or mortality rates when analyzing the data. Clustering of cases in space in Maxcy's spot maps showed the focal distribution of endemic typhus, thus providing the evidence that finally incriminated a reservoir and mode of infection.

Space-time clustering data were valuable in unraveling the etiology of infectious diseases, so it is not surprising that interest has now developed in studying the clustering of cases of diseases of unknown etiology to determine whether they may be of infectious origin. Similarly, there have been many studies of clusters of cases of leukemia and other forms of cancer where an infectious agent is considered to be a possible etiological factor (18). These studies have resulted in the development of a variety of complex statistical techniques to determine whether or not these "clusters" could have arisen by chance alone. A review of these studies indicates that the determination of statistically significant findings varies with the different statistical methods used in the analysis (10, 19, 21, 26, 28).

A major problem in many of these studies is that they deal only with clusters of cases and, generally, do not take into consideration the varying concentrations of the population in the communities where these cases appear. One should view the occurrence of a cluster as only a lead to the possible common exposure of a segment of the population to an etiological agent that may possibly be infectious. If the search for an infectious agent is of major interest, these studies should be followed by epidemiologic studies comparing population groups such as families, neighborhoods, and schools whose members have been exposed to a case with similar population groups that have not been so exposed. Secondary attack rates can then be computed and compared as has been done most recently for Hodgkin's disease (30). If the clusters are limited to families, it becomes necessary to consider the possible influence of genetic factors as well as environmental factors that are common to family members.

D. PERSONS

Epidemiologists are interested in the occurrence of morbidity by such personal characteristics as age, sex, color, and social status. The number of personal characteristics available for study—as already mentioned—is not as limited as in analyses of mortality, where the information must be obtained from death certificates. Routinely collected morbidity statistics share some of the limitations of mortality data but the variables included in the National Health Survey or in disease registers are generally more extensive than those on death certificates.

An epidemiologist who wishes to determine the incidence or prevalence of a disease entity in a community by means of a morbidity survey can include any factor he considers relevant to his investigation, such as demographic, physiological, biochemical, immunological characteristics and personal living habits. This would permit him to analyze the relationship of these factors to the disease within the surveyed population in terms of individual characteristics (see Chap. 1, p. 14). However, he is also interested in the distribution of the relevant factors in the community as a whole. Consistency in the distribution of a set of these factors with that of morbidity in the population clearly strengthens the evidence upon which an etiological inference can be based; this will be discussed in Chapter 12.

The few personal characteristics already reviewed in Chapter 5

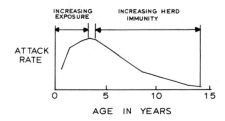

Figure 7–10. Changes in incidence rate from measles by age, reflecting changes in degree of exposure and in increasing immunity in the population

in the context of mortality statistics are also pertinent to morbidity studies. These will be discussed together with several additional factors.

Age

Many infectious diseases such as measles and chickenpox are considered childhood diseases; that is, their highest frequency of occurrence is in the younger age groups. In the United States, the incidence rate of measles increases sharply from about one to four years

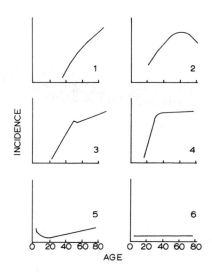

Figure 7–11. Frequently observed patterns of age-specific cancer incidence rates in humans

Source: Higginson and Muir (17).

of age, probably as a result of increasing socialization of the child. This age group also has a low proportion of immune individuals because they have had no previous exposure to the virus. After age four, the incidence rate gradually decreases until it approaches zero at about 12–15 years of age. Since an attack of measles confers lifelong immunity, the increasing incidence rate up to age four results in a high frequency of immune individuals in the age group from four to about thirteen years and few susceptibles remain to be infected (Fig. 7–10).

Different forms of cancer have varying patterns of age-specific incidence rates, which have provided a basis for suggested etiological interpretations by Higginson and Muir (17). Some of the more frequent ones are shown in Figure 7–11. Graph 1 represents a pattern frequently observed when an exogenous agent, acting continuously throughout life, is believed to be the major etiological stimulus, as in carcinoma of the esophagus or lung. The shape of the curve in graph 2 suggests that the etiological stimuli are the strongest in early life. The decrease in incidence in the very old age groups could be explained by:

1. Diminished exposure to an exogenous stimulus or a birth cohort effect (see Chap. 5, p. 117);
2. Elimination of a susceptible population subgroup;
3. Changes in the host occurring in middle age, as at menopause;
4. Serious underreporting in old age.

The bimodal curve in graph 3, as seen in breast cancer, suggests differing stimuli in early and later life. Graph 4 shows a curve with an increasing rate until age forty, after which the rate remains the same for the remainder of life. It is seen in liver carcinoma in Africa, suggesting a strong stimulus in childhood, with either reduced exposure or decreased susceptibility to the stimulus in adult life. The curved peak in childhood and slow increase in later life shown in graph 5 is seen in certain leukemias. This may indicate a viral etiology with an increased incidence in immunodeficient children and a lesser increase in immunologically competent adults. The pattern is also observed in certain sarcomas and, in this case, exposure to two different carcinogens—the first acting in the neonatal period or in infancy and the second in adult life—has been hypothesized. The curve in graph 6 shows a minimal increase with

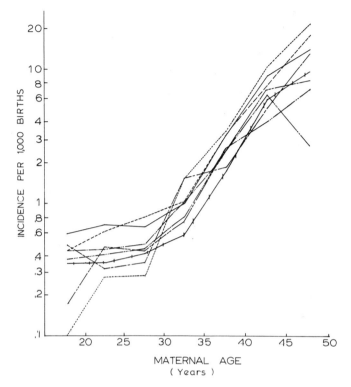

Figure 7–12. Incidence rates of mongolism by maternal age at birth from selected studies, 1923–1964.

Source: Lilienfeld (20). Copyright © 1969, The Johns Hopkins University Press.

age, as in chronic lymphatic leukemia in Japan and in certain soft tissue sarcomas. Because of the small number of cases upon which this curve is based, however, it may not be very reliable. The interpretations of these patterns by Higginson and Muir are quite specific, probably reflecting the availability of specific etiological hypotheses for the various types of malignancies.

Maternal Age

One aspect of age that has not yet been considered is the relationship of maternal age at the time of birth to disorders in the offspring. The relationship of maternal age to infant mortality and prematurity has been known for years, although there have been no widely accepted biological explanations. Perhaps the classic and

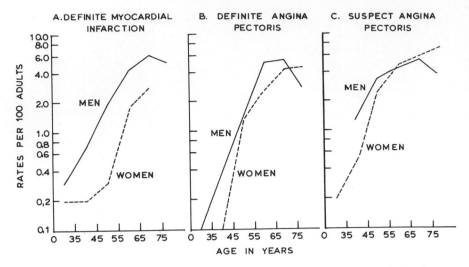

Figure 7–13. Age-specific prevalence rates of definite myocardial infarction, definite angina pectoris, and suspect angina pectoris by sex, National Health Examination Survey, United States, 1960–1962

Source: Gordon and Garst (15).

most consistently observed relationship is the markedly increased incidence of Mongolism with increasing maternal age (Fig. 7–12) (20). Biological reasons for this pattern have not been elucidated.

Sex

Differences in the prevalence of myocardial infarction, definite and suspect angina pectoris by sex are shown in Figure 7–13, which is based on data collected by the National Health Examination Survey during 1959–1962 from a nationwide sample of about 7000 adults, 18–79 years of age (15). Up to 75 years of age, the prevalence of these three forms of coronary disease increases with age for both sexes. Definite cases of myocardial infarction and angina pectoris are more prevalent among men than women at all ages, but the sex differential is less marked in angina. In contrast, suspect angina is more common in men until 55 years of age, after which it becomes more prevalent in women. The variation in sex pattern suggests that these components of coronary heart disease have different sets of etiological factors, or perhaps, that they are different diseases. It is also possible that the sexes differ in their exposure to whatever

Table 7-1. Prevalence of Definite and Suspect Heart Disease in White and Black Adults by Heart Disease Diagnosis: United States, 1960–1962

	Percent Prevalence	
Heart Disease Diagnosis	White	Black
*Definite Heart Disease**		
Hypertensive	8.2	20.8
Coronary	2.9	2.6
Rheumatic	1.1	1.7
Congenital	0.2	0.2
Syphilitic	0.1	0.7
Other†	0.3	0.2
Total	12.0	24.4
Suspect Heart Disease		
Hypertensive	3.9	4.9
Coronary	2.2	2.6
Other†	6.4	8.3
Total	11.3	14.8

* Percents for the specified heart diseases are not exclusive.
† Percents exclude persons with any of the specified heart diseases.

Source: Gordon (14).

etiological factors underlie the different components of the disease spectrum of coronary artery disease. In any epidemiologic study of coronary heart disease, the investigator must differentiate between these three manifestations and analyze them separately.

Color

Differences in the prevalence of various forms of heart disease by color were observed in the National Health Examination Survey (Table 7–1) (14). Clearly, hypertensive heart disease is markedly more prevalent among blacks. This is true for both definite and suspect hypertensive disease, and it confirms clinical impressions. The higher prevalence among blacks is a significant lead in a search for etiological factors in hypertension, although the difference has not been explained. It seems more likely to be the result of environmental rather than genetic factors. Definite coronary heart disease is more prevalent among whites than blacks, but suspect coronary disease is more prevalent among blacks, although only slightly more

Table 7–2. Age-specific Frequencies (per 1,000) of Cervical Cancer Found on First Examination among Amish and Non-Amish Women in Holmes County, Ohio, Compared to Other Studies

Age	Holmes County, Ohio		San Diego, California	Floyd County, Georgia	Memphis,* Tennessee	Washington County, Maryland
	Amish	Non-Amish				
<20	0.0	4.7	6.8	1.1	—	—
20–29	2.1	14.4	7.3	1.3	2.23	—
30–39	3.9	17.7	13.6	4.5	5.75	14.4
40–49	3.9	12.1	9.4	7.0	6.27	6.9†
50–59	0.0	12.5	11.8	5.3	3.84	—
60–69	0.0	0.0	14.1	13.6‡	7.42	—
70+	4.5	23.0	10.0	—	7.05	—
All ages	2.9	12.4	10.1	4.2	4.58	7.2

* Limited to clinically unsuspected cases and Caucasians.
† Limited to 40–45-year age group.
‡ Includes all women over 60 years old.

Source: Cross, Kennel, and Lilienfeld (8).

so. The higher prevalence of syphilitic heart disease among blacks would be expected since they have a higher frequency of syphilis.

Religion and Other Characteristics

Religion is a very interesting population characteristic because it is usually related to an individual's living habits or environmental exposures. Morbidity data for the Amish strongly suggest that they have a lower frequency of both *in situ* and invasive carcinoma of the cervix (Table 7–2) (8). These data were not obtained in a total population morbidity survey but were derived from an analysis of a cervical cancer screening program in a county where the population was composed of both Amish and non-Amish groups. Confirmation of the finding by mortality analyses and, perhaps, by a more systematic morbidity survey would be desirable. Still, it is an interesting finding because a low frequency of cancer of the cervix has been consistently observed among Jewish women and had been attributed to the practice of circumcision (34). The fact that the Amish do not practice circumcision casts doubt on this interpretation. The very strict sexual mores of the Amish suggest another explanation.

Religion was judged as a factor in disease in a study of ulcerative colitis conducted in Baltimore during 1960–1963 (23). This survey

Table 7–3.   Number and Annual Rates of Total and First Hospitalizations of Ulcerative Colitis Cases among Whites by Sex and Religion, Baltimore, Maryland, 1960–1963

Patients	Total Hospitalizations				First Hospitalizations (Definite Ulcerative Colitis)	
	Definite Ulcerative Colitis		Possible Ulcerative Colitis			
	Number	Rate	Number	Rate	Number	Rate
Males						
Jews	23	23.78	9	9.31	9	9.31
non-Jews	59	5.74	40	3.89	35	3.40
ratio						
Jews/Non-Jews		4.14		2.39		2.74
Females						
Jews	34	31.82	4	3.74	18	16.85
non-Jews	77	6.87	53	4.73	46	4.10
ratio						
Jews/Non-Jews		4.63		0.79		4.11

Source: Monk et al. (23). Copyright © 1967, Williams and Wilkins Co.

of all hospitalized cases in a community confirmed previous reports of an incidence of ulcerative colitis that was about two to four times higher among Jews than in the general population (Table 7–3). As part of the survey, efforts were made to determine whether certain social and demographic factors such as occupation, education, marital status, and birthplace (foreign, urban) could explain this difference (24). An attempt was also made to determine whether a variety of events that could be regarded as emotionally or psychologically disruptive might explain the higher frequency of ulcerative colitis among Jews. Such events included social and cultural discontinuities (e.g., differences between spouse's and patient's religion and education), geographic mobility, job changes, and stressful events occurring three to four months before the patient's hospitalization. None of these factors could account for the differences in disease incidence between Jews and non-Jews (25).

STUDY PROBLEMS

1. M. Clarke et al. compiled information from the register of reports of tuberculosis cases made to the Leicestershire Health

Authority in Great Britain, which included the name, sex, age, site of tuberculosis, and whether the patient was Asian or non-Asian. Ethnic group was essentially ascertained from the patients' surnames. When the disease was reported as being present in the respiratory system in addition to other sites, the case was classified as respiratory tuberculosis. The compiled data are presented in the following two tables:

Tuberculosis notification rate (per 100,000) by age, site of disease, and ethnic group in Leicestershire, 1975

	Asian				Non-Asian			
	Respiratory		Nonrespiratory		Respiratory		Nonrespiratory	
Age	Rate	No.	Rate	No.	Rate	No.	Rate	No.
0–4	42.1	2	42.1	2	–	0	–	0
5–14	106.0	10	74.2	7	–	0	0.8	1
15–24	633.0	51	198.6	16	9.5	11	–	0
25–34	486.3	34	300.4	21	4.1	4	4.1	4
35–44	508.0	27	413.9	22	8.8	8	–	0
45–64	650.3	28	534.1	23	7.2	13	4.4	8
65+	487.3	5	292.4	3	10.1	10	6.1	6
Total	393.7	157	238.2	95	6.0	46	2.5	19

Tuberculosis notification rate (per 100,000) by sex, site of disease, and ethnic group in Leicestershire, 1975

	Respiratory		Nonrespiratory		Total	
	Rate	No.	Rate	No.	Rate	No.
Male						
Asian	420.1	90	172.7	37	592.8	127
Non-Asian	7.4	28	1.6	6	9.0	34
Female						
Asian	363.1	67	314.3	58	677.4	125
Non-Asian	4.6	18	3.3	13	7.9	31
Total						
Asian	393.7	157	238.2	95	632.0	252
Non-Asian	6.0	46	2.5	19	8.5	65
Total	25.4	203	14.3	114	39.6	317

a) How do you interpret these findings?
b) Discuss any limitations in interpreting these data that you can think of.

c) What additional information, if any, would you desire to strengthen your interpretation of these data?

2. In 1930, as part of a program of epidemiologic studies of poliomyelitis, an index of immunity to poliomyelitis virus was developed in the form of a neutralization test, in which the virus was neutralized by blood serum. Such neutralization had been observed in (1) individuals who had passed through an attack of the disease, (2) monkeys surviving experimental poliomyelitis, and (3) immunized monkeys.

   The blood sera of 75 normal individuals, who gave no history of having had an attack of poliomyelitis and who either resided in a large city or had spent all their lives in a rural area, were collected and tested. The frequency of positive neutralization tests by age and urban-rural residence was compared with the results of previously published data on the results of Schick testing for diphtheria in urban and rural areas. (Note: Positive Schick test indicates susceptibility to diphtheria.) The comparison was made according to age and urban-rural residence.

Age	Percent with Negative Neutralization Test for Poliomyelitis		Percent with Positive Schick Test for Diphtheria	
	Rural	Urban	Rural	Urban
0–4*	100	59	100	63
5–9	100	20	80	30
10–14	75	34	75	27
15–19	50	16	65	25
20–64	60	12	72	20

* Does not include anyone under 6 months of age.

Disregarding possible issues conecrning sampling, including sample size, discuss the epidemiologic inferences that can be derived from these data. Take into account the urban-rural differences and age patterns as well as the comparison between the test results for poliomyelitis and diphtheria.

3. What are the major differences between the analysis of morbidity statistics and the analysis of mortality statistics?

4. In the United States National Health Interview Survey, information was obtained from a sample of households on whether or not anyone in the household had diabetes. Additional informa-

tion was also obtained regarding several aspects of diabetes, such as treatment and disability, for the periods July 1964–June 1965 and during 1973. The prevalence rate per 1,000 population obtained at these two times by age group and sex are shown in the following table.

Age (years)	1964–1965		Age (years)	1973	
	Male	Female		Male	Female
All ages	10.5	13.8	All ages	16.3	24.1
<25	1.2	1.3	<17	1.1	1.6
25–44	6.2	6.2	17–44	6.9	10.8
45–54	15.4	20.0 ⎱	45–64	40.6	44.4
55–64	32.0	41.4 ⎰			
65–74	47.1	60.6 ⎱	65+	60.3	91.3
75+	47.0	50.8 ⎰			

a) What inferences would you derive from these data?
b) Would you desire any additional information? If so, what?
c) List a few types of studies that are suggested by the data.

5. The Third National Cancer Survey was conducted in seven metropolitan areas and two entire states of the United States during the three year period 1969–71 to obtain information on the incidence of different forms of cancer according to a variety of population characteristics. For all areas combined, the following average annual age-specific incidence rates (per 100,000 population) for cancer of the esophagus as a primary site were observed for white and black males.

Age (years)	Whites	Blacks
35–39	0.3	1.8
40–44	0.7	8.8
45–49	2.6	22.6
50–54	6.0	40.3
55–59	12.2	59.5
60–64	18.4	59.0
65–69	22.6	66.1
70–74	24.1	108.2
75–79	34.2	57.7
80–84	37.6	46.7
85+	32.1	43.3

Discuss possible reasons for the difference in rates between the two groups.

6. On St. Lawrence Island, in the Bering Sea, an epidemic of mumps occurred in 1956. A survey demonstrated the following age-specific incidence rates, which were compared with those observed among families in Baltimore during an epidemic in 1959–60.

Age	Incidence rate per 100 exposed susceptibles	
	St. Lawrence Island	Baltimore
<1	17	12
1–4	56	60
5–9	86	54
10–19	82	18
20–49	68	19
50+	21	0

What are the reasons for the differences in age-specific incidence rates between these two areas?

7. In 1964, Cohen and colleagues reported the following staphylococcal postoperative wound infection rates for selected operations at the Johns Hopkins Hospital:

Operation	Number of		Percent Infected
	Infections	Operations	
Thyroidectomy	0	227	0.0
Herniorrhaphy	4	540	0.7
Appendectomy	3	348	0.9
Vein stripping	1	50	2.0
Laminectomy & other vertebral surgery	8	368	2.2
Cardiac surgery	5	209	2.4
Mastectomy	2	78	2.6
Intracranial neurosurgery	13	224	5.8
Amputations	8	136	5.9
Gastrectomy	8	126	6.3
Cholecystectomy	9	139	6.5
Lobotomy (segmental resection)	5	62	8.1
Radical neck dissection	5	43	11.6
Colectomy	7	24	29.2
Abdomino-perineal resection	8	18	44.4
All operations	143	8,952	1.6

a) What other information is necessary for the epidemiologic analysis of these data?

b) What types of surgical procedures have a higher percentage of postoperative staphylococcal infections? Why might they be at such high risk?

c) What do these data suggest about other types of postoperative infections? About infections, in general?

d) How might the conclusions from these data be applied to other hospitals? To similar studies in other hospitals?

REFERENCES

1. Booth, K., Burkitt, D.P., Bassett, D.J., Cooke, R.A., and Biddulph, J. 1967. "Burkitt lymphoma in Papua, New Guinea." *Brit. J. Cancer* 21:657–664.

2. Burkitt, D. 1958. "A sarcoma involving the jaws in African children." *Brit. J. Surg.* 46:218–223.

3. ———. 1961. "Observations on the geography of malignant lymphoma." *East Afr. Med. J.* 38:511–514.

4. ———. 1962. "A 'Tumour Safari' in East and Central Africa." *Brit. J. Cancer* 16:379–386.

5. ———. 1967. "Burkitt's lymphoma otuside the known endemic areas of Africa and New Guinea." *Int. J. Cancer* 2:562–565.

6. ———. 1969. "Etiology of Burkitt's lymphoma–an alternative hypothesis to a vectored virus." *J. Natl. Cancer Inst.* 42:19–28.

7. Center for Disease Control. 1974. *Reported Morbidity and Mortality in the United States 1973. Vol. 22, No. 53.* Washington, D.C.: United States Department of Health, Education and Welfare.

8. Cross, H.E., Kennel, E.F., and Lilienfeld, A.M. 1968. "Cancer of the cervix in the Amish population." *Cancer* 21:102–108.

9. Dalldorf, G., Linsell, C.A., Barnhart, F.E., and Martyn, R. 1964. "An epidemiologic approach to the lymphomas of African children and Burkitt's sarcoma of jaws." *Perspect. Biol. Med.* 7:435–449.

10. Ederer, F., Myers, M.H., and Mantel, N. 1964. "A statistical problem in space and time: Do leukemia cases come in clusters?" *Biometrics* 20:626–638.

11. Edwards, P.Q., and Palmer, C.E. 1957. "Prevalence of sensitivity to coccidioidin with special reference to specific and nonspecific reactions to coccidioidin and histoplasmin." *Dis. Chest* 31:35–60.

12. Epstein, M.A. 1978. "An assessment of the possible role of viruses in the aetiology of Burkitt's lymphoma." *Prog. Exp. Tumor Res.* 21:72–99.

13. ———, and Achong, B.G. 1970. "The fine structure of cultured Burkitt lymphoblasts of established in vitro strains." In *Burkitt's Lymphoma*, D.P. Burkitt and D.H. Wright, eds. Edinburgh and London: E. and S. Livingstone, pp. 118–133.

14. Gordon, T. 1964. *Heart Disease in Adults United States, 1960–1962*. National Center for Health Statistics, Department of Health, Education and Welfare, PHS Pub. No. 1000, Series 11, No. 10, Washington, D.C.: United States Government Printing Office.

15. ————, and Garst, C.C. 1965. *Coronary Heart Disease in Adults United States, 1960–1962*. National Center for Health Statistics, Department of Health, Education and Welfare, PHS Pub. No. 1000, Series 11, No. 10, Washington, D.C.: United States Government Printing Office.

16. Henle, W., Henle, G., and Lennette, E.T. 1979. "The Epstein-Barr virus." *Scientific American* 241:48–59.

17. Higginson, J., and Muir, C.S. 1973. Epidemiology. In *Cancer Medicine,* J.F. Holland and E. Frei, III, eds. Philadelphia: Lea and Febiger, pp. 241–306.

18. Kessler, I.I., and Lilienfeld, A.M. 1969. "Perspectives in the epidemiology of leukemia." *Adv. Cancer Res.* 12:225–302.

19. Knox, G. 1964. "Epidemiology of childhood leukemia in Northumberland and Durham." *Brit. J. Prev. Soc. Med.* 18:17–24.

20. Lilienfeld, A.M. 1969. *Epidemiology of Mongolism*. Baltimore: The Johns Hopkins Press.

21. Mantel, N. 1967. "The detection of disease clustering and a generalized regression approach." *Cancer Res.* 27:209–220.

22. Maxcy, K.F. 1926. "An epidemiological study of endemic typhus (Brill's disease) in the Southeastern United States with special reference to its mode of transmission." *Pub. Health Reps.* 41:2967–2995.

23. Monk, M., Mendeloff, A.I., Siegel, C.I., and Lilienfeld, A.M. 1967. "An epidemiological study of ulcerative colitis and regional enteritis among adults in Baltimore. I. Hospital incidence and prevalence, 1960 to 1963." *Gastroenterology* 53:198–210.

24. ————. 1969. "An epidemiological study of ulcerative colitis and regional enteritis among adults in Baltimore. II. Social and demographic factors." *Gastroenterology* 56:847–857.

25. ————. 1970. "An epidemiological study of ulcerative colitis and regional enteritis among adults in Baltimore. III. Psychological and possible stress-precipitating factors." *J. Chron. Dis.* 22:565–578.

26. Mustacchi, P., David, F.N., and Fix, E. 1967. "Three tests for space-time interaction: A comparative evaluation." In *Proceedings of the Fifth Berkeley Symposium on Mathematical Statistics and Probability,* Berkeley and Los Angeles: University of California Press, pp. 229–235.

27. Pike, M.C., Morrow, R.H., Kisuule, A., and Mafigiri, J. 1970. "Burkitt's lymphoma and sickle cell trait." *Brit. J. Prev. Soc. Med.* 24:39–41.

28. ————, and Smith, P.G. 1968. "Disease clustering: A generalization of Knox's approach to the detection of space-time interactions." *Biometrics* 24:541–556.

29. Roe, D.A. 1973. *A Plague of Corn: The Social History of Pellagra*. Ithaca: Cornell University Press.

30. Vianna, N.J., and Polan, A.K. 1973. "Epidemiologic evidence for transmission of Hodgkin's disease." *N. Engl. J. Med.* 289:499–502.

31. Wedderburn, N. 1970. "Effect of concurrent malarial infection on development of virus-induced lymphoma in balb/c mice." *Lancet* 2:1114–1116.

32. Werner, S.B., Pappagianis, D., Heindl, I., and Mickel, A. 1972. "An epidemic of coccidioidomycosis among archeology students in Northern California." *New Eng. J. Med.* 286:507–512.

33. Woodward, T.E. 1970. "President's address: Typhus verdict in American history." *Transactions Amer. Clin. Climatol. Assoc.* 82:7–8.
34. Wynder, E.L., Cornfield, J., Shroff, P.D., and Doraiswami, K.R. 1954. "A study of environmental factors in carcinoma of the cervix." *Amer. J. Obstet. Gynec.* 68:1016–1052.

8 Observational Studies: I. Retrospective and Cross-Sectional Studies

> Is your study to be retrospective or prospective?
> If the former, the replies will be general, vague,
> and I fear of little value.
>
> WILLIAM FARR, 1837

A. THE EPIDEMIOLOGIC STUDY

From the mortality and/or morbidity studies in a community or population group described in Chapters 4 to 7, the epidemiologist may observe a statistical association between a population characteristic and the occurrence of a disease. It should be recalled, though, that such associations may be subject to an "ecological fallacy," as noted in Chapter 1 (p. 14). Clinical and/or experimental observations may also suggest an association. The epidemiologist attempts to confirm such associations by conducting "epidemiologic studies," which determine whether these associations are also present in individuals with the characteristic(s) of interest as compared to those without it.

There are two types of epidemiologic studies: **experimental** and **observational** (Fig. 8–1). The major difference between these two is that in an experimental setting, the epidemiologist *can specify the conditions* under which the study is to be conducted, while in an observational setting, he is *not able* to control these conditions. In experiments, the epidemiologist controls the method of assigning subjects to either the exposed or nonexposed groups. A commonly used means of assignment is to *randomly* allocate similar individuals to the exposed or nonexposed group; such an experimental study is termed a "clinical trial" and is discussed in Chapter 10. Most of the other types of experiments are known as "community trials" and are further explored in Chapter 11. Clearly, if the epidemiolo-

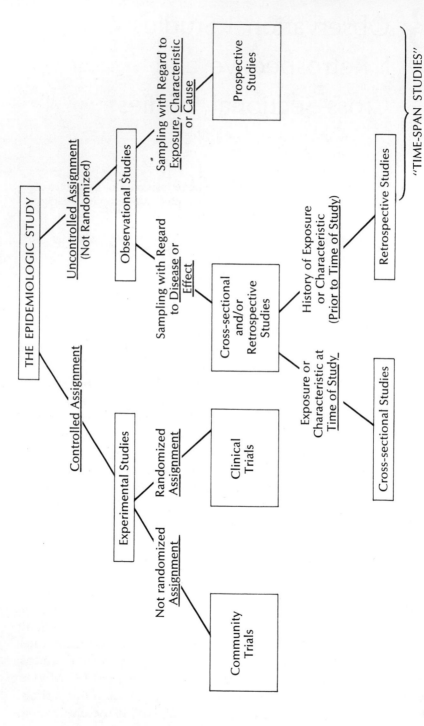

Figure 8–1. The Anatomy of the Epidemiologic Study.

gist is able to conduct either an experimental or an observational study, he would prefer experimental studies, as he could then control the conditions under which the study is carried out. Experiments are not, however, always feasible. For example, consider conducting an experiment on the effects of cigarette smoking; one would have to randomly assign persons to either a group that would be required to smoke, or one that would not be allowed to smoke, until the experiment was concluded.

Data collected in an observational study can be tabulated in the form of a fourfold table, as shown in Table 8–1. If two similar

Table 8–1. The Distinction between Retrospective and Prospective Studies

PROSPECTIVE STUDY →		RETROSPECTIVE STUDY ↓	
	Etiological Characteristic or Exposure	Diseased Group (cases)	Nondiseased Group (controls)
	Present (exposed)		
	Absent (not exposed)		

groups can be identified that differ only in whether or not they were *exposed* to a given environmental factor, e.g., use of oral contraceptives, or had a characteristic, e.g., a specific blood group, the study is a "prospective" one; such studies are further discussed in Chapter 9. In many situations, however, it is impractical for the epidemiologist to identify groups of individuals based upon their exposure histories or characteristics. He can more readily identify those individuals who have or do not have the *disease* of interest. From these individuals, he may obtain a history of their past exposure to the factor or characteristic of interest; such studies are "retrospective." If the characteristic and/or exposure of the two groups is limited to their current situations, the study is "cross-sectional." In actual practice, retrospective and cross-sectional studies are often used together because of their similarities. The remainder of this chapter will deal with these two types of studies.

Briefly, then, epidemiologic studies may be divided into experimental (e.g., clinical trials) and observational studies, the distinction being whether or not the epidemiologist has control over the assignment of individuals into the study groups. Observational studies can be divided into three categories: 1) prospective, 2) cross-sectional, and 3) retrospective; the former involves selection of individuals based upon exposure to an agent, while the latter two involve selection based upon the presence or absence of the disease. The distinction between cross-sectional and retrospective studies is that in the former, the exposure or characteristic is current, while in the latter, it had occurred at some time in the past.

B. RETROSPECTIVE AND CROSS-SECTIONAL STUDIES
General Description of Method

In cross-sectional and retrospective studies, comparisons are made between a group of persons who have the disease and a group that does not. Usually, those with the disease are called "cases" and those without the disease are called "controls." (For this reason, such studies are generally referred to as "case-control studies"; however, as will become clear after the discussion of prospective studies in Chapter 9, the term "case-control" can also be applied to prospective studies.) Cross-sectional studies have also been called "prevalence" studies, and retrospective studies called "case-history" studies.

Whether the characteristic or factor of interest is (or was) present in the two groups is usually determined by interview and/or a review of records. In both retrospective and cross-sectional studies, the proportion of cases exposed to the agent or possessing the characteristic (or factor) of etiological interest is compared to the corresponding proportion in the control group. If a higher frequency of individuals with the characteristic is found among the cases than the controls, an association between the disease and the characteristic may be inferred.

To illustrate the difference in inferences that can be derived from cross-sectional and retrospective studies, assume that one is interested in the relationship between cerebrovascular disease (stroke) and the level of serum cholesterol. A group of stroke cases and appropriate controls are selected, and blood is drawn to determine their serum cholesterol levels. If the levels are significantly higher among the cases than the controls, a statistical association is said to exist between stroke and elevated cholesterol levels. In this cross-sectional approach, however, one does not know whether the elevated serum cholesterol preceded the onset of the stroke or followed it. If the latter were true, obviously the elevated serum cholesterol could not be regarded as being etiologically important in the development of stroke. On the other hand, in a retrospective study, one would seek information on the level of serum cholesterol that was present before the onset of the stroke. If a statistical association is then established, a causal relationship can be inferred with greater confidence.

Since the difference between cross-sectional and restrospective studies depends upon the factor of time, a natural issue concerns the length of time that differentiates these two types of studies, i.e., should it be one month, one year, five years, etc. There is no general answer to this question, since it depends upon the nature and pathogenesis of the disease under investigation. In acute communicable diseases, the time period will be relatively short. In diseases where the pathogenesis is more prolonged, the time period would be longer. In many instances, particularly where knowledge of the pathogenesis and natural history is minimal, the differentiation between cross-sectional and retrospective studies is difficult and sometimes impossible to make. Although the remainder of this chapter will be expressed in terms of retrospective studies, the issues discussed also apply to cross-sectional studies.

This distinction between cross-sectional and retrospective studies is most important when the factor is a physiological or biochemical characteristic of the individual, as these are likely to have been influenced by the disease process itself. Of course, one cannot eliminate the possibility that the disease may have changed a person's environment after its onset. Therefore, the distinction between cross-sectional and retrospective studies must be kept in mind even when environmental factors are studied.

When interested in determining whether prior exposure to an environmental factor is etiologically important, the epidemiologist will attempt to obtain a history of such exposure by interviewing the cases and controls. In practice, information on both current *and* past characteristics is usually obtained. One must constantly be aware that the derivation of inferences depends upon the temporal sequence between the characteristic and the disease. In contrast to cross-sectional studies, retrospective studies should be regarded as "time-span studies."

The data for a retrospective study are generally tabulated in the form of a fourfold table, as shown in Table 8–2. If $\dfrac{a}{a+c}$ is statisti-

Table 8–2.   Framework of a Retrospective Study

| Characteristic | Number of Individuals | | Total |
	With Disease (cases)	Without Disease (controls)	
With	a	b	a + b
Without	c	d	c + d
Total	a + c	b + d	a + b + c + d = N

cally significantly different from $\dfrac{b}{b+d}$, a statistical association can be said to exist between the disease and the characteristic. The study by Mann et al. of the relationship between oral contraceptive use and myocardial infarction, initiated at the same time as the oral contraceptive–myocardial infarction study mentioned in Chapter 1, illustrates this (41). Cases were defined as married women under 45 years of age who were treated for myocardial infarction in two hospital regions in England and Wales during 1968–72. For each case, three controls from among other patients not being treated for a myocardial infarction in the same hospitals were ran-

Table 8–3. Number of Hospitalized Married Female Patients With and Without Myocardial Infarction Under 45 Years of Age By Oral Contraceptive Practice

| Oral Contraceptive Practice | Number of Patients | |
	With Myocardial Infarction	Without Myocardial Infarction
Used	23	34
Never used	35	132
Total	58	166

Source: Adapted from Mann et al. (42)

Table 8–4. Different Sources of Cases and Controls in Retrospective Studies

Cases	Controls
All cases diagnosed in the community (in hospitals, other medical facilities, including physicians' offices)	Sample* of the general population in a community
All cases diagnosed in a sample of the general population	Non-cases in a sample of the general population, or subgroup of a sample of general population
All cases diagnosed in all hospitals in community	Sample of patients in all hospitals in the community, who do not have the disease or related diseases being studied
All cases diagnosed in a single hospital	Sample of patients in same hospital where cases were selected
All cases diagnosed in one or more hospitals	Sample of individuals who are residents in same block or neighborhood of cases
Cases selected by any of the above methods	Spouses, siblings, or associates of cases; accident victims

* When the term "sample" is used, it means a probability sample.

domly selected. The data presented in Table 8–3 shows that the percentage of oral contraceptive users among the myocardial infarction cases is 40 percent $(\frac{23}{58})$, as compared to 20 percent $(\frac{34}{166})$ among the controls. A method for determining whether these different percentages are statistically significant can be found in Appendix 1 (p. 338).

The Selection of Cases and Controls

Various methods have been used to select cases and controls for retrospective studies (Table 8–4). Sometimes investigators select cases from one source and controls from a variety of sources, permitting comparisons with different control groups. Consistency of findings among different types of control groups as compared to the cases increases the validity of inferences that may be derived from the findings.

In developing guidelines for the selection of controls, any factors already known or strongly suspected to be related to the disease should be taken into account if unbiased data on the specific characteristics being studied are desired. If the samples of cases and controls are drawn at random from the populations of cases and controls, some of the extraneous factors may be equally distributed in the two groups, but others will not. The case and control groups, for instance, will usually differ in age, sex, and color, since many diseases differ in these factors.

To avoid any biases in comparing groups that might differ in their composition, various methods of selection and analysis are available (2, 5, 10, 16, 17, 49). Adjustment procedures similar to age-adjustment (see Chap. 4) can be useful in making group comparisons. It is also possible to make a series of specific comparisons for each level of the extraneous factor, i.e., for each age, sex, and color group (29, 30, 43). To ensure the equality of the distribution of cases and controls for each level of these extraneous factors (i.e., their comparability), one may "group match" the cases and controls by stratifying them for each factor level. For example, the cases can be stratified into different 10 year age groups, 25–34, 35–44, 45–54, etc. The control group can then be similarly stratified and samples of controls within each stratum can be randomly selected to provide the same number of controls as cases. Comparisons can then be made at each factor level between cases and controls by the usual statistical significance tests (9, 43).

As an alternative to group matching, individual cases and controls can be matched for various factors so that each case essentially has a pairmate. Ideally, these pairmates should be chosen to be alike on all factors except the particular characteristic under investigation. In practice, if many factors are chosen for matching, or if many levels are chosen for each factor, it becomes difficult to find matching controls for each of the cases. In epidemiologic studies, there are usually a small number of cases and a large number of controls to select (or sample) from. Each case is then classified by the extraneous characteristics that are not of primary interest, and a search is made for a control with the same set of characteristics. If the factors are not too numerous and there is a large reservoir of persons from which the controls can be chosen, case-control pair matching may be readily carried out. However, if several factors and/or levels are considered and there are not many more potential controls than cases, matching can be difficult. It is quite likely that for many cases, no control will be found; indeed, it may be necessary to either eliminate some of the factors from consideration or reduce the number of levels for some of them. With age matching, for example, it is unlikely that pairs can be formed using one year age intervals, but five- or ten-year age groups make matching feasible.

The number of factors or levels where matching is desirable and practical is actually rather small. It is usually sensible to match cases and controls only for factors, such as age and sex, whose association with the disease under study is already known or has been observed in available mortality statistics, morbidity surveys, or other sources (10, 45). In addition, when cases and controls are matched on any selected factor, the influence of that factor on the disease can no longer be studied. Hence, caution must be exercised in determining the number of variables or factors selected for matching, even when feasible. If the effect of a factor is in doubt, the preferable strategy is not to match but to adjust for these extraneous factors in the statistical analysis. While the logical absurdity of attempting to measure the effect of a factor when cases and controls are matched for it is obvious, it is surprising how often investigators must be restrained from attempting this. A more detailed discussion of these issues is presented in Appendix 1.

A method commonly used in conducting retrospective studies is to select the cases from one or more hospitals. The control groups usually consist of patients with other diseases admitted to the same hospital. This is a popular method for the initial studies that explore a suspected relationship because the data can generally be obtained quickly, easily, and inexpensively. But several assumptions and sources of bias must be considered in analyzing the findings from such studies.

SELECTION BIAS
Selection is one of the major methodological problems encountered when hospital patients are used in retrospective studies. W. A. Guy (see Chapter 2) was the first to suggest that a spurious association could be obtained between diseases or between a characteristic and a disease because of the different probabilities of admission to a hospital for those with the disease, without the disease, and with the characteristic of interest (27). This possibility was actually first demonstrated by Berkson (4).

The influence of these differences on the study group in the hospital can be illustrated with a hypothetical example.

Let:

   X = Etiological factor or characteristic
   A = Disease group designated as cases
   B = Disease group designated as controls

Assume that there is no real association between disease A and X in the general population, as indicated in Table 8–5; that is, the per-

Table 8–5.   Frequency of Characteristic X in Disease Groups A and B in the General Population

	Number of Individuals in Disease Groups	
Characteristic	A (cases)	B (controls)
With X	200	200
Without X	800	800
Total	1,000	1,000
Percent of total with X	20	20

centage of those with A who have X and the percentage of those with B who have X is equal. Assume also that there are different rates or probabilities of admission to the hospital for persons with X, A, and B, each of which acts independently, as follows: X = 50 percent; A = 10 percent; B = 70 percent. Now consider the actual numbers of people in these groups who are admitted to the hospital:

a) *For those with A and X:*
   10 percent of the 200 in this category are
   admitted because they have A   = 20
   50 percent of the remaining 180 in this
   category are admitted because they have X   = 90

                                                            Total admitted   = $\overline{110}$

b) *For those with A and without X:*
10 percent of the 800 in this category are
admitted because they have A   = 80
c) *For those with B and X:*
70 percent of the 200 in this category are
admitted because they have B   = 140
50 percent of the remaining 60 in this category
with B are admitted because they have X   = 30
Total admitted   = 170
d) *For those with B and without X:*
70 percent of the 800 in this category are
admitted because they have B   = 560

These numbers are then inserted into the four cells of Table 8–6, allowing a comparison of disease A (cases) and disease B (controls) with respect to those who do and do not have the characteristic in our hypothetically constructed hospital population. The result is that 58 percent of those with disease A have X as compared to 23

Table 8–6. An Hypothetical Hospital Population Based on Differential Rates of Hospital Admission

Characteristic	Number of Individuals in Disease Groups	
	A (cases)	B (controls)
With X	110	170
Without X	80	560
Total	190	730
Percent of total with X	$(\frac{110}{190}) = 58$	$(\frac{170}{730}) = 23$

percent of those with disease B. This indicates that an association exists between A and X, even though this association is not present in the general population, which is the source of the hospital population. This spurious association results from the different rates of admission to the hospital for people with the different diseases and X. However, spurious associations such as this will not arise if either (31):

1. X does not affect hospitalization, that is, no person is hospitalized simply because he has X; or
2. the rate of admission to the hospital for those persons with A is equal to those with B.

One can never be absolutely certain that the first condition is met in any given study. For example, if X represents eye color, it might be assumed that this would not influence the probability of hospitalization. It is possible, however, that persons with a particular eye color belong to an ethnic group whose members are mainly of a low social class, which, in turn, may influence the probability of their hospitalization. It should be clear that the likelihood of a spurious association is greater if the factor under investigation (i.e., X) is another disease. The second condition is, of course, the exception rather than the rule since persons with different diseases usually have different probabilities of hospitalization. In any event, one cannot assume that these differences do not exist unless it is demonstrated that there are no differences in the hospitalization rates for individuals regardless of the disease.

In hospital studies, the same factors that may produce a spurious association, also termed "Berksonian" or "selection" bias, can have the reverse effect. The differences in hospital admission rates may conceal an association in a study although one actually does exist in the population.

REPRESENTATIVENESS

A basic assumption underlying the analysis of retrospective studies is that the selected cases are representative of persons with the disease. This implies that all cases with the disease or a representative sample of them have been ascertained. This assumption might be correct if:

1. all patients with the disease received medical attention;
2. all medical facilities used by these patients are thoroughly canvassed; and
3. an effective system for ascertaining the cases is in operation.

In actual practice, these requirements may not be adequately satisfied. Not all patients seek medical attention, and studies are generally confined to the most convenient medical facility, the hospital.

That this is not sufficient can be seen from the experiences of several excellent registers of cancer cases in various countries of the world (57). For cancer cases registered during the early 1970s, the percentage of cases initially brought to the attention of the registers by reviewing the death certificates varied from 0 to 58 percent for different countries or regions of countries. These represent cases who had not received hospital care or were not reported.

A parallel assumption that requires careful examination is that the sample of individuals without the disease—the control or comparison group—is representative of the nondiseased population or that the prevalence of the characteristic under study is the same in the control group as in the general population. Investigators conducting retrospective studies are generally content to select a control group consisting of persons with some disease other than the one under study and to assume that the frequency of the characteristic in the control group is an unbiased estimate of its frequency in the nondiseased population.

An illustration that this can be a dangerous assumption is given by Pearl's study of the association between cancer and tuberculosis (46). In the first 7,500 autopsies performed at the Johns Hopkins Hospital, Pearl identified 816 individuals with a malignant tumor and 816 control patients who did not have a malignant tumor, matched at death by age, sex, color, and date of death. At autopsy, 16.3 percent of the control group showed active tuberculous lesions, while in the cancer group only 6.6 percent showed such lesions. A difference in the same direction and of the same magnitude persisted when the two groups were divided into white and nonwhite males and females, and the subgroups were analyzed separately. Numerous additional analyses of other subgroups confirmed the negative association, or as Pearl called it, "antagonism" between the diseases. The possibility that this negative association was causal was further investigated by animal experiments, with negative results. One may ask whether this negative association can be accepted as evidence that a population group with active tuberculous lesions will, at some point in time, subsequently have a lower risk of developing cancer than a group without the lesions (46, 58–60). If the control group of autopsied cases provides a biased estimate of the prevalence of active tuberculous lesions among all noncancerous individuals in the population, the answer may be negative.

A recent examination of Pearl's original records in the Department of Biostatistics of The Johns Hopkins University showed that the control group included a considerable number of individuals who had died from tuberculosis, and, therefore, would necessarily have had a higher prevalence of active tuberculous lesions than the population of living, noncancerous individuals. Had the same negative association been found using a control group that consisted of persons who had died of some specific disease other than malignancy and tuberculosis, it could not have been so readily attributed to a selection bias. Attempting to confirm Pearl's interpretation, Carlson and Bell selected as controls persons who had died from heart disease, and found the same prevalence of tuberculous lesions among them as in a cancer group (8). Pearl's findings, therefore, resulted not so much from the use of autopsies, but rather from using it in a way that provided a grossly biased estimate of the prevalence of tuberculous lesions in a living population. It illustrates the earlier statement that a spurious negative association can result from a biased selection of study groups.

Selection bias is not limited to the analysis of hospital patients. It may be present in any situation when persons with different diseases or characteristics in any type of population enter a study group at different rates or probabilities. For example, in studying an autopsy series from a specified hospital population where the autopsy rates differ for the diseases and characteristics being studied in the manner described, the inferred associations will be spurious or biased (40, 41, 54).

Selection biases, however, do not necessarily invalidate study findings. This issue should be resolved on its own merits for any particular investigation, and the following means are available to increase the likelihood that an observed association is real:

1. The strength of the association can be evaluated to see if it could result from the type of selection bias described above. In general, it can be shown numerically that only small degrees of association, resulting in relative risks (to be discussed later in this chapter) of about two or three, could result from selection bias. It would be difficult to explain a complete association of a disease and a characteristic as the result of such bias.

2. Depending on the disease and the personal characteristic (such as serum cholesterol level) or the possible etiological factor (such as cigarette smoking), it may be possible to classify the characteristic or factor into a gradient from low to high levels. If the degree of

Table 8–7. Average Amount of Tobacco* Smoked Daily over the Ten Years Preceding Onset of the Present Illness among Male Lung Cancer Patients and Matched Control Patients with Other Diseases

Disease Group	Total Number	Percent and Number† of Nonsmokers	Percent Smoking Daily Average of Cigarettes				
			<5	5–14	15–24	25–49	50+
Lung cancer patients	1,357	0.5 (7)	4.0 (55)	36.0 (489)	35.0 (475)	21.6 (293)	2.8 (38)
Control patients with other diseases	1,357	4.5 (61)	9.5 (129)	42.0 (570)	31.8 (431)	11.3 (154)	0.9 (12)

* Ounces of tobacco have been expressed as being equivalent to so many cigarettes.
† Parentheses contain number of cases.

Source: Doll and Hill (14).

association between the disease and the characteristic or factor increases with increasing levels of the characteristic or factor, it decreases the likelihood that the association is a result of selection bias. For selection bias to occur, it would be necessary to hypothesize the unlikely occurrence of a similar gradient of rates of entry into the study group or of hospitalization in a study of hospitalized patients for the characteristic and the disease. This can be illustrated with some data from the retrospective study of lung cancer and tobacco smoking conducted by Doll and Hill among patients in a number of hospitals in several English cities (14). Information was obtained on the smoking habits of both male and female lung cancer patients and control patients with other diseases. Table 8–7 presents the results of a comparison of male lung cancer patients and controls according to the average amount of tobacco smoked daily over a ten-year period preceding the onset of the illness. Not only is there a higher proportion of tobacco users (predominantly cigarette smokers) among the lung cancer patients than the controls, but the lung cancer patients tended to smoke more tobacco than the control patients. A gradient showing an increase in lung cancer with increased tobacco use is evident.

Another illustration is provided by Antunes and his colleagues, who examined the possible relationship between estrogen use and endometrial cancer (1). Their results are shown in Table 8–8. A

Table 8–8. Percent Distribution of Endometrial Cancer Cases and Controls According to Daily Estrogen Dose and Duration of Estrogen Use

Estrogen Use	Endometrial Cancer Cases		Controls	
	No.	Percent	No.	Percent
Dose (mg):				
None	274	83	390	96
<1	23	7	9	2
1–2	27	8	5	1
>2	6	2	2	1
Total	330	100	406	100
Duration of use (yr):				
None	274	81	390	95
<1	11	3	7	2
1–5	17	5	8	2
>5	36	11	3	1
Total	338	100	408	100

Source: Antunes et al. (1). Reprinted by permission from *The New England Journal of Medicine* (300:9–13, 1979).

distinct gradient of estrogen use and endometrial cancer is evident.

3. A precaution to avoid the influence of selection biases that can be built into studies within the limitations imposed by the study hypothesis is to draw controls from a variety of disease categories or admission diagnoses. These should be diseases that have different hospital admission rates. Should the frequency of the study characteristic be similar in each control group and differ from the case group, selection bias would not be a likely explanation.

The use of several different control groups protects against two other sources of error: a) mistaking an association (positive or negative) between a factor or characteristic and the disease from which the controls were drawn from one between the factor and the disease under investigation; and b) failure to detect a positive relationship because both the study and the control diseases are associated with the same suspected etiological factor. The latter situation is far from impossible. Both tuberculosis and bronchitis, for example, are associated with cigarette smoking and the use of patients with either disease as a control group in a study of the cigarette smoking–lung cancer relationship could result in misleading findings.

Table 8–9. Comparison between Smoking Habits of Male Patients Without Cancer of the Lung (Control Group) and of Those Interviewed in the Social Survey: London, 1951

Subject	Percent Nonsmokers	Most Recent Amount Smoked: Percent Smoking Cigarettes				Number Interviewed
		1–4	5–14	15–24	25+	
Patient with diseases other than lung cancer	7.0	4.2	43.3	32.1	13.4	1,390
General population sample (Social Survey)	12.1	7.0	44.2	28.1	8.5	199

Source: Doll and Hill (14).

4. Another method of evaluating the influence of selection is to compare hospital control groups with a sample of the general population. This was accomplished by Doll and Hill in their study of lung cancer and smoking (14). They obtained information on the smoking habits of a sample of the general population from a social survey that was conducted in Great Britain during 1951. The smoking habits of patients in their control group were compared with those of persons in the Social Survey who were residents of Greater London, after adjusting for the age differences between the two groups. Table 8–9 shows the distribution of smoking habits among males in these two groups. The smaller proportion of nonsmokers and the higher proportion of heavy smokers among the controls than in the general population may result from the fact that patients in the control group had diseases that were also related to smoking habits. Thus, the degree of relationship between smoking and lung cancer shown in Table 8–9 is actually underestimated by the use of hospital controls.

BIAS IN OBTAINING INFORMATION

Another bias that may distort the findings from retrospective studies develops from the interviewer's awareness of the identity of cases and controls. This knowledge may influence the structure of the questions and the interviewer's manner, which in turn may influence the response. Whenever possible, interviews should be conducted without prior knowledge of the identity of cases and controls, although administrative matters often prevent such "blind" interviews. In special circumstances, hospital patients may be interviewed by lay persons at the time of admission and information of epidemiologic interest is obtained before the patient is seen by a physician and a diagnosis is made establishing the identity of cases and controls. This requires a comprehensive, general-purpose interview routinely administered to all admissions, which could restrict the method to publicly supported institutions. Several epidemiologic studies have used the unique set of data from the Roswell Park Memorial Institute, where such a procedure is used (6, 7, 35–37, 50, 61). Comparing their results with those of studies that depend on more conventional sources of controls provides a means for evaluating possible interviewer bias and related issues.

Patients interviewed as diagnosed cases in studies occasionally have had their diagnoses changed later. If data obtained from the erroneously diagnosed group resemble that of the control rather than the case series, interviewer bias can be discounted (Table 8–10).

The association of a factor and a disease may often be restricted to a specific histologic type or other component of the disease spectrum, as determined by objective means. For example, the fact that squamous cell and undifferentiated pulmonary carcinoma is more positively related to smoking history than adenocarcinoma of the lung more firmly establishes the relationship. When such diagnostic details and their significance are unknown to the interviewer, another check on possible interviewer bias is provided.

The response on interview can also be directly validated by comparison with other records. This was recently shown in a study of the accuracy of recall of the history of contraceptive use. Retrospective studies of the relationship between oral contraceptive use and a variety of diseases assumed that women recalled their use of oral contraceptives with reasonable accuracy (11, 42, 52, 53). This assumption was tested by comparing oral contraceptive histories of seventy-five women attending family planning clinics with information available in the clinic records. It was found that the type of information obtained in the retrospective studies was likely to be remembered with reasonable accuracy (22). This finding has been confirmed by Stolley et al. (51).

Table 8–10.   The Smoking Habits of Patients in Different Disease Groups, 45–74 Years of Age, Standardized According to the Age Distribution of the Population of England and Wales as of June 30, 1950

Disease Group	Percentage of Nonsmokers	Percent Smoking Daily Average of Cigarettes				Number of Patients Interviewed
		<5	5–14	15–24	25+	
Males						
Cancer of lung	0.3	4.6	35.9	35.0	24.3	1,224
Patients incorrectly thought to have cancer of lung	5.3	9.9	35.5	37.8	11.4	202
Other respiratory diseases	1.9	9.9	38.3	38.7	11.2	301
Other cancers	4.6	9.4	47.2	26.0	12.8	473
Other diseases	5.6	9.0	44.8	26.9	13.7	875
Females						
Cancer of lung	40.6	13.7	22.0	9.5	14.2	90
Patients incorrectly thought to have cancer of lung	66.9	16.4	12.7	4.2	0.0	45
Other respiratory diseases	66.5	22.4	0.0	11.1	0.0	25
Other cancers	68.4	14.3	11.0	5.0	1.3	294
Other diseases	55.9	22.1	17.5	3.6	0.9	157

Source: Doll and Hill (14).

Methods of Measuring Association in Retrospective Studies

RELATIVE RISK

Several statistical methods have been developed for measuring the degree of association in epidemiologic studies (2, 17, 23, 24, 28, 43, 62). The usual measure of association between the characteristic and the disease in an observational study is the *relative risk* (RR) (12):

$$\text{Relative Risk} = \frac{\text{Incidence rate of disease in exposed group}}{\text{Incidence rate of disease in nonexposed group.}}$$

Although incidence rates are not determined in a retrospective study, the relative risk can be estimated by the cross product of the entries in Table 8–2, $\frac{ad}{bc}$ (see Appendix 1, p. 342), first used by Guy in 1843 (26). Two assumptions are necessary in making this estimate: a) the frequency of the disease in the population must be small, and b) the study cases should be representative of the cases in the population and the controls representative of the noncases in the population. This cross product estimate can be made with either actual numbers or percentages (12). Using the numerical data in Table 8–3 the relative risk would be estimated as follows:

$$\frac{ad}{bc} = \frac{23 \times 132}{35 \times 34} = \frac{3,036}{1,190} = 2.55$$

Another term for this cross product is the "odds ratio." The variances, standard errors, confidence limits, and significance tests for the relative risk can be computed by the fairly simple procedures presented in Appendix 1.

Relative Risk for Multiple Categories. As has been shown, inferences about the association between a disease and a factor are considerably strengthened if information is available to support a gradient of relationship between the degree of exposure (or "dose") to a characteristic and a disease. Relative risks can be computed for each dose of the characteristic or factor. The general approach is to treat the data as a series of 2 × 2 tables, comparing controls and cases at different levels of exposure, and then calculating the relative risk for each level. The data from Table 8–7 are presented in Table 8–11, together with the computed relative risks.

Table 8–11. Relative Risk for Smokers and Nonsmokers, Using Data from Table 8–7

Daily Average Cigarettes Smoked	Patients		Relative Risk of Different Categories of Smokers to Nonsmokers
	Lung Cancer	Controls	
0	7	61	1.0
1–4	55	129	3.7
5–14	489	570	7.5
15–24	475	431	9.6
25–49	293	154	16.6
50+	38	12	27.6

The different degrees or levels of cigarette smoking are to be compared with the nonsmokers and, therefore, the relative risk of lung cancer for nonsmokers is defined to be 1.0. The risks for smokers relative to nonsmokers are:

$$\text{RR (1–4 cigarettes daily)} = \frac{55 \times 61}{7 \times 129} = \frac{3,355}{903} = 3.7$$

$$\text{RR (5–14 cigarettes daily)} = \frac{489 \times 61}{7 \times 570} = \frac{29,829}{3,990} = 7.5$$

$$\text{RR (15–24 cigarettes daily)} = \frac{475 \times 61}{7 \times 431} = \frac{28,975}{3,017} = 9.6$$

A significance test for these relative risks as a group was developed by Cochran and a method for calculating a summary relative risk for all the categories was developed by Mantel and Haenszel (9, 43). If several studies of the same epidemiologic problem have been carried out at different times and in different places it may be useful to combine the estimates and then determine whether they are homogeneous; methods for such calculations are available (9, 13, 18–20, 43, 44, 47, 48).

Matched Cases and Controls. When cases and controls are matched in pairs in order to make the two groups comparable with regard to one or more factors, the fourfold (2 × 2) table takes a form different from that shown in Table 8–2. The status of the cases with regard to the presence or absence of the characteristic is compared with its presence or absence in their respective controls (Table 8–12). The cell in the upper left-hand corner of Table 8–12 contains r number of pairs in which both cases and controls possess the characteristic of interest. The marginal totals (a, b, c, d) represent the entries in the cells of Table 8–12 and the total for the entire table is $\frac{1}{2}N$ pairs where N represents the total number of paired

Table 8–12. Symbolic Representation of Matched Cases and Controls with and without a Characteristic

Cases	Controls With Characteristic	Controls Without Characteristic	Total
With characteristic	r	s	a*
Without characteristic	t	u	c*
Total	b*	d*	$\frac{1}{2}N$

* a, b, c, and d are the entries in the cells of Table 8–2.

individuals. The calculation of the relative risk for this table is simple (32):

$$RR = \frac{s}{t} \text{(provided } t \neq 0\text{)}$$

Both a test of significance and a method of calculating the standard error is presented in Appendix 1 (p. 352).

Interrelationships Between Risk Factors. Relative risks can also be used to determine whether interrelationships exist between various factors of characteristics. A study of leukemia in children who were exposed to multiple risk factors provides an example of this (21, 25). In different areas in three states containing a population of approximately 13,000,000, the mothers of all children diagnosed as having leukemia from 1959 to 1962 were interviewed. Within these areas, a sample was selected from a census of households with a sampling fraction of approximately 1 in 3000 persons. This sample provided approximately 3 child controls for each case of childhood leukemia. Interviews were completed on 319 children with leukemia and 884 child controls.

The four factors studied included:

1. Irradiation of the mother before conception of the subject.
2. Reproductive wastage—mother's history of miscarriages and stillbirths before conception of the subject.
3. In utero irradiation of the mother while she was pregnant.
4. History of childhood virus diseases, such as measles, rubella, chickenpox, mumps, poliomyelitis, herpes zoster, encephalitis, and infectious mononucleosis, which were contracted by the subject in the period prior to one year before the diagnosis of leukemia.

The analysis suggested that each of these four factors was related to the development of leukemia in children. The data were further analyzed as combinations of risk factors, with reproductive wastage and preconceptional radiation considered as preconceptional factors and in utero radiation and history of childhood virus diseases as postconceptional factors (21, 38). The results are presented in Table 8–13, where the relative risk in the absence of any factor is

Table 8–13.   Estimated Relative Risks for Leukemia in Children 1–4 Years of Age, Depending on a Combination of Factors Arranged by Sequence of Occurrence

Number of Preconceptional Factors	Number of Postconceptional Factors		
	None	1	2
None	1.0	1.1	1.8
1	1.2	1.6	2.7*
2	1.9	3.1*	4.6*

* Significant at 0.05 level.

Source: Lilienfeld (38).

taken to be 1.0. From these data, it appears that the relative risk increases with an increase in the number of factors. When the four factors are combined the relative risk rises sharply. This suggests that these factors are synergistic in their effect.

Effect of Misclassification. There are two areas in which misclassification of individuals in the study groups can occur. The first is that in which erroneous diagnoses may result in having the cases misclassified as controls or having the controls misclassified as cases, or including within the controls those persons with a subclinical component of the spectrum of disease. In any of these occurrences, the calculated relative risk would underestimate the true biological situation because of a dilution effect. The other misclassification area concerns errors in determining the exposure factor or the etiological characteristic of interest. In this situation, the computed relative risk may either be higher or lower than the true relative risk, depending upon the direction and extent of misclassification (3, 17). In such cases, relative risks greater than two or three, however, are probably not spurious, although they may be overestimated.

These effects of misclassification emphasize the need for the epidemiologist to verify the information obtained in a study by every means at his disposal. Information with respect to previous exposures or characteristics of study individuals may be verified by obtaining records from another independent source, such as hospitals, physicians, schools, military services, industries, on either all or a

Table 8–14. Hypothetical Data for Annual Incidence Rates and Relative Risks* of Slipped Discs in Population A with 25 Percent Frequent Automobile Drivers and Population B with 90 Percent Frequent Automobile Drivers

	Number of Persons			Annual Incidence Rate of Slipped Discs (Percent)
Characteristic	With Slipped Discs	Rest of Population	Total	
Population A				
Frequent automobile drivers†	75	2,425	2,500	3
Infrequent automobile drivers	75	7,425	7,500	1
Total	150	9,850	10,000	
Population B				
Frequent automobile drivers	270	8,730	9,000	3
Infrequent automobile drivers	10	990	1,000	1
Total	280	9,720	10,000	

* Relative Risk for Populations A and B $= \dfrac{\text{Incidence Rate Among Frequent Drivers}}{\text{Incidence Rate Among Infrequent Drivers}} = \dfrac{3}{1} = 3.0$

† Frequent = driving an automobile more than 20,000 km annually.

sample of individuals in the study. Disease diagnoses should be verified whenever possible by independent review of medical records, histological slides, electrocardiograms, etc. The degree of verification possible depends upon the factors and the diseases being studied. For example, verification of alcohol consumption or of the content of an individual's diet over a period of time poses some problems.

An example of misclassification and its possible effects on a retrospective study is provided by Lilienfeld and Graham, who were examining the relationship between cancer of the cervix and circumcision (39). They found that at the Roswell Park Memorial Institute, 33 percent of the males interviewed could not state correctly whether or not they were circumcised as compared to physicians' examinations. This finding was later confirmed by both

Table 8–15. Hypothetical Data from Retrospective Studies of a Relationship Between Frequent Automobile Driving and Slipped Discs Conducted in Populations A and B

	Number of Persons	
Characteristic	Cases	Probability Sample Controls
	Population A	
Frequent automobile drivers*	75	243
Infrequent automobile drivers	75	743
Total	150	986
	Population B	
Frequent automobile drivers	270	873
Infrequent automobile drivers	10	99
Total	280	972

* Frequent = driving an automobile more than 20,000 km annually.

Wynder et al. in New York City and Dunn et al. in California (15, 63).

Relative Risk Versus Absolute Differences. The use of relative risks to indicate associations rather than absolute differences between the percent of cases and controls with the factor or characteristic under study has one major advantage, which is illustrated with hypothetical data. Assume that populations A and B, each of 10,000 persons, have a proportion of persons who annually drive an automobile more than 20,000 km of 25 and 90 percent, respectively (Table 8–14). Also, assume that the annual incidence rate of lumbar disc herniation ("slipped disc") in each population among persons driving more than 20,000 km yearly is 3 percent in contrast to 1 percent for those driving less than 20,000 km, resulting in a relative risk of three. In each population, a retrospective study is carried out in which all cases of "slipped discs" are ascertained and a 10 percent sample of the population without this condition is selected to determine if an association exists between excessive driving and herniated lumbar discs. The findings for each population are presented in Table 8–15. From these data, absolute differences in the percentage of individuals driving more than 20,000 km yearly in the

Table 8–16. Absolute Difference in Percent of Frequent Drivers Among Cases and Controls in Hypothetical Retrospective Studies of Populations A and B

	Percentage	Estimated Relative Risk
	Population A	
Percent frequent drivers* in patients with slipped discs	$\frac{75}{150} = 50$	
Percent frequent drivers in controls	$\frac{243}{986} = 25$	$\frac{75 \times 743}{75 \times 243} = 3.06$
Differences in percent = 25		
	Population B	
Percent frequent drivers in patients with slipped discs	$\frac{270}{280} = 96$	
Percent frequent drivers in controls	$\frac{873}{972} = 90$	$\frac{270 \times 99}{10 \times 873} = 3.06$
Difference in percent = 6		

* Frequent = driving an automobile more than 20,000 km annually.

disease and control groups are computed and compared with the relative risks. The results are summarized in Table 8–16.

The estimated relative risks are the same in populations A and B and are similar to the relative risks based on the incidence rates in the populations (Table 8–14), but the absolute differences in the percentage of persons driving more than 20,000 km yearly among cases and controls differ markedly in the two populations. The reason for this discrepancy is that the absolute difference varies according to the frequency of the characteristic in a particular population, while estimates of relative risk are not influenced in this manner. In an attempt to infer a biological relationship between a disease and a population characteristic from a statistical association, it would be undesirable to have the measure of association influenced by the frequency of the characteristic in the population. This is particularly true for population groups since they usually differ in the frequency of a characteristic or their exposure to a particular agent.

ATTRIBUTABLE RISK

Another measure of association, influenced by the frequency of a characteristic in the population, is the *attributable risk*. Levin originally defined it in terms of lung cancer and smoking as the "maximum proportion of lung cancer attributable to cigarette smoking" (33, 34). More generally, it is the maximum proportion of a disease that can be attributed to a characteristic or etiological factor; alternatively, it is considered the proportional decrease in the incidence of a disease if the entire population were no longer exposed to the suspected etiological agent.

It is expressed as:

$$\text{Attributable Risk (AR)} = \frac{b\,(r-1)}{b\,(r-1)+1} \times 100$$

where r = the relative risk and b = proportion of the total population classified as having the characteristic; the derivation of this formula can be found in Appendix 1. Standard errors and confidence limits have been derived for the attributable risk by Walter (see Appendix 1, p. 347) (55, 56).

The effect of various values of the relative risk (r) and various proportions of those with a characteristic in the population (b) on the values of the attributable risk are shown in Table 8–17. When the freqeuncy of a characteristic in a population is low and the rela-

Table 8–17. Attributable Risks as a Proportion for Selected Values of Relative Risk and Proportion of Population with the Characteristic*

b = Proportion of Population with Characteristic (percent)	r = Relative Risk			
	2	4	10	12
10	.09	.23	.47	.52
30	.23	.47	.73	.77
50	.33	.60	.82	.84
70	.41	.67	.86	.89
90	.47	.73	.89	.91
95	.49	.74	.90	.92

* Attributable risk $= \dfrac{b(r-1)}{b(r-1)+1}$.

tive risk for that characteristic in a given disease is also low, only a small proportion of the cases of disease can be attributed to that characteristic. However, with a high relative risk and a high proportion of the population having the characteristic, a much larger percentage of cases can be attributed to it. Of course, it is assumed that other etiological factors are equally distributed among those with and without the characteristic.

The measurement of attributable risk becomes particularly noteworthy when a characteristic or factor has already been inferred to be etiologically important (see Chap. 12). The attributable risk is also useful in planning disease control programs. It enables health administrators to estimate the extent to which a particular disease is due to a specific factor and to predict the effectiveness of a control program in reducing the disease by eliminating exposure to the factor.

Computations of attributable risk are also helpful in developing strategies for epidemiologic research, particularly if there are multiple etiological factors (55). For example, in the United States, it is estimated that in certain age groups, 80–85 percent of lung cancer can be attributed to cigarette smoking. Other etiological factors apparently play a relatively minor role and, therefore, the investigator interested in ascertaining these factors may decide to limit his studies to nonsmoking lung cancer patients. In general, if close to 100 percent of a disease is attributable to one or more factors, a search for additional etiological agents may not be profitable unless one is interested in studying other characteristics that influence those already exposed to a high-risk factor.

STUDY PROBLEMS

1. What is a "Berksonian Bias"? Why is it important to the epidemiologist?
2. Many hypotheses concerning the etiology of gastric cancer involve the consumption of food. Usually, a retrospective study is conducted in which the type and amount of food consumed by gastric cancer cases and their corresponding controls is obtained by interview and compared. Discuss possible problems in the design of these studies.
3. Assume that John Snow (see Chap. 2, p. 36) was unable to conduct a "natural experiment." Describe the design of a retrospective study that would yield the same information.

4. Under what conditions would the epidemiologist conduct
   a) An experiment?
   b) A prospective study?
   c) A cross-sectional study?
   d) A retrospective study?
5. It has often been stated that the Standardized Mortality Ratio (SMR) and the Relative Risk are equivalent. Are they? Why might such a statement be made?
6. During the mid-1970s, three reports appeared in the literature indicating that an association existed between exogenous estrogen use and endometrial cancer. However, the following specific objections were raised about the design of these studies:
   a) The association may be spurious owing to the increased diagnostic surveillance that women on estrogens are assumed to receive.
   b) As estrogen use can produce endometrial hyperplasia, it is supposed that women with endometrial hyperplasia are classified as having endometrial cancer; hence, the association is spurious.
   c) It is possible that the early symptoms of the tumor were being treated by the estrogens.
   In attempting to evaluate the hypothesized association between estrogen use and endometrial cancer, Antunes et al. (25) conducted a study, the results of which were presented in part in Table 8–8. There were two control groups, both chosen from hospital services: one from the gynecology service and the other from services other than gynecology, obstetrics, and psychiatry services.
   a) Why would two distinct control groups be selected?
   b) Why were the patients from gynecology, obstetrics, and psychiatry services excluded from the second control group?
   c) Why was one control group selected from patients in the gynecology service? (*Hint:* What bias does the choice of this control group attempt to avoid?)
   d) The overall results for the study were that the relative risk using the nongynecology controls was 6.0 and that for the gynecology controls was 2.1. How would you interpret these results, recalling the objections listed above?
7. In Table 8–8, data on the relationship of estrogen use and endometrial cancer are presented. (a) Calculate the relative risks for each category. Are they statistically significant? (b) Compute

the percentage of women with endometrial cancer that would be attributed to the use of exogenous estrogens.

8. What routinely obtained data could be analyzed to determine if they are consistent with the findings reported by Antunes et al.?

9. How useful is the attributable risk to the epidemiologist?

10. In the 1950s, retrospective studies were carried out regarding the relationship between a history of prior tonsillectomy and poliomyelitis. In one such study, Paffenbarger compared the history of prior tonsillectomy among all reported cases of poliomyelitis in Olmsted County and neighboring counties with that of the adult members of a random sample of 588 households who were surveyed in the same area; these data are presented in the following table. All tonsillectomies reported in these groups had been performed two months or more before the onset of disease or an equivalent point of reference.

Age	Number of Poliomyelitis Cases		Number in Survey Population	
	With Tonsillectomy	Without Tonsillectomy	With Tonsillectomy	Without Tonsillectomy
0–4	2	65	3	233
5–9	12	41	34	203
10–19	18	17	130	234
20–29	20	17	154	184
30+	14	19	421	588
Total	$\overline{66}$	$\overline{159}$	$\overline{742}$	$\overline{1,442}$

a) Determine whether the frequency of history of prior tonsillectomy differs significantly between poliomyelitis cases and the survey population. (*Hint:* See Appendix 1.)

b) Compute relative risks for each age group.

c) Is there a relationship between a history of prior tonsillectomy and poliomyelitis?

11. Between 1969 and 1971 the Collaborative Group for the Study of Stroke in Young Women conducted a retrospective study in 12 university hospitals of cerebrovascular disease in 598 non-

pregnant women 14 to 44 years of age, with matched (age, sex, and race) hospital and neighborhood control groups, studying the relationship between cerebral ischemia (stroke) and oral contraceptive use. The results were:

Oral Contraceptive Use by Matched Controls	Oral Contraceptive Use by Cases With								
	Thrombotic Stroke			Hemorrhagic Stroke			Other Types of Stroke		
	No	Yes	Total	No	Yes	Total	No	Yes	Total
Hospital controls:									
No	50	38	88	95	26	121	44	9	53
Yes	4	6	10	13	7	20	8	3	11
Total	54	44	98	108	33	141	52	12	64
Neighborhood controls:									
No	55	44	99	107	30	137	35	16	51
Yes	5	2	7	13	5	18	16	4	20
Total	60	46	106	120	35	155	51	20	71

a) Why should two types of control groups be used?
b) Calculate the relative risk for each fourfold table. What can you say about oral contraceptive use and stroke?

Later, the following analysis of the data was performed as if the case and control groups were not matched:

Oral Contraceptive Use	Thrombotic Stroke			Hemorrhagic Stroke		
		Controls			Controls	
	Cases	Hospital	Neighbor-hood	Cases	Hospital	Neighbor-hood
User	59	53	69	44	53	69
Nonuser	81	340	382	152	340	382
Total	140	393	451	196	393	451

c) Why do the cell-frequencies in the unmatched analysis not equal the margin totals in the matched analysis?

d) Calculate the relative risk for each fourfold table. What can you say about oral contraceptive use and stroke? What can you say about the effect of matching on estimating the relative risk? Why?

12. An investigator suspects that a certain pharmaceutical P causes disease D. He is told by a physician that she has records of users of P (for whom she prescribed it) dating back 30 years. The physician also has records of patients for whom she considered prescribing P, but did not. She also has addresses of all these patients, which were provided to the investigator. At the same time, the physician agrees to provide the investigator with the names and addresses of everyone for whom she presently prescribes P and those for whom she considered prescribing P in the past 5 years, but did not. The physician is in charge of a hospital as well, and agrees to identify cases of D that were diagnosed during the past two years. Another physician has agreed to give an inert substance to every other hospitalized patient for whom he was going to prescribe P. If you are the investigator, identify the various types of studies that could be conducted.

REFERENCES

1. Antunes, C.M.F., Stolley, P.D., Rosenshein, N.B., Davies, J.L., Tonascia, J.A., Brown, C., Burnette, L., Rutledge, A., Pokempner, M., and Garcia, R. 1979. "Endometrial cancer and estrogen use." *New Engl. J. Med.* 300:9–13.
2. Armitage, P. 1971. *Statistical Methods in Medical Research.* New York: John Wiley and Sons.
3. Barron, B.A. 1977. "The effects of misclassification on the estimation of relative risk." *Biometrics* 33:414–418.
4. Berkson, J. 1946. "Limitations of the application of fourfold table analysis to hospital data." *Biometrics* 2:47–53.
5. Bross, I.D.J. 1966. "Spurious effects from an extraneous variable." *J. Chron. Dis.* 19:637–647.
6. ———. 1968. "Effect of filter cigarettes on the risk of lung cancer." *Natl. Cancer Inst. Monogr.* 28:35–40.
7. ———, and Tidings, J. 1973. "Another look at coffee drinking and cancer of the urinary bladder." *Prev. Med.* 2:445–451.
8. Carlson, H.A., and Bell, E.T. 1929. "Statistical study of occurrence of cancer and tuberculosis in 11,195 post-mortem examinations." *J. Cancer Res.* 13:126–135.
9. Cochran, W.G. 1954. "Some methods of strengthening the common χ^2 tests." *Biometrics* 10:417–451.
10. ———. 1965. "The planning of observational studies of human populations." *J. Roy. Stat. Soc., Series A.* 128:234–265.

11. Collaborative Group for the Study of Stroke in Young Women. 1973. "Oral contraception and increased risk of cerebral ischemia or thrombosis." *N. Engl. J. Med.* 288:871–878.
12. Cornfield, J. 1951. "A method of estimating comparative rates from clinical data. Applications to cancer of the lung, breast and cervix." *J. Natl. Cancer Inst.* 11:1269–1275.
13. ———. 1956. "A statistical problem arising from retrospective studies." *Proc. Third Berkeley Symp. Math. Stat. Prob.* 4:135–148.
14. Doll, R., and Hill, A.B. 1952. "A study of the aetiology of carcinoma of the lung." *Brit. Med. J.* 2:1271–1286.
15. Dunn, J.E., Jr., and Buell, P. 1959. "Association of cervical cancer with circumcision of sexual partner." *J. Natl. Cancer Inst.* 22:749–764.
16. Fisher, L., and Patil, K. 1974. "Matching and unrelatedness." *Amer. J. Epid.* 100:347–349.
17. Fleiss, J.L. 1973. *Statistical Methods for Rates and Proportions.* New York: John Wiley and Sons.
18. Gart, J.J. 1972. "On the combination of relative risks." *Biometrics* 18:601–610.
19. ———. 1970. "Point and interval estimation of the common odds ratio in the combination of 2 × 2 tables with fixed marginals." *Biometrika* 57:471–475.
20. ———. 1971. "The comparison of proportions: A review of significance tests, confidence intervals, and adjustments for stratification." *Rev. Internat. Statist. Institute* 39:148–169.
21. Gibson, R.W., Bross, I.D.J., Graham, S., Lilienfeld, A.M., Schuman, L.M., Levin, M.L., and Dowd, J.E. 1968. "Leukemia in children exposed to multiple risk factors." *N. Engl. J. Med.* 279:906–909.
22. Glass, R., Johnson, B., and Vessey, M. 1974. "Accuracy of recall of histories of oral contraceptive use." *Brit. J. Prev. Soc. Med.* 28:273–275.
23. Goodman, L.A., and Kruskal, W.H. 1954. "Measures of association for cross classifications." *J. Amer. Stat. Assoc.* 49:732–764.
24. ———, and ———. 1959. "Measures of association for cross classifications. II. Further discussion and references." *J. Amer. Stat. Assoc.* 54:123–163.
25. Graham, S., Levin, M.L., Lilienfeld, A.M., Dowd, J.E., Schuman, L.M., Gibson, R., Hempelmann, L.H., and Gerhardt, P. 1963. "Methodological problems and design of the Tristate Leukemia Survey." *Ann. New York Acad. Sci.* 107:557–569.
26. Guy, W.A. 1843. "Contributions to a knowledge of the influence of employments upon health." *J. Roy. Stat. Soc.* 6:197–211.
27. ———. 1856. "On the nature and extent of the benefits conferred by hospitals on the working classes and the poor." *J. Roy. Stat. Soc.* 19:12–27.
28. Haldane, J.B.S. 1956. "The estimation and significance of the logarithm of a ratio of frequencies." *Ann. Hum. Genet.* 20:309–311.
29. Kalton, G. 1968. "Standardization: A technique to control for extraneous variables." *Appl. Statistics* 17:118–136.
30. Kitagawa, E.M. 1964. "Standardized comparisons in population research." *Demography* 1:296–315.
31. Kraus, A.S. 1954. "The use of hospital data in studying the association between a characteristic and a disease." *Pub. Health Reps.* 69:1211–1214.
32. ———. 1958. *The Use of Family Members as Controls in the Study of the Possible Etiologic Factors of a Disease.* Sc.D. Thesis, Graduate School of Public Health, University of Pittsburgh.

33. Levin, M.L. 1953. "The occurrence of lung cancer in man." *Acta Unio. Internat. Contra Cancrum* 9:531–541.

34. ———, and Bertell, R. 1978. Re: "Simple estimation of population attributable risk from case-control studies." *Amer. J. Epid.* 108:78–79.

35. ———, Goldstein, H., and Gerhardt, P.R. 1950. "Cancer and tobacco smoking: A preliminary report." *JAMA* 143:336–338.

36. ———, Kraus, A.S., Goldberg, I.D., and Gerhardt, P.R. 1955. "Problems in the study of occupation and smoking in relation to lung cancer." *Cancer* 8:932–936.

37. Lilienfeld, A.M. 1956. "The relationship of cancer of the female breast to artificial menopause and marital status." *Cancer* 9:927–934.

38. ———. 1973. "Epidemiology of infectious and non-infectious disease: Some comparisons." *Amer. J. Epid.* 97:135–147.

39. ———, and Graham, S. 1958. "Validity of determining circumcision status by questionnaire as related to epidemiological studies of cancer of the cervix." *J. Natl. Cancer Inst.* 21:713–720.

40. McMahan, C.A. 1962. "Age-sex distribution of selected groups of human autopsied cases." *Arch. Path.* 73:40–47.

41. Mainland, D. 1953. "Risk of fallacious conclusions from autopsy data on incidence of diseases with applications to heart disease." *Amer. Heart J.* 45:644–654.

42. Mann, J.I., Vessey, M.P., Thorogood, M., and Doll, R. 1975. "Myocardial infarction in young women with special reference to oral contraceptive practice." *Brit. Med. J.* 2:241–245.

43. Mantel, N., and Haenszel, W. 1959. "Statistical aspects of the analysis of data from retrospective studies of disease." *J. Natl. Cancer Inst.* 22:719–748.

44. McKinlay, S.M. 1975. "The design and analysis of the observational study —a review." *J. Amer. Stat. Assoc.* 70:503–523.

45. ———. 1977. "Pair matching—A reappraisal of a popular technique." *Biometrics* 33:725–735.

46. Pearl, R. 1929. "Cancer and tuberculosis." *Amer. J. Hyg.* 9:97–159.

47. Sheehe, P.R. 1966. "Combination of log relative risk in retrospective studies of disease." *Amer. J. Pub. Health* 56:1745–1750.

48. Seigel, D.G., and Greenhouse, S.W. 1973. "Validity in estimating relative risk in case-control studies." *J. Chron. Dis.* 26:219–225.

49. Snedecor, G.W., and Cochran, W.G. 1967. *Statistical Methods.* 6th ed., Ames, Iowa: The Iowa State University Press.

50. Solomon, H.A., Priore, R.L., and Bross, I.D.J. 1968. "Cigarette smoking and periodontal disease." *J. Amer. Dent. Assoc.* 77:1081–1084.

51. Stolley, P.D., Tonascia, J.A., Sartwell, P.E., Tockman, M.S., Tonascia, S., Rutledge, A., and Schinnar, R. 1978. "Agreement rates between oral contraceptive users and prescribers in relation to drug use histories." *Amer. J. Epid.* 107:226–235.

52. Thomas, D.B. 1972. "Relationship of oral contraceptives to cervical carcinogenesis." *Obstet. Gynec.* 40:508–518.

53. Vessey, M.P., and Doll, R. 1968. "Investigation of relation between use of oral contraceptives and thromboembolic disease." *Brit. Med. J.* 2:199–205.

54. Waife, S.O., Lucchesi, P.F., and Sigmond, B. 1952. "Significance of mortality statistics in medical research: Analysis of 1,000 deaths at Philadelphia General Hospital." *Ann. Intern. Med.* 37:332–337.

55. Walter, S.D. 1975. "The distribution of Levin's measure of attributable risk." *Biometrika* 62:371–374.

56. ———. 1978. "Calculation of attributable risk from epidemiological data." *Int. J. Epid.* 7:175–182.

57. Waterhouse, J., Muir, C., Correa, P., and Powell, J. 1976. *Cancer Incidence in Five Continents*. Lyon, France: International Agency for Cancer Research, pp. 70–81.

58. Wijsman, R.A. 1958. "Contribution to the study of the question of association between two diseases." *Hum. Biol.* 30:219–236.

59. Wilson, E.B. 1930. "Morbidity and the association of morbid conditions." *J. Prev. Med.* 4:27–28.

60. ———, and Maher, H.C. 1932. "Cancer and tuberculosis with some comments on cancer and other diseases." *Amer. J. Cancer* 16:227–250.

61. Winkelstein, W. Jr., Stenchever, M.A., and Lilienfeld, A.M. 1958. "Occurrence of pregnancy, abortion, and artificial menopause among women with coronary artery disease: A preliminary study." *J. Chron. Dis.* 7:273–286.

62. Woolf, B. 1955. "On estimating the relation between blood group and disease." *Ann. Hum. Genet.* 19:251–253.

63. Wynder, E.L., and Licklider, S.D. 1960. "The question of circumcision." *Cancer* 13:442–445.

9 Observational Studies: II. Prospective Studies

> Tables of sickness for the entire population would be formed by taking 100,000 persons of given ages, indiscriminately, and observing them for one, two, three, &c., years.
>
> WILLIAM FARR, 1839

A. THE PROSPECTIVE APPROACH
General Description of Method

The limitations of inferences derived from retrospective studies (discussed in Chap. 8) make it desirable, in many instances, to confirm any association observed in a retrospective study by means of a *prospective* one. The general concept of the prospective study is relatively simple, although such studies can be conducted in several ways. A sample of the population is selected and information is obtained to determine which persons either have a particular characteristic (such as a certain living habit or physiological trait) that is suspected of being related to the development of the disease being investigated, or have been exposed to a possible etiological agent. These individuals are then followed for a period of time to observe who develops and/or dies from that disease. The necessary data for assessing the development of the disease can be obtained either directly (by periodic examinations of everyone in the sample) or indirectly (by reviewing physician and hospital records, disease registration forms, and/or death certificates). Incidence or death rates for the disease are then calculated, and the rates compared for those with the characteristic of interest and those without it. If the rates are different (either relatively or absolutely), an association can be said to exist between the characteristic and the disease. It is important to obtain information on other general characteristics of the study groups, including age, sex, color, and occupation, in addition to the specific characteristic of interest, in order to be able to account for an influence of any factors that are known to be related to the disease. Statistical methods are available for such analyses (4, 6–8, 18, 28, 47).

This type of study has been described by a variety of terms: "cohort," "incidence," "longitudinal," "forward-looking," and "follow-up," of which the most widely used is "cohort." "Prospective" rather than "cohort" is used here in an effort to limit the use of the term "cohort" to the cohort method of analysis of mortality data discussed in Chapter 5. A distinction between these two types of studies is necessary because individuals are followed or traced in prospective studies, whereas there is no actual follow-up of individuals in a cohort analysis of mortality data; the follow-up is *artificially constructed* by the analysis of mortality in successive age groups over a series of time periods.

Types of Prospective Studies

Prospective studies can be classified as follows:

1. Concurrent studies
   a) General population sample
   b) Select groups of the population
      i) Special groups—professional, veteran, etc.
      ii) Exposed groups—occupational, etc.
2. Nonconcurrent studies
   a) Population census taken in the past—usually special and unofficial
   b) Select groups of the population
      i) Special groups—professional, veteran, etc.
      ii) Exposed groups—occupational, etc.

Concurrent and nonconcurrent prospective studies are contrasted in Figure 9–1. In a concurrent study, those with and without the characteristic or exposure are selected at the start of the study (1980 in Fig. 9–1) and *followed* over a number of years by a variety of methods. In a nonconcurrent study, the investigator goes back in time (to 1950 in Fig. 9–1), selects his study groups, and *traces* them over time, usually to the present, by a variety of methods. These

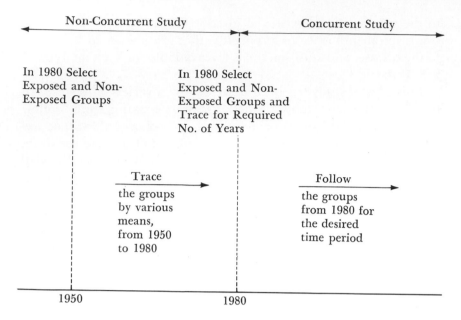

Figure 9–1.   Diagrammatic representation of concurrent and nonconcurrent prospective studies

two types of prospective studies must be distinguished because they involve different methodological problems.

A simple example of a nonconcurrent prospective study is the investigation of a food-poisoning outbreak discussed in Chapter 1 (p. 15). After such an outbreak, investigators usually locate members of the groups in which the epidemic occurred and obtain histories of their food intake. Then they compute attack rates for those exposed and not exposed to the various food items to determine the cause of the epidemic. In food-poisoning outbreaks, the incubation periods of the disease are very short, usually days or weeks. Therefore, they are not usually regarded as prospective studies; however, the reasoning used in studying these outbreaks is that of a prospective study. The lengthy incubation periods of some (usually noninfectious) diseases introduce methodological complexities, which affect the inferences derived from the data collected in a prospective study (see Chap. 1, p. 5 for another example).

CONCURRENT STUDIES

In concurrent studies, the investigator begins with a group of individuals and follows them for a number of years. This was Ham-

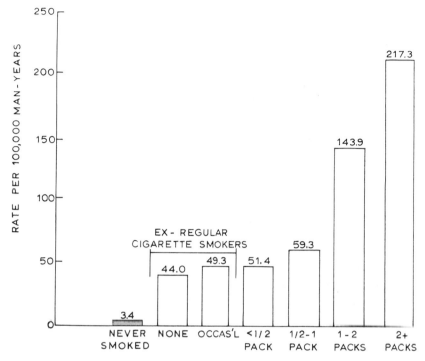

Figure 9–2. Age-adjusted death rates from malignant neoplasm of lung (exclusive of adenocarcinoma) by amount of cigarette smoking at beginning of prospective study in 1952

Source: Hammond and Horn (25). Reprinted from *The Journal of the American Medical Association,* 166:1159–1308, 1958. Copyright 1958, American Medical Association.

mond and Horn's approach to studying the relationship between cigarette smoking and lung cancer (25). For this study, sponsored by the American Cancer Society, 22,000 volunteers were recruited in 1952. Each volunteer was asked to record on forms the smoking histories of ten white men, 50–60 years of age, whom he/she knew and were not seriously ill and with whom he/she expected to remain in contact for a number of years. Annually, the volunteers reported on each individual, indicating whether he was "alive," "dead," or "status unknown." Death certificates were obtained for each reported death. About 190,000 completed forms were received on persons residing in 394 counties in nine states. Forty-four months later, 92.7 percent of the men were reported to be alive, 6.2 percent had died, and 1.1 percent could not be traced. Age-cause-specific

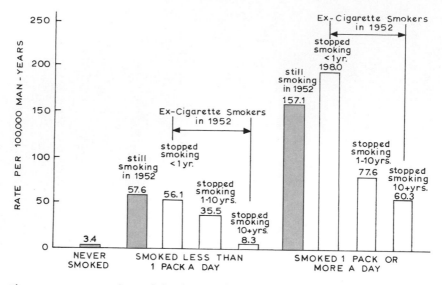

Figure 9–3. Age-adjusted death rates from malignant neoplasm of lung (exclusive of adenocarcinoma) among men who had never smoked, who had stopped smoking, and who were still smoking at beginning of prospective study in 1952

Source: Hammond and Horn (25). Reprinted from *The Journal of the American Medical Association,* 166:1159–1308, 1958. Copyright 1958, American Medical Association.

and age-standardized mortality rates by history of tobacco use were computed from the collected data. Figures 9–2 to 9–4 illustrate some of the interesting findings of this classic study.

Figure 9–2 shows an increasing risk of mortality from bronchogenic (or lung) cancer with increasing number of cigarettes smoked and lower mortality rates among ex-regular cigarette smokers than among current smokers. Figure 9–3 shows that the mortality rate among ex-regular cigarette smokers decreases as the period of time since they had stopped smoking increases, except for those who had stopped smoking within a year of entry into the study. This exception may reflect the fact that some of the men gave up cigarette smoking because they had already been diagnosed as having lung cancer. The interesting fact that there are marked differences in lung cancer mortality rates between cigarette and non-cigarette smokers living in different sized cities and in rural areas is illustrated in Figure 9–4. Although the mortality rates increase with increasing degree of urbanization for both smokers and nonsmokers,

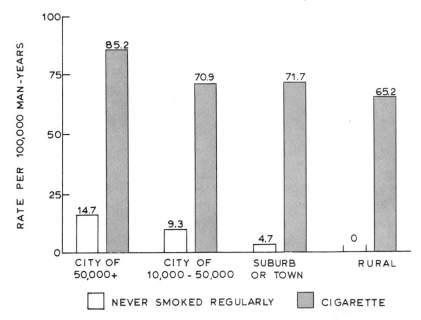

Figure 9–4. Age-adjusted death rates from malignant neoplasm of lung (exclusive of adenocarcinoma) among men who were cigarette smokers compared to those who had never smoked regularly by degree of urbanization of their residence at beginning of prospective study in 1952

Source: Hammond and Horn (25). Reprinted from *The Journal of the American Medical Association,* 166:1159–1308, 1958. Copyright 1958, American Medical Association.

the urban-rural differences are much smaller than those between cigarette and non-cigarette smokers. Such differences are important in deriving etiological inferences from prospective studies (a subject that will be discussed in detail in Chap. 12). The groups in Hammond and Horn's study were not probability samples of the general population, which would have been preferable, but a probability sample of the required size would have been almost impossible to obtain.

Another example comes from a study by Peritz and his colleagues of the effects of oral contraceptive use (41). These investigators followed a group of 17,942 women, 18–58 years of age, during the period December 1968 through February 1972. The results in Table 9–1 show both a gradient of an increasing risk of cervical cancer with longer oral contraceptive use and an overall relative risk for cervical cancer of 5.41 for those who used oral contraceptives for more than four years.

Table 9–1. Age-adjusted Incidence Rates and Relative Risks of Cervical Carcinoma and Dysplasia by Duration of Oral Contraceptive Use

Duration of Oral Contraceptive Use	Cervical Cancer	Cervical Dysplasia
	Incidence Rate per 100,000	
0	32	24
<1 year	63	129
1–4 years	97	72
>4 years	173	117
	Relative Risks*	
0	1.00	1.00
<1 year	1.97	5.38
1–4 years	3.03	3.00
>4 years	5.41	4.88

* Incidence for each group is compared with nonusers i.e., duration of use = 0, whose relative risk = 1.0.

Source: Peritz et al. (41).

In some situations, a prospective study can be conducted in a population selected from a well-defined geographical, political, or administrative area. This is particularly feasible when the disease or cause of death is fairly frequent in the population and does not require recruiting a large number of persons for the study. The Framingham Heart Study is a good example of this type of prospective study (12–14, 24). It was initiated in 1948 by the United States Public Health Service in order to study the relationship of a variety of factors to the subsequent development of heart disease. The town of Framingham, Massachusetts, with a population of 28,000 in 1948, was chosen for its population stability, cooperation with prior community studies, availability of a local community hospital, and proximity to a large medical center. The initial population sample was a group of persons 30–62 years of age that, when followed over a period of twenty years, would result in enough new cases and/or deaths of cardiovascular disease to insure statistically reliable findings. The town's population in this age group was approximately 10,000 and a sample of 6,500 persons of both sexes was selected. After the first examination, each person was re-examined at two year intervals for a twenty-year period. Information was obtained on several factors that could be related to heart disease, such as serum cholesterol level, blood pressure, weight, and history of cigarette smoking.

During the course of the study, some of the findings were reported. Table 9–2 presents the incidence rates and relative risks of coronary heart disease (CHD) among males and females during the first eighteen years of follow-up by initial serum cholesterol levels and age (45). There is an increasing risk of CHD with increasing initial serum cholesterol levels in the 45–54 age group from a relative risk of 1.14–3.25 (1.13–2.89 for females), a gradient of CHD disease which, though still present, is slightly less steep in the older male age groups (2.46–4.41 and 3.31–4.12, respectively) though it was steeper for the females (2.87–10.29 and 4.05–18.43, respectively).

The Framingham Study became a prototype for similar studies in Tecumseh, Michigan, and other areas (30, 36, 40). However, the difficulties in selecting general population samples for such studies tend to make investigators utilize special groups that for one reason or another are easy to follow: certain professional groups, people enrolled in medical care programs, veterans, and others. In Doll and Hill's prospective study of cigarette smoking and lung cancer, for instance, a questionnaire was sent to all physicians on the British Medical Register who were living in the United Kingdom (15, 16) (see Chap. 1, p. 10). Follow-up was simplified because the subjects were physicians and, therefore, maintained contact with several professional organizations. Information from death certificates where "physician" was the stated occupation was obtained from the Registrar General's Office. Lists were also obtained from the General Medical Council or the British Medical Association for deaths that had occurred abroad or in the military service. Similarly, Dorn studied a group of 293,658 veterans who held United States Government Life Insurance policies in 1953 (17, 29). In 1954 and 1957, questionnaires were sent to these policyholders to ascertain the respondents' smoking habits. When a claim was filed at the death of a policyholder, a copy of the death certificate was sent to the Veterans Administration (VA). Information was obtained when a policy was terminated, usually by death, and the VA made available additional mortality information on those veterans who received other medical and social services. Thus, the VA system served as a means for determining the mortality status of these veterans. The results of this study corroborated previous retrospective and pro-

spective studies that indicated an association exists between cigarette smoking and lung cancer (11).

A more recent example of the use of a unique population is the
Oral Contraception Study of the Royal College of General Practi-

Table 9–2. Average Annual Incidence Rate and Relative Risk from Coronary
Heart Disease per 10,000 Population at Risk for Males and Females, by Ages
45–74 Years and Levels of Serum Cholesterol at First Examination

Framingham, 18-year Follow-up

Initial Serum Cholesterol	Years of Age		
Level (mg/100 ml)	45–54	55–64	65–74
		MALES	
	Incidence Rates		
62–179	40.6	99.7	134.5
180–199	46.3	106.5	137.8
200–219	54.9	113.7	141.2
220–239	60.3	121.3	144.6
240–259	68.7	129.5	148.2
260–279	78.3	138.2	151.8
280–299	89.3	147.5	155.5
300–319	101.7	157.3	159.2
320–339	115.8	167.8	163.1
340–968	131.8	179.0	167.1
	*Relative Risks**		
62–179	1.00	2.46	3.31
180–199	1.14	2.62	3.39
200–219	1.35	2.80	3.48
220–239	1.48	2.99	3.56
240–259	1.69	3.19	3.65
260–279	1.93	3.40	3.74
280–299	2.20	3.63	3.83
300–319	2.50	3.87	3.92
320–339	2.85	4.13	4.02
340–968	3.25	4.41	4.12
		FEMALES	
	Incidence Rates		
62–179	6.3	18.1	25.5
180–199	7.1	20.9	30.2
200–219	8.0	24.1	35.8
220–239	9.0	27.7	42.4
240–259	10.1	32.0	50.2
260–279	11.4	36.8	59.4
280–299	12.8	42.4	70.3
300–319	14.4	48.9	83.1
320–339	16.2	56.3	98.3
340–968	18.2	64.8	116.1

| Initial Serum Cholesterol | Years of Age | | |
Level (mg/100 ml)	45–54	55–64	65–74
	Relative Risks†		
62–179	1.00	2.87	4.05
180–199	1.13	3.32	4.79
200–219	1.30	3.83	5.68
220–239	1.43	4.40	6.73
240–259	1.60	5.08	7.97
260–279	1.81	5.84	9.43
280–299	2.03	6.73	11.16
300–319	2.29	7.76	13.19
320–339	2.57	8.94	15.60
340–968	2.89	10.29	18.43

* Incidence in each group is compared with that of males 45–54 years of age and with initial serum cholesterol levels under 190 mg. per 100 ml. where relative risk = 1.0.
† Incidence in each group is compared with that of females 45–54 years of age and with initial cholesterol levels under 180 mg. per 100 ml. where relative risk = 1.0.

Source: Adapted from Shurtleff (45).

tioners in England (42, 43). Between May 1968 and July 1969, 23,000 oral contraceptive users and an equal number of nonusers, matched only for age and marital status, were recruited by physicians from among their patients. Oral contraceptive users were selected as the first two women in each calendar month for whom the physicians wrote a prescription for an oral contraceptive. A nonuser was selected by the following procedure: starting with the user's

Table 9–3. Standardized Relative Risks for Oral Contraceptive Users to Non-Users for Acute Myocardial Infarction, Chronic Ischaemic Heart Disease, Deep Thrombosis of the Leg, and Subarachnoid Hemorrhage

Disease (ICD Category)	Relative Risk (Oral Contraceptive User to Nonuser)
Nonrheumatic heart disease and hypertension (400–429)	4.7
Acute myocardial infarction (410)	3.2
Subarachnoid hemorrhage (430)	>10.0
Deep thrombosis of leg (451, 453)*	5.68†

* Recoded
† 1974 Progress Report

Source: Adapted from Royal College of General Practitioners' Oral Contraception Study (42, 43).

Table 9–4. Relation Between EBV Antibody Status on Entrance to College, Clinical History, and Subsequent Development of Infectious Mononucleosis

Antibody Status	Number Studied	Percent Positive	
		Past History of Mononucleosis	Development of Clinical Mononucleosis During Next 4 Years
Positive	94	6.4	0.0
Negative	268	0.0	14.9

Source: Evans et al. (19). Reprinted by permission from *The New England Journal of Medicine* (279:1121–1127, 1968).

record, returned to its correct place in the doctor's file, each subsequent record was examined in alphabetical order until the next record was found for a woman whose year of birth was within three years either side of that of the user and who had never used an oral contraceptive. Both the user and nonuser had to be either married or known to be "living as married." These 46,000 women were followed with regard to their morbidity and/or mortality experience. In both 1974 and 1977, progress reports were issued, showing associations between oral contraceptive use and 1) deep venous thrombosis, 2) acute myocardial infarction, and 3) subarachnoid hemorrhage (Table 9–3). The latter association, which was first found in this study, has stimulated other investigations.

Concurrent prospective studies are not limited to noninfectious diseases. An illustration of the application of this method to infectious diseases is afforded by the studies implicating the Epstein-Barr Virus (EBV) as the etiological agent of infectious mononucleosis (19). Blood samples were taken from Yale University freshmen on entry into college from 1958–63. A sample of 362 of these freshmen was studied to ascertain the relationship of the incidence of infectious mononucleosis to EBV-antibody status. Information about prior histories of mononucleosis was provided by college-entry health records. Using information from university health records, the attack rates for infectious mononucleosis over a four-year period were calculated. As shown in Table 9–4, 6 students (6.4 percent) whose sera contained EBV antibodies had a recorded prior history of infectious mononucleosis. In none of these did infectious mononucleosis develop during their stay in college. Of the 268 students with no EBV antibodies in their sera, none had a past history of infectious mononucleosis; however 40 (14.9 percent) of these students developed the disease during their college years. Thus, the presence of EBV antibodies was associated with immunity and their absence with susceptibility to the development of infectious mononucleosis over a period of time.

In the concurrent prospective studies discussed so far, the study groups were divided into those with and those without one or more possible etiological factors. The groups were sometimes classified according to different degrees of exposure or to levels of a characteristic such as the concentration of serum antibodies. The incidence and/or mortality rates of these subgroups were then compared. The study groups were selected because they offered particular advantages for follow-up and information about a specific factor was obtainable from them. In a different type of concurrent prospective study, a specific group that has been exposed to a possible etiological factor is selected and followed to determine the effects of this exposure. This method has been especially useful in studies of the effects of exposure to substances in occupational environments. The United States Public Health Service's (USPHS) study of uranium mine workers exposed to airborne radiation provides an example of this strategy.

A high frequency of lung cancer deaths among miners was first observed by Harting and Hess in 1879 (26). In the early 1900s, it was assumed that pneumoconioses, in combination with arsenic and cobalt (also present in the mines), were etiologically important. By 1950, as a result of pathological studies and animal experiments, several investigators had begun to attribute the increased mortality to radioactive materials, chiefly radon daughters (22, 33). In the USPHS study, which began in 1950, about 3,400 white uranium miners with underground mining experience were examined every three years. These miners were followed through an annual census of the uranium mining industry and mail questionnaires. Credit bureaus, vital statistics bureaus, and Social Security claims were additional sources of follow-up information. Approximately 95 percent of the study group was successfully traced (34, 49).

It was necessary to estimate the miners' degree of exposure to radioactivity. The principal radiation hazard for uranium is not radon itself but its radioactive daughters. Using available field methods, about 12,000 measurements were made of these radon daughters by various federal and state agencies. Although these measurements were not complete, their overall quality was good.

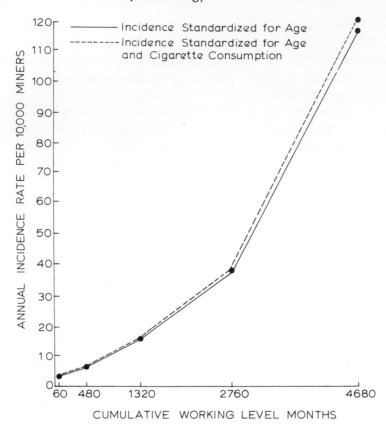

Figure 9–5. Annual age-standardized and age-cigarette consumption-standardized incidence rates of malignant neoplasm of lung among uranium mine workers by cumulative working level months

Source: Wagoner et al. (49). Reprinted by permission of *The New England Journal of Medicine,* 273:181–188, 1965.

They were recorded as fractions of the working level (WL), which is defined as 1.3×10^5 million electron volts (Mev) of potential alpha energy from radon daughters per liter of air; this represents the radiation dose from alpha particles. It was possible to obtain occupational histories and exposure measurements for each miner. Radiation exposure values for each miner were expressed as working-level months (WLM), which is the number of months an individual was exposed to a particular amount of radiation. These were added to provide an estimate of each miner's total amount of radiation exposure until 1963, the cutoff date for the initial analysis of the data (49). Incidence rates for respiratory cancer were then calculated and standardized for factors such as age, number of years since the beginning of exposure, and cigarette consumption and were found to increase with the degree of exposure (Figure 9–5). A more recent report with additional follow-up information to 1974 has indicated that in addition to the radiation exposure, cigarette smoking influenced the mortality from lung cancer (2).

Estimates of the degree of exposure permit internal comparisons; that is, comparisons between subgroups of the study population. In many situations, however, where information on different degrees of exposure is not available or the entire study group was equally exposed, it is necessary to use an external comparison or control group. If none is available, the mortality experience of the exposed group is usually compared with the death rates in the same geographical area as the exposed group, with statistical adjustments for age, sex, and calendar time of exposure and follow-up. In the study of the uranium mine workers, comparisons were made with data on lung cancer mortality from the four-state area where the miners resided.

Another group that had a unique exposure to radiation is being studied by the Atomic Bomb Casualty Commission in Hiroshima and Nagasaki (see Chap. 3, p. 52). A variety of effects of exposure to the atom bomb have been reported from this study (1, 39).

NONCONCURRENT STUDIES

In nonconcurrent prospective studies, the period of observation starts from some date in the past, as illustrated in Figure 9–1. These studies cannot be conducted with samples of the general population unless the investigator has access to a census of a community, usually unofficial, which was conducted in the past. Samples of the population covered by the census can then be selected and traced from the time of the census (9).

Nonconcurrent studies usually involve specially exposed groups or industrial populations because of the usual unavailability of such past census information and the availability of employment, medical, or other types of records. This is illustrated by the study of the relationship between polycythemia vera (PV) and leukemia, which had been clinically observed since 1905 (38). The increased medical use of radiation treatment for PV and the observations on

Table 9–5. Number and Percentage of Patients Who Developed Acute Leukemia, by Diagnostic Group and Method of Treatment, among All Patients and in the "Subgroup"

Method of Treatment	Polycythemia Vera			Questionable Polycythemia			Secondary Polycythemia		
		Acute Leukemia			Acute Leukemia			Acute Leukemia	
	Total	Number	Percent	Total	Number	Percent	Total	Number	Percent
All Patients									
N.R.*	133	1	0.8	301	0	0.0	211	0	0.0
X-ray	79	7	8.9	48	1	2.1	11	1	9.1
P^{32}	228	25	11.0	102	10	9.8	8	0	0.0
X-ray + P^{32}	72	12	16.7	25	2	8.0	4	0	0.0
Total	512	45	8.8	476	13	2.7	234	1	0.4
The Subgroup†									
N.R.	99	1	1.0	267	0	0.0	199	0	0.0
X-ray	37	3	8.1	19	0	0.0	5	0	20.0
P^{32}	102	9	8.8	35	5	14.3	4	0	0.0
X-ray + P^{32}	30	5	16.7	9	2	22.2	0	0	0.0
Total	268	18	6.7	330	7	2.1	208	1	0.5

* No radiation treatment.
† Patients first seen and treated during the year of their diagnosis.

Source: **Modan and Lilienfeld (38). Copyright © 1965, Williams and Wilkins Co.**

the leukemogenic effect of ionizing radiation in various studies raised the question as to whether the development of leukemia in patients with PV was part of the disease's natural history or a result of treatment with X-ray and/or of P^{32}. A study was undertaken to estimate the risk of developing leukemia among patients with PV and to determine whether it was increased as a result of P^{32} and/or X-ray treatment. Medical records of patients with PV who had been seen during 1947–55 in seven medical centers were obtained at the same time as those of two comparison groups: a) patients with polycythemia secondary to lung disease and b) patients with questionable polycythemia. These groups were then classified by method of treatment into four categories:

1. No radiation treatment
2. X-ray alone
3. P^{32} only
4. A combination of X-ray and P^{32}.

The patients were traced through December 31, 1961. The major results are presented in Table 9–5. It is clear that leukemia occurred predominantly in patients who had received some form of radiation.

A similar type of study was conducted by Coombs and her colleagues, who examined the relationship between benign breast diseases (BBD) and breast cancer (10). The study group consisted of women between 15 and 69 years of age, residing in New York State, having been discharged from the Roswell Park Memorial Institute in Buffalo, New York, who were diagnosed as having BBD between 1957 and 1965; this group comprised 747 women. An equal number of controls who were also New York State residents and who had been seen at Roswell Park Memorial Institute between 1957 and 1965, with discharge diagnoses of nonmalignant conditions exclusive of the reproductive sites, were selected. (It is clear that the study, using BBD cases as the exposed group and non-BBD controls as the nonexposed group, is a case-control study. As was indicated in Chapter 8, p. 194, both prospective *and* retrospective studies can be case-control.) The groups were matched for date of admission, age at admission, and color. In December 1977, both groups were mailed questionnaires to determine their status with respect to breast cancer. The results are shown in Table 9–6. A distinct relationship between BBD and the development of breast cancer is evident.

Table 9–6. Age-Adjusted Mortality Rates by Cause per 1,000 Person-Years of Follow-up and Relative Risks for Women with Benign Breast Diseases Compared with Women with Nonmalignant Conditions

Cause of death	Benign breast diseases	Nonmalignant conditions	Relative risk
All causes	6.68	9.04	0.7
All cancers	2.84	2.03	1.4
Breast cancer	0.93	0.20	4.7
All other cancers	1.91	1.84	1.0

Source: Coombs et al. (10).

Nonconcurrent prospective studies of industrial exposures to possible etiological agents of disease can only be carried out by using company records of past and present employees that include information on the date they began their employment, age at hiring, the date of departure, and whether they were living or dead. The mortality experience can be determined and compared with that of another industry or with the mortality rates of the state where the industry is located or of the country as a whole. Lee and Fraumeni adopted this approach in their study of the role of arsenic in human carcinogenesis (31). They determined the mortality experience of 8,047 white male smelter workers who had been exposed to arsenic trioxide, sulfur dioxide, and other chemicals during 1938–63, and compared it with that of the white male population in the same states where these industries were located. It was possible to classify the workers by duration and degree of exposure, and increased mortality from lung cancer with increasing duration of exposure to sulfur dioxide and arsenic trioxide was observed.

Study Procedures

A major source of difficulty in carrying out prospective studies is to maintain follow-up of the selected group of persons. This is least troublesome in concurrent prospective studies for obvious reasons. At the very start of a study, methods can be adopted for keeping in contact with the population, including periodic home visits, telephone calls, and mailed questionnaires, preferably all three on an annual basis. The names and addresses of several friends and relatives can be obtained at the beginning of a study so that they may be contacted if the person moves out of the community. (Geographic mobility of people, particularly in the United States, does pose a problem.) Although the Social Security Administration (SSA) does not divulge information on the current employment of people who have moved, Social Security numbers are useful because the SSA will, for legitimate research purposes, inform investigators if and where a person has died. Social Security numbers also help to identify individuals on records from other sources.

Despite the best efforts, a certain percentage of individuals will always be lost to follow-up, although even for this group, information on mortality status can be obtained from state vital statistics bureaus. Then, their mortality experience can be compared with that of the individuals not "lost to follow-up" to determine if there are any differences between the two groups. In addition, the successfully traced group can be compared to the "lost" group with respect to several known characteristics. To the extent that they show similar frequencies of a variety of characteristics of interest in the study, one's confidence is increased that no bias has been introduced into the findings by the lost group.

In a nonconcurrent prospective study, when one goes back perhaps twenty to thirty years to select a study group, the problem of tracing becomes more difficult. Every available source of information must be used. Table 9–7 presents the various means used by Modan in determining the survivorship status of patients in his study of polycythemia vera and leukemia (37). In all prospective studies, it is desirable to trace as high a percentage of the study group as possible. Questions are usually raised about the possibility of bias in the results if the degree of follow-up is less than 95 percent. This issue has been considered in several studies. Modan found that a very good estimate of the total mortality rate was obtained from the first 77 percent of the patients he traced, although the group that was reached first had a somewhat higher leukemia mortality rate than those traced later (38). In a study of the outcome of neurosis, on the other hand, Sims found considerable differences between the patients who were easily contacted and those who were traced with more effort (46). Only three deaths had occurred among the first 110 successfully traced patients (59 percent of the study group), but eighteen additional deaths were discovered in the sixty-six patients (36 percent of the study group) who were found by more intensive tracing. Thus, it appears that the pattern varies in differ-

Table 9–7.   Distribution of Sources of Information on Patient's Survivorship Status in the Study of Polycythemia Vera and Leukemia

Source of Information	Patients	
	Number	Percent
Patient	158	12.9
Local physician	201	16.4
Relative	103	8.4
Hospital	540	44.2
Neighbors	49	4.0
Postmaster	18	1.5
Town/County clerk	20	1.6
Health department	89	7.3
Other	24	2.0
Untraced	20	1.6
Total	1,222	100.0

Source: Modan (37).

ent studies and, perhaps, with different types of disease entities so that a general rule cannot be established about the degree of follow-up necessary to ensure unbiased conclusions. The safest course is to achieve as complete a follow-up as possible.

Analysis of Results

It has already been made clear that the results of prospective studies are preferably analyzed in terms of relative risks, which provide a relatively simple expression of the relationship between the incidence or mortality rates from different diseases in the groups being compared. This is particularly true if the time when the follow-up observations that are made are the same for all the study groups.

Many prospective studies, however, whether concurrent or non-concurrent, involve lengthy and varying periods of observations. Persons are lost to follow-up or die at different times during the course of the study and, consequently, they are under observation for different time periods. In some studies, persons are enlisted or enter the study at different times and, if the follow-up is terminated at a specific time, they will have been observed for different lengths of time. Three related methods are available for analyzing the results of such studies (4, 6–8, 18, 23, 27, 28, 44, 47, 50):

1. actuarial, or life tables;
2. the calculation of person-years or months of observation as the denominator for the computation of incidence or mortality rates; and
3. using statistical models, such as the logistic or log-linear.

Many consider using life tables the preferred method of analyzing such data (6–8, 18, 23, 28). They provide direct estimates of the probability of developing or dying from a disease for a given time period and relative risks can be computed as the ratio of these probabilities.

Difficulties develop when the study group has to be divided into several subgroups such as age, sex, color, socioeconomic status, with small numbers of persons in each or when the persons enter the study group at different times. A detailed description of the statistical methods used in analyzing life tables is beyond the scope of this text.

Person-years of observation are frequently used as denominators in the computation of rates in prospective studies. They are particularly useful when several factors, such as age, sex, and varying periods of observation, which result from persons entering and leaving the study at different ages and times, make the computation of an actuarial life table difficult or impossible. They take into consideration both the number of persons who were followed and the duration of observation of each person. For example, five persons who remain under observation for twenty years contribute one hundred person-years, and one hundred persons who are observed for one year also contribute one hundred person-years. The use of person-years makes it possible to express in one figure the period when a varying number of persons is exposed to the risk of the occurrence of an event such as death or the development of a disease. In addition, the age distribution of the groups under observation changes as a study progresses, as do the mortality and morbidity rates with chronological time (35). Sheps has pointed out that the use of person-years is limited by the assumption that the risk of occurrence of an event per unit time is constant during the period of observation for the individual (44). This limitation is diminished when the size of the sample is large and the risk is low, but is increased when the period of observation used for analysis is long. The overall effect of this limitation is modest and usually acceptable in most prospective studies.

More recently, various statistical methods based on logistic or log-linear models have been put to increasing use in the analysis of prospective studies. These may be useful in taking into account and adjusting for factors of secondary interest that may have had an influence on the endpoint in the study. Expert statistical advice should be sought before they are used (4, 27, 47, 50).

B. PROSPECTIVE VS. RETROSPECTIVE STUDIES
Advantages and Disadvantages of Prospective Studies

It is natural to compare prospective and retrospective studies in considering the utility of either type; the advantages of one often represent the disadvantages of the other. Compared to retrospective studies, prospective studies have the following advantages:

1. They provide a direct estimate of the risk of developing a disease in individuals with a specific characteristic relative to those without the characteristic. In a retrospective study, the estimate of the relative risk is obtained indirectly. No estimate of the risk of developing a disease is possible in a retrospective study.

2. If the criteria and procedures of the study are established in advance, they decrease the possibility of subjective bias in obtaining the necessary information. In a retrospective study, one has to depend upon the individual's memory for information on the occurrence of an event far in the past or on the availability of some record. There may also be a selective recall for certain events by people with certain diseases. In a prospective study, one starts with individuals who have the characteristic under study. The information obtained cannot be biased by knowledge of the result since it is recorded before the outcome is known. This also diminishes the chances of misclassifying individuals by their characteristics.

3. Depending upon the disease and the characteristic being studied, one can obtain information on people whose status has changed with regard to the characteristic. In the cigarette smoking–lung cancer studies, for example, information was obtained on individuals who stopped smoking during the course of the studies.

4. Information can be obtained on the relationship of the characteristic to other diseases. In a retrospective study, one disease is usually selected for study; in a prospective study, the entire spectrum of morbidity and/or mortality experience can be investigated.

5. Even the best-designed retrospective study is limited to those individuals who have survived for a period of time after the exposure to the possible etiological agent or the initial event has occurred. During the period between the initial event and the occurrence of the disease—at which time the retrospective study is conducted—some individuals in this group will have died. If the characteristic or exposure under study is related to mortality, the deaths that had occurred during the interval will have a disproportionately higher percentage of those with the characteristic or exposure and will not be represented in the groups selected for the retrospective study. This may result in underestimating the degree of association between the characteristic and the disease, which would not occur in prospective studies.

Prospective studies also have several disadvantages:

1. They are usually more difficult and expensive to execute, requiring large study populations and long periods of observation for definite results. It is sometimes possible to reduce the expense of a prospective study by incorporating some features of retrospective studies. In a prospective study of the relationship of hormonal factors to the subsequent development of female breast cancer, for instance, women could be selected and blood specimens collected and frozen. The women would then be followed and the blood specimens of those who developed breast cancer could be retrieved, examined for hormonal or other components, and compared to the blood specimens of women selected from the original group who had not developed breast cancer. Such a study was conducted to examine the relationship between female breast cancer and certain hormonal metabolites in the urine (5).

2. In a prospective study involving the periodic examination of people, it is possible that participation in the study may influence the development of disease in individuals. For exam-

Table 9–8. Estimated Number of Individuals Required in Each Group for Detecting Statistically Significant Relative Risks between Groups in a Prospective Study by Relative Risk and Incidence of Disease in a Control Group*

Relative Risk	Incidence Rate in Control Group for Period of Study			
	1 per 10,000	1 per 1,000	1 per 500	1 per 100
2	100,000	10,000	5,000	1,000
3	70,000	7,000	3,500	700
4	40,000	4,000	2,000	400
5	25,000	2,500	1,250	250
10	10,000	1,000	500	100

* Based on the probability of detecting a difference between the two groups of 80 percent and a significance level of 5 percent.

 ple, participants in a study of diet and heart disease may voluntarily change their dietary habits simply because of their interest in the study.

3. It has been shown that sampling selection, in which different groups of the population are enlisted in a prospective study with different probabilities, may also result in biased estimates of relationships, as in retrospective studies (see Chap. 8, p. 199) (3).

4. Prospective studies are very inefficient, if not impossible, in studying rare diseases. Table 9–8 shows the estimated number of individuals required in each group (exposed and nonexposed) for detecting a statistically significant relative risk in a prospective study by relative risk and the incidence rate of disease in the control (nonexposed) group. In the United

Table 9–9. Number of Woman-Years of Users of Oral Contraceptives Required to Detect Significant Results for Several Diseases

Disease	Woman-Years
Diabetes	8,000
Liver disease	11,000
Myocardial infarction	57,500
Pulmonary embolism	125,000

Source: Royal College of General Practitioners (42).

States, with a population of over 200 million, male breast cancer is so rare that only about 600 deaths occur annually. A prospective study of the relationship of various factors to the development of this disease would require such a large study group that it would be virtually impossible to conduct. Similarly, when the Royal College of Physicians began its oral contraceptive study, it determined the number of woman-years of observation needed to detect possible associations with specific diseases (Table 9–9); for some disorders, the number is quite large (42).

Conclusions

Some investigators contend that prospective studies have no particular advantage over well-executed retrospective studies. It is true that in several instances where both types of studies have been done on the same problem, the overall results were similar. Retrospective and prospective studies of the relationship between cigarette smoking and lung cancer, for example, have had similar results, as have studies of the relationship between artifical menopause and female breast cancer and those of diseases associated with oral contraceptive use (20, 32, 48). On the other hand, there are those who feel that the only way to definitely establish an association between a disease and a characteristic is by performing a prospective study (21). The general consensus is that prospective studies are not always necessary. When feasible, however, they do provide another, and more direct, view of the association; there is also value in testing any scientific hypothesis in different ways.

In general, prospective studies are not desirable for the exploration of a hypothesis or for the examination of a large number of factors of doubtful significance, for which retrospective studies are particularly suitable. They are most valuable when a specific hypothesis has already been developed, usually from the findings of a retrospective study, and additional evidence is needed to support or refute it.

STUDY PROBLEMS

1. Ulcerative colitis (UC) is an inflammatory disease of the colon. It is frequently diagnosed by radiologic examination and, since the disease is chronic, its course is monitored by periodic radio-

logic examinations, usually biannually. Two consistent observations have been made: 1) Jews have a higher incidence of UC and 2) sometimes, at least ten years after the diagnosis of UC, the patients develop colon cancer. It has been suggested that the cancer is the result of the periodic radiologic examinations. Outline a study to examine this hypothesis. Include a discussion of the selection of the sample.

2. A chemotherapy regimen for disease X was developed and used on several patients. It was noted that all patients lived until the start of the fourteenth year after diagnosis, when deaths began to occur. A study was undertaken to determine if chemotherapy had increased the survivorship of those with the disease. A group of 2,168 patients with the disease, but no chemotherapy, was selected from the hospital population and compared to a group of patients with the same disease who had received chemotherapy and who were similar with respect to age, sex, and color. All those in the study had had the disease for at least fourteen years. The numbers of deaths in the following years, for both groups, were as follows:

Years after diagnosis	No chemotherapy	Chemotherapy
14	70	10
15	61	201
16	119	150
17	225	80
18	231	270
19	437	70
20	365	120
21	230	141
22	177	163
23	54	157
24	63	292
25	71	221
26	46	131
27	5	13
28	1	60
29	2	0
30	7	45
31	0	41
32	4	3
Total	2,168	2,168

a) List at least 3 methods that can be used to analyze these data.
b) Analyze these data using person-years.
c) What assumptions are made in using person-years? Are they satisfied? Explain.
d) Analyze these data using life-tables. Are the results different from those obtained from the person-years analysis? Explain. (Note: See Reference 28 for a method of life table analysis.)

3. Consider Paffenbarger's study of tonsillectomy and poliomyelitis (Chap. 8, p. 220). Outline a prospective study that would explore a similar hypothesis.

4. In his study of polycythemia vera (PV) (see p. 239), Modan collected the following data, showing the number of persons alive at each year after diagnosis:

| Years after diagnosis | Diagnostic group and method of treatment | | | | | |
| | PV | | Questionable PV | | PV + Questionable PV | |
	Not radiated	P32 and/or x-ray	Not radiated	P32 and/or x-ray	Not radiated	P32 and/or x-ray
1	99	169	267	63	366	232
2	88	164	231	62	379	226
3	82	157	209	59	291	216
4	72	150	188	55	260	205
5	68	141	175	52	243	193
6	63	131	163	50	226	181
7	60	123	156	46	216	169
8	54	114	145	44	199	158
9	51	105	136	42	187	147
10	39	85	116	33	155	118
11	28	62	97	28	125	90
12	24	46	84	17	108	63
13	18	34	64	13	82	47
14	14	21	53	10	67	31
15	9	12	44	6	53	18
16	8	9	34	4	42	13
17	8	6	29	2	37	8
18	5	5	28	1	33	6
19	5	3	20	0	25	3
20	3	2	12	0	15	2

a) Analyze these data using person-years. What assumptions have been made in this analysis? Are they valid?
b) Analyze these data using life-tables. Are the results different from those obtained from the person-years analysis? Explain.

5. A certain virus V is suspected of being the cause of infectious disease D. Design a prospective study to elucidate the relationship between V and D. How does the design change if (a) V is a "slow virus"? (b) D is currently viewed as a non-infectious disease?

6. Several prospective studies have addressed the relationship of food consumption and certain diseases. Usually, for a one-week or one-month period, a spouse is asked to list in a diary his/her food consumption. Then, the spouse is followed along with members of his/her family for a period of time. Death rates or incidence rates can then be calculated by the type of foodstuff consumed. Compare this type of study design with that of a retrospective study (see Chap. 8, Problem 2, p. 218). What biases are removed? What biases remain? What biases are introduced? What methods can be used to remove remaining and introduced biases?

REFERENCES

1. Advisory Committee on the Biological Effects of Ionizing Radiation. 1972. *The Effects on Populations of Exposure to Low Levels of Ionizing Radiation.* Washington, D.C.: Division of Medical Sciences, National Academy of Sciences—National Research Council.
2. Archer, V.E., Gillam, J.D., and Wagoner, J.K. 1976. "Respiratory disease mortality among uranium miners." *Ann. N.Y. Acad. Sci.* 271:280–293.
3. Berkson, J. 1955. "The statistical study of association between smoking and lung cancer." *Proc. Mayo Clinic* 30:319–348.
4. Bishop, Y.M.M., Fienberg, S.E., and Holland, P.W. 1975. *Discrete Multivariate Analysis.* Cambridge: M.I.T. Press.
5. Bulbrook, R.D., Hayward, J.L., and Spicer, C.C. 1971. "Relation between urinary androgen and corticoid excretion and subsequent breast cancer." *Lancet* 2:395–398.
6. Chiang, C.L. 1960. "A stochastic study of the life table and its applications: I. Probability distributions of the biometric functions." *Biometrics* 16:618–635.
7. ——. 1960. "A stochastic study of the life table and its applications. II. Sample variance of the observed expectation of life and other biometric function." *Hum. Biol.* 32:221–238.
8. ——. 1961. "A stochastic study of the life table and its applications. III. The follow-up study with the consideration of competing risks." *Biometrics* 17:57–78.
9. Comstock, G.W., Abbey, H., and Lundin, F.E., Jr. 1970. "The nonofficial census as a basic tool for epidemiologic observations in Washington County, Maryland." In *The Community as an Epidemiologic Laboratory: A Casebook of Community Studies.* I.I. Kessler and M.L. Levin, eds. Baltimore, Md.: The Johns Hopkins Press, pp. 73–99.

10. Coombs, L.J., Lilienfeld, A.M., Bross, I.D.J., and Burnett, W.S. 1979. "A prospective study of the relationship between benign breast diseases and breast carcinoma." *Prev. Med.* 8:40–52.
11. Cornfield, J., Haenszel, W., Hammond, E.C., Lilienfeld, A.M., Shimkin, M.B., and Wynder, E.L. 1959. "Smoking and lung cancer: Recent evidence and a discussion of some questions." *J. Natl. Cancer Inst.* 22:173–203.
12. Dawber, T.R., Kannel, W.B., and Lyell, L.P. 1963. "An approach to longitudinal studies in a community: The Framingham Study." *Ann. N.Y. Acad. Sci.* 107:539–556.
13. ———, ———, and McNamara, P.M. 1963. *The prediction of heart disease.* Seventy-second Annual Meeting of Association of Life Insurance Medical Directors of America. New York City: Recording and Statistical Company.
14. ———, Meadors, G.F., and Moore, F.G., Jr. 1951. "The epidemiological approach to heart disease: The Framingham Study. *Am. J. Pub. Health* 41:279–286.
15. Doll, R., and Hill, A.B. 1964. "Mortality in relation to smoking: Ten years' observation of British doctors." *Brit. Med. J.* 1:1399–1410; 1460–1467.
16. ———, and Peto, R. 1976. "Mortality in relation to smoking: Twenty years' observations on male British doctors." *Brit. Med. J.* 2:1525–1536.
17. Dorn, H.F. 1959. "Tobacco consumption and mortality from cancer and other diseases." *Pub. Health Reps.* 74:581–593.
18. Elveback, L. 1958. "Estimation of survivorship in chronic disease: The 'Actuarial' method." *J. Amer. Stat. Assoc.* 53:420–440.
19. Evans, A.S., Niederman, J.C., and McCollum, R.W. 1968. "Seroepidemiologic studies of infectious mononucleosis with EB virus." *New Eng. J. Med.* 279:1121–1127.
20. Feinleib, M. 1968. "Breast cancer and artificial menopause: A cohort study." *J. Natl. Cancer Inst.* 41:315–329.
21. Feinstein, A.R. 1974. "Clinical biostatistics. 20. The epidemiologic trohoc, the ablative risk ratio, and 'retrospective' research." *Clin. Pharmacol. Ther.* 11:291–307.
22. Furth, J., and Lorenz, E. 1954. "Carcinogenesis by ionizing radiation." In *Radiation Biology.* A Hollaender, ed. *High Energy Radiation, Part 2,* Vol. 1. New York: McGraw-Hill.
23. Gehan, E.A. 1969. "Estimating survival functions from the life table." *J. Chron. Dis.* 21:629–644.
24. Gordon, T., and Kannel, W.B. 1970. "The Framingham, Massachusetts, Study, twenty years later." In *The Community as an Epidemiologic Laboratory: A Casebook of Community Studies.* I.I. Kessler and M.L. Levin, eds. Baltimore, Md.: The Johns Hopkins Press, pp. 123–146.
25. Hammond, E.C., and Horn, D. 1958. "Smoking and death rates—Report on forty-four months of follow-up of 187,783 men. Part I. Total mortality. Part II. Death rates by cause." *JAMA* 166:1159–1172; 1294–1308.
26. Härting, F.H., and Hesse, W. 1879. "Der Lungenkrebs die Bergkrankheit in den Schneebergen Gruben." *Vrtljschr f. Gerichtl. Med. N.F.* 30:296–309; 31:102–132, 313–337.
27. Hartz, S.C., and Rosenberg, L.A. 1975. "The computation of maximum likelihood estimates for the multiple logistic risk function for use with categorical data." *J. Chron. Dis.* 28:421–429.
28. Hill, A.B. 1971. *Principles of Medical Statistics.* 9th Ed., New York: Oxford University Press.

29. Kahn, H.A. 1966. "The Dorn study of smoking and mortality among U.S. veterans: Report on eight and one-half years of observations." In *Epidemiological Approaches to the Study of Cancer and Other Chronic Diseases.* W. Haenszel, ed. Natl. Cancer Inst. Monogr. 19, Washington, D.C.: United States Government Printing Office, pp. 1–125.

30. Keys, A., ed. 1970. *Coronary Heart Disease in Seven Countries.* Amer. Heart Assoc. Monog. No. 29. New York: The American Heart Association.

31. Lee, A.M., and Fraumeni, J.F., Jr. 1969. "Arsenic and respiratory cancer in man: An occupational study." *J. Natl. Cancer Inst.* 42:1045–1052.

32. Lilienfeld, A.M. 1956. "The relationship of cancer of the female breast to artificial menopause and marital status." *Cancer* 9:927–934.

33. Lorenz, E. 1944. "Radioactivity and lung cancer: A critical review of lung cancer in the miners of Schneeberg and Joachimsthal." *J. Natl. Cancer Inst.* 5:1–15.

34. Lundin, F.E., Jr., Wagoner, J.K., and Archer, V.E. 1971. *Radon Daughter Exposure and Respiratory Cancer: Quantitative and Temporal Aspects.* National Institute for Occupational Safety and Health, National Institute of Environmental Health Services Joint Monogr. No. 1. Washington, D.C.: United States Department of Health, Education and Welfare, Public Health Service.

35. Matanoski, G.M., Seltser, R., Sartwell, P.E., Diamond, E.L., and Elliott, E.A. 1975. "The current mortality rates of radiologists and other physician specialists: Deaths from all causes and from cancer." *Amer. J. Epidem.* 101:188–198.

36. McGee, D., and Gordon, T. 1976. *The Framingham Study: The Results of the Framingham Study Applied to Four Other U.S.-based Epidemiologic Studies of Cardiovascular Disease.* Washington, D.C.: U.S. Government Printing Office.

37. Modan, B. 1966. "Some methodological aspects of a retrospective follow-up study." *Amer. J. Epidem.* 82:297–304.

38. ———, and Lilienfeld, A.M. 1965. "Polycythemia vera and leukemia—The role of radiation treatment." *Medicine* 44:305–344.

39. Moriyama, I.M., Steer, A., Hamilton, H.B., Russell, W.J., Shimizu, K., and Dock, D.S. 1970. "Radiation effects on atomic bomb survivors." *Atomic Bomb Casualty Commission Tech. Rep. 6–73.*

40. Napier, J.A., Johnson, B.C., and Epstein, F.H. 1970. "The Tecumseh, Michigan Community Health Study." In *The Community as an Epidemiologic Laboratory: A Casebook of Community Studies.* I.I. Kessler and M.L. Levin, eds. Baltimore, Md.: The Johns Hopkins Press, pp. 25–46.

41. Peritz, E., Ramcharan, S., Frank, J., Brown, W.L., Huang, S., and Ray, R. 1977. "The incidence of cervical cancer and duration of oral contraceptive use." *Amer. J. Epidem.* 106:462–469.

42. Royal College of General Practitioners. 1974. *Oral Contraceptives and Health.* London: Pittman Medical.

43. Royal College of General Practitioners' Oral Contraception Study. 1977. "Mortality among oral contraceptive users." *Lancet* 2:727–731.

44. Sheps, M.C. 1966. "On the person-years concept in epidemiology and demography." *Milbank Mem. Fund Q.* 44:69–91.

45. Shurtleff, D. 1974. *The Framingham Study: Some Characteristics Related to the Incidence of Cardiovascular Disease and Death: Framingham Study, 18-Year Follow-up.* Washington, D.C.: U.S. Government Printing Office.

46. Sims, A.C.P. 1973. "Importance of a high tracing-rate in long-term medical follow-up studies." *Lancet* 2:433–435.

47. Truett, J., Cornfield, J., and Kannel, W. 1967. "A multivariate analysis of the risk of coronary heart disease in Framingham." *J. Chron. Dis.* 20:511–524.
48. Vessey, M.P., and Mann, J.I. 1978. "Female sex hormones and thrombosis." *Brit. Med. Bull.* 34:157–162.
49. Wagoner, J.K., Archer, V.E., Lundin, F.E., Jr., Holaday, D.A., and Lloyd, J.W. 1965. "Radiation as the cause of lung cancer among uranium miners." *N. Eng. J. Med.* 273:181–188.
50. Walker, S.H., and Duncan, D.B. 1967. "Estimation of the probability of an event as a function of several independent variables." *Biometrika* 54:167–179.

10 Experimental Epidemiology: I. Clinical Trials

> When we can produce a phenomenon artificially
> . . . and observe it in circumstances . . . with
> which we are accurately acquainted . . . , we
> may produce . . . variations to any extent, and
> of such kinds as we think best calculated to bring
> the laws of the phenomenon into clear light.
>
> J. S. MILL, 1876,
> *A System of Logic*

A. THE EXPERIMENTAL METHOD

The strength of the experimental method lies in the investigator's **direct control** over the assignment of individuals to study groups. In observational studies, by contrast, the investigator essentially accepts the conditions as they are. Broadly considered, there are two forms of epidemiologic experiments: 1) *clinical trials* and 2) *community trials* or *experiments* (the latter are also referred to as *field experiments*). In **clinical trials,** the efficacy of a preventive or therapeutic agent or procedure is tested in *individual subjects*. In **community trials,** as the term implies, *a group of individuals as a whole* is used to determine the efficacy of a drug or procedure. One example of such a community trial is the evaluation of fluorides in preventing dental caries, discussed in Chapter 1 (p. 5). Studies in which epidemics are experimentally produced in groups of animals in order to determine what factors influence such epidemics may also be considered as community experiments. This chapter deals with clinical trials; community trials are discussed in the next one (Chap. 11).

B. THE CLINICAL TRIAL

In order to simplify the discussion, we will consider clinical trials in terms of evaluating the efficacy of a drug in the treatment of a disease. However, they can also be used to evaluate a prophylactic agent, such as a vaccine, or a public health procedure, such as a screening method. Specific conditions of the trial may have to be changed depending upon its purpose, but the general methods and principles, for the most part, remain the same.

The clinical trial is an experiment in which individuals are randomly allocated to two groups, known as the "experimental" and the "control" groups. The experimental group is given the drug being tested and the control group is given the drug in current use; if no such drug exists, then a placebo, an inert substance such as a sugar pill or a saline injection, is used.

Randomization

The major difference between a clinical trial and a prospective study is the randomized nature of the clinical trial (7, 12, 16, 17, 20, 23). The experimental and control groups must be comparable in all factors except the one being studied, i.e., the drug (24, 26, 29, 31). The epidemiologist can achieve comparability on factors that are known to have an influence on the outcome, such as age, sex, race, or severity of disease, by matching for these factors. But one cannot match individuals for factors whose influence is not known or cannot be measured. This problem can be resolved by the random allocation of individuals to the experimental and control groups, which assures the comparability of these groups with respect to *all* factors—known and unknown, measurable and not measurable—except for the one being studied. In addition, randomization is the means by which the investigator avoids introducing conscious or subconscious bias into the process of allocating individuals to the experimental or control groups, thereby increasing the degree of comparability. A phrase that expresses this concept of comparability is *ceteris paribus*, meaning "all other things being equal."

Types of Clinical Trials

Within this basic framework there are several types of clinical trials:

1. **Therapeutic trials,** in which a therapeutic agent or procedure is given in an attempt to *relieve* the symptoms and/or *improve* the survivorship of those with the disease.

2. **Intervention trials,** in which the investigator *intervenes* before a disease has developed in individuals with characteristics that increase their risk of developing the disease.

3. **Preventive trials,** in which an attempt is made to determine the efficacy of a *preventive* agent or procedure; these are also referred to as **prophylactic** trials.

Table 10–1 provides examples of these three kinds of studies.

Table 10–1. Types and Examples of Clinical Trials

Type	Example
Therapeutic	1. Laser treatment for diabetic retinopathy
	2. Simple mastectomy for breast cancer
Intervention	1. Antihypertensive drugs to reduce the risk of developing a stroke
	2. Physical exercise for decreasing the risk of myocardial infarction
Preventive	1. BGG vaccination for tuberculosis
	2. Isoniazid for prevention of tuberculosis

If, in a randomized clinical trial of the first type, the therapeutic agent successfully relieves the symptoms of the disease or increases the survivorship, then that agent may be used to treat the disease. One such trial was that of Anturane for individuals who had suffered a myocardial infarction (2). Those who received this drug had approximately a 70 percent decrease in mortality from sudden death during the first six months after the infarction.

The second type of study, the treatment of risk factors by intervention, is illustrated by evaluations of drugs intended to reduce hypercholestrolemia and thus decrease the risk of developing coronary heart disease. If, in a randomized controlled trial, a drug successfully lowers serum cholesterol levels and this, in turn, reduces the incidence of coronary heart disease, not only has the utility of the drug been demonstrated but also a strong link has been added to the chain of evidence showing a causal relationship between elevated serum cholesterol levels and coronary heart disease. Such studies are currently in progress (28). The **cessation experiment** is also included in this category. Such a study differs from the others in that, instead of the addition of a mode of treatment, an attempt is made to evaluate the termination of a living habit considered to be of etiological importance. To confirm the causal association between cigarette smoking and lung cancer, one could select a group of cigarette smokers and randomly allocate them to two groups; the first continues to smoke and the second stops. If lung cancer mortality in the second group is lower than in the first, the causal implication is obvious.

The last type of study, the testing of a preventive agent, is illustrated by the evaluation of a vaccine for a given disease or of some form of chemoprophylaxis, such as isoniazid for tuberculosis. If a randomized clinical trial shows that the vaccine or chemoprophylactic agent lowers the incidence of the disease, then that vaccine or agent may be used as a preventive measure against the disease.

Of course, randomized clinical trials provide information relevant to the etiology and/or natural history of a disease. And one should note that a very fine line exists between the three types of clinical trials; indeed, intervention studies can be viewed as special types of either a therapeutic or preventive trial.

The general principles are essentially the same in conducting clinical trials for infectious and noninfectious diseases, but the spectrum of noninfectious diseases (see Fig. 3–10) is more complex. Each stage in the course of a chronic disease usually lasts a number of years, varying with the disease and the individual, and the distinctions between the stages are often difficult to make. In addition, the etiological agent is often unknown. In many chronic diseases, however, something is usually known about factors that are associated with an increased risk of a person developing the disease. These "risk factors" include such characteristics as elevation of serum cholesterol in the case of coronary heart disease and high blood pressure in cerebrovascular disease. Thus, in diagramming

Table 10–2. Spectrum of Selected Diseases Divided into Three Categories

Etiological Factor	Predisease State or Risk Factor	Disease
Diet?	Elevated serum cholesterol	Coronary heart disease
Virus??	*In situ* cancer of the cervix	Invasive cancer of the cervix
???	Elevated blood pressure	Stroke

RISK FACTOR OR PRE-DISEASE STATE	PATHOLOGIC CHANGES	SYMPTOMS	DIAGNOSIS	DISEASE	DEATH

the natural history of a chronic disease, we can replace "etiologic factor" in Figure 3–10 with "risk factor" (Fig. 10–1). The relationship between the risk factors and possible etiological factors for three diseases are shown in Table 10–2.

General Plan of a Clinical Trial

The plan of a clinical trial is formally stated in a **protocol,** which contains the *objectives* and *specific procedures* to be used in the trial. It must be written before the start of the trial and should contain such information as the methods for selecting the study groups and details for the performance of any laboratory tests. During the course of the trial, if any questions arise because of a given contingency, the protocol is referred to as the guide for what the investigator is to do. An outline for a typical protocol is presented in Table 10–3. Bearman's description of how to write such a protocol is an excellent guide (6).

Table 10–3.   General Outline of a Protocol for a Clinical Trial

1. Rationale and background for study
2. Specific objectives of study
3. Concise statement of the study design (masking, randomization schemes, types and duration of treatment, number of patients)
4. Criteria for including and excluding subjects
5. Outline of treatment procedures
6. Definition of all clinical, laboratory, etc., methods
7. Methods of assuring the integrity of the data
8. Major and minor endpoints (e.g., death, myocardial infarction)
9. Provisions for observing and recording side effects
10. Procedures for handling problem cases
11. Procedures for obtaining informed consent of subjects
12. Procedures for analyzing results
13. Appendices: Forms

Source: Adapted from Bearman (6).

Selection of the Study Groups

At the beginning of a clinical trial, a decision regarding the characteristics of the population to be studied must be made; that is, what
age and sex groups, disease characteristics, etc. are eligible for inclusion in the experiment. For example, in the Veterans Administration Cooperative Study on Antihypertensive Agents, the criteria
for inclusion in the study population was "hospitalized . . . male
patients whose diastolic blood pressures from the fourth through
sixth day of hospitalization averaged 115 through 129 mm Hg without treatment" (33). In brief, the investigator selects a reference or
"target" population that may be composed of persons with a certain
disease or set of characteristics related to a disease, or persons in
specific age groups, geographic areas, or occupations that would suggest their inclusion in the study. The type of reference population
selected depends on the purpose of the study, as well as the difficulties involved in reaching the individuals.

Once the "target population" has been selected, the participants
in the trial must be recruited. Several strategies have evolved for
enrolling the individuals and can generally be classified into two
types:

1. *Accrual,* in which the subjects needed for the trial are recruited during the course of the study.
2. *Nonaccrual,* in which all of the subjects needed for the trial
   are recruited before the study begins.

In both instances, the number of persons (the sample size) necessary
to detect an effect of the drug or procedure must be computed from
various statistical formulae that have been developed (3, 4).

Use of Historical Controls

At this point, one type of control group should be mentioned because of its frequent use in evaluating preventive and therapeutic
agents (17, 29). **Historical controls** are selected from patients who
had been treated in the past in one way so that their outcome can
be compared with that of patients treated with a new method. The
term is also used to describe a group of patients treated with a new
drug and compared to a much broader prior experience with a
standard form of treatment. Clearly, there is no random allocation

of patients to treatment and control groups. Such a comparison may provide acceptable evidence if prior experience with a disease indicates that the standard method of treatment had resulted in a very high case fatality rate, such as 95 percent, while the new treatment has a marked effect, resulting in, say, a 50 percent fatality rate. This was the case with penicillin. Before its introduction, the case-fatality rate from some infectious diseases was 100 percent, and this was sharply reduced when the diseases were treated with penicillin. In most instances, however, the difference between new and old treatment methods is not so marked. When a new treatment results in small improvements in the course of a disease, or a large number of known and/or unknown factors influence the outcome of the disease, it is necessary to conduct a well-planned controlled study in an explicitly defined group where the treatment(s) or absence of treatment (control) can be allocated to subgroups in a systematic manner.

Allocation

The subjects, once recruited, are randomly allocated to either the experimental (or "treatment") or control groups. Simple random allocation can be refined by using such methods as the "randomized block" design to increase the efficiency of a study (10). This design takes advantage of some of the factors that are known to influence the disease being studied. For instance, participants are often classified by sex and age, usually in five- or ten-year age groups known as "blocks" or "strata," since matching by individual years of age is impractical. When an individual is of the desired sex and within a certain age stratum, he or she is randomly assigned to a treatment or control group by a method that does not permit a difference of more than a few cases between the number treated and the number of controls within that stratum. It may also be desirable to use severity of disease as one of the strata, since severity generally has an effect on the outcome of the disease. Participants classified by severity of disease can *then* be randomly allocated to treatment and control groups by methods assuring approximately equal numbers in the treatment and control groups within each category of severity. The study group receives the new treatment, preventive agent, or whatever type of intervention is under investigation, and the control group receives the usual, accepted treatment.

Table 10–4. Mean Percent Change in Middle-Aged Men's Serum Cholesterol Level, National Diet–Heart Study

Diet	Minneapolis–St. Paul	Oakland
B	−14.7	−11.0
C	−15.5	−10.9
D	− 7.3	− 1.8

Source: Adapted from Ederer (16).

MULTICENTER CONTROLS

If the study is a collaborative one involving many hospitals (which is often necessary to obtain a sufficient number of subjects), a control group is needed at each center. Each of these centers represents a separate stratum; one center's control group *cannot* serve as a control for the other centers. This is illustrated in Table 10–4, with the results from two of the centers in the National Diet–Heart Study, a randomized clinical trial that attempted to determine the influence of several different diets on serum cholesterol (1, 16).

The data in Table 10–4 show the mean percent change in middle-aged men's serum cholesterol level for two experimental diets (B and C) and one control diet (D) at the Minneapolis–St. Paul and Oakland centers. Consider what one would conclude from using the Minneapolis–St. Paul diet D as the control for Oakland—that there was a 3 percent to 4 percent change in the serum cholesterol level in Oakland men. Yet, by subtracting each center's diet D from the diets B and C, it is clear that the net effect obtained is the same in each center, i.e., an 8 percent–9 percent decrease in serum cholesterol levels. Without a control group at each center, one might also be tempted to conclude that the diets were more effective at Minneapolis–St. Paul than at Oakland. The allocation of subjects to a control group at each center is necessary since hospitals vary in their admission policies and in the characteristics of the patients they serve.

Compliance (Reliability)

Epidemiologists cannot be certain that a treatment is or is not effective unless they can be assured that the experimental group is actually receiving the treatment; thus, it is necessary to determine compliance or reliability (22). A common strategy for assessing the compliance of patients in taking their medication, when it is a pill, is to give them more pills than they need. They are instructed to return the unused pills, which are then counted. A comparison is made between the number of pills returned and the amount that should have been returned if the patient had taken the proper number.

Other ways of assessing reliability have been used. In the previously mentioned Veterans Administration antihypertensive study, patients had to pass certain reliability tests before they could be included in the trial. For example, patients of "dubious reliability," such as vagrants and alcoholics, were excluded from the trial. A biological method was used in the Anturane Reinfarction Trial (2). It was known that Anturane had the pharmacologic effect of lowering serum uric acid levels. The investigators determined the serum uric acid levels in both the experimental and control groups. The uric acid levels decreased in the experimental group and did not in the control group, thereby indicating that those in the experimental group had been reliable in taking their medication.

Determination of the Effect

The clinical trial requires that observations be made for each participant concerning the effect of the treatment being evaluated. In some situations, the individual participant is essentially the "observer" of the effect, as in the assessment of pain; in other situations a physician must determine if the individual's disease status has been altered or if the disease has been prevented. Unfortunately, knowledge of whether the participant was in the treatment or control group can influence the observation, resulting in *biased inferences,* either consciously or subconsciously. Of course, if death is the outcome or effect being measured, the possibility of bias is considerably diminished. To remove these sources of bias in the observations, three procedures for making the necessary observations have evolved (4, 5, 16, 18, 23):

1. *Single blind* (or "single masked")
2. *Double blind* (or "double masked")
3. *Triple blind* (or "triple masked").

Single blinding. In a single blind study, the participants are not given any indication whether they are in the experimental or control group. The object of single blinding is to prevent the participant from introducing bias into the observations, and is usually accomplished by means of a placebo. An example of the need for a placebo can be found in the mammary artery coronary bypass surgery trials of the 1950s for the treatment of angina pectoris; the control group underwent a sham procedure in which only the skin was cut (15). In one particular trial, 10 of 13 patients who were operated on showed marked improvement in the degree of angina pectoris; however, *all five* of the patients who had only a skin incision also reported marked improvement! This suggested that an individual's perception of pain was influenced by knowing that he had been operated on.

Double blinding. Double blinding seeks to remove biases that occur as a result of *either the subject or the observer of the subject* being influenced by knowledge that the subject is in the control or experimental group. The bias due to the subject's knowledge of his allocation can be eliminated by single blinding, as already described; to eliminate the bias that may result from the observer's knowledge requires that the observer also be "blind" with respect to the subject's allocation. Thus, in a "double blind" study, both the subject and the observer (or assessor) of the subject are "blind" regarding the subject's group allocation.

When examination of the subjects is not necessary to measure the outcome and an objective test such as an electrocardiogram or laboratory procedure is available, it is a simple matter to assemble the records and have them interpreted by someone not involved in the study. In addition, it is often considered desirable to use mortality as the end point of a study since this leaves little room for subjective judgment. Even so, when specific causes of death are used as an end point, their determination can be biased by knowing in which group the subject belongs.

Triple blinding. Triple blind studies carry the concept of blinding one step further than does a double blind study; *the subject, the observer of the subject, and the person analyzing the data* are all "blind" with regard to the group to which a specific individual belongs. Two examples of the bias that can occur in a double blind

Table 10–5. Overview of the Various Types of Blinding Used in Clinical Trials

	Type of blinding		
	Single	Double	Triple
Subject	⊠	⊠	⊠
Observer	—	⊠	⊠
Data analyst	—	—	⊠

⊠ = blind with respect to subject's allocation

— = may be aware of subject's allocation

trial when the data analyst is conscious of which group is the experimental one and which is the control are given in references 31 and 32.

Double blinding is the most frequently used method when a blind trial is conducted. Ideally, of course, triple blinding should be used, as it eliminates more possibilities of bias, but, unfortunately, it is not very popular today. An overview of the various types of blinding is schematically presented in Table 10–5.

Some Problems

VOLUNTEERS

In many studies, only volunteers can be used. This limits the inferences that can be derived from their results, since several investigations have shown that volunteers differ in several significant ways from nonvolunteers.

The design of the National Diet–Heart Study made it possible to compare the characteristics of those who volunteered and those who did not (1, 13). The volunteers were more frequently found to be non-cigarette smokers, more concerned about health, members of community organizations, more active in community affairs, possessed of more formal education, and employed in professional and skilled positions. A larger proportion of volunteers than nonvolunteers were Protestants or Jews and lived in households with children. If any of these characteristics were related to the outcome being measured, the investigator would have to limit his inferences from the study's results and generalize cautiously. Of course, the degree of limitation also would depend on the percentage of participants who volunteered.

The problem of differences between volunteers and nonvolunteers can be dealt with, to some extent, by following the nonvolunteers in the same way as the volunteers to determine their outcome. Even if such follow-up is limited to mortality data, comparisons between the volunteer and nonvolunteer groups will provide valuable information on the generalizability of the results.

REFUSALS TO CONTINUE IN THE STUDY (WITHDRAWALS)

In any follow-up study, there will be those who, at some point, withdraw from the study. In the National Diet–Heart Study, Crocetti found that the long-term participants were more aware of the relationship of diet to heart disease and more active in community organizations than the short-term participants (13). The presence of withdrawals could bias the results of a study. As with nonvolunteers, this problem can be partially solved by obtaining whatever information is possible on the characteristics of the withdrawals in addition to determining their outcome. It may be advisable to select a random sample of withdrawals for intensive follow-up depending on their number and the difficulty of obtaining information about them.

LOST TO FOLLOW-UP

The need to keep the proportion of persons lost to follow-up at a minimum was discussed in the context of prospective studies (see Chap. 9, p. 242). Attempts should be made to obtain such minimal information on this group as mortality data. It may be necessary to randomly select a sample on which to focus these efforts.

INTERVENTION STUDIES

In the treatment of risk factors and cessation experiments, there is a special problem which reflects the biological features of some chronic, noninfectious diseases. Does a negative result in the examples cited earlier—the coronary disease and lung cancer trials— indicate that no causal relationship exists between the risk factors that were experimentally modified and the specific disease? The answer is a negative one since it is quite conceivable that the underlying pathological process could represent the cumulative effect of exposure to the etiological agent over many years and that this process had already reached an irreversible state in those studied. Thus, either type of study may lead to a negative finding from which a negative inference cannot be drawn. There is no general rule for interpreting negative results of cessation and risk-factor treatment studies of chronic disease. The results of each study must be evaluated in terms of the current knowledge of the particular disease.

Integrity of the Data

One of the most frequently overlooked aspects in the design of a clinical trial is maintaining the integrity of the data; this issue is critical to the success of a multi-center trial and is of general importance in any trial (2, 12). The epidemiologist must be certain that the data from the trial are accurately recorded, as well as accurately transferred from one medium to another. All forms should be clear in their instructions.

Perhaps the easiest way of assuring that the integrity of the data has not been violated is by having a group of epidemiologists and/or biostatisticians not involved with the trial conduct an audit of the data. This was done in the Anturane Trial discussed above. An independent audit of the completed trial that was done on a sample of the collected data indicated errors in less than 1 percent of the data.

Analysis of Results

Although many statistical methods of analyzing clinical trials have been developed, the actual statistical analysis of the data is probably the least important aspect (14). If the trial has been conducted in an uncomplicated manner, then the analysis of the data should be straightforward.

Several tools are available for the analysis of clinical trial data, but the epidemiologist should first compare the characteristics of the two groups in order to assure their comparability. The Veterans Administration Cooperative Study on Anti-hypertensive Medication is a good example of this (Table 10–6 and 10–7) (33). Clearly, the two groups were comparable on a large number of characteristics.

After ascertaining the comparability of the experimental and

Table 10–6. Comparison of Patient's Qualitative Characteristics Present at Beginning of Veterans Administration Cooperative Study on Antihypertensive Agents

Characteristic	Number of Patients Who Received	
	Placebo	Drug
Total randomized	70	73
White	35	31
Negro	35	42
Family history of hypertension		
None	19	23
Present	48	49
Unknown	3	1
Cardiac symptoms		
None	48	52
Present	22	21
Heart size by roentgenogram		
Ungerleider normal	39	44
Ungerleider enlarged	31	29
Electrocardiogram		
Left ventricular hypertrophy absent	48	49
Left ventricular hypertrophy present	22	24
Prior cardiovascular thrombosis	5	6
Occipital headaches	12	10
Diabetes absent	65	65
Diabetes present	5	8

Source: Veterans Administration Cooperative Study Group on Anti-hypertensive Agents (33). Reprinted from *The Journal of the American Medical Association*, 202:1028–1034, 1967. Copyright 1967, American Medical Association.

control groups, the investigator must determine whether the treatment was effective. Several methods have been developed to do this; the one most commonly used is the *life-table*. Another is known as *sequential analysis* (4). In this method, the endpoint of the trial is not fixed. Rather, the investigator analyzes the data at intervals to determine whether a statistical difference exists. If it does, the trial stops; if it does not, the trial continues. Details on several other methods of analysis that are available are provided in some of the references (3, 8, 10, 14, 17, 19). Many of the methods are very specific in their area of application, and newer methods are constantly being devised (21, 24, 25, 27, 30).

When analyzing results, it is worthwhile to compare the information obtained early in a study on the withdrawals and persons lost

Table 10–7. Comparison of Patient's Characteristics at Beginning of Veteran's Administration Cooperative Study on Anti-hypertensive Agents

Characteristic	Placebo Mean	Placebo SD	Drug Mean	Drug SD
Age (yr)	51.4	10.8	50.0	8.7
Height (in)	69.0	2.6	68.7	2.9
Weight (lb)	182.9	34.5	185.2	36.7
Duration known hypertension (yr)	5.4	4.4	5.3	4.7
Average hospital diastolic pressure (mm Hg)	105.8	8.4	106.5	8.4
Average clinic systolic (mm Hg)	186.8	17.2	185.6	15.4
Average clinic diastolic (mm Hg)	121.0	4.7	121.2	5.0
Severity grades (0–4)				
Fundi (hypertensive)	1.2	—	1.3	—
Fundi (sclerotic)	1.3	—	1.4	—
Cardiac	1.2	—	1.0	—
Central nervous system	0.4	—	0.3	—
Renal	0.5	—	0.3	—
Blood glucose, fasting (mg/100 cc)	96.8	20.6	97.7	18.9
Blood glucose, 2-hr postprandial	118.0	41.5	116.1	54.3
Cholesterol (mg/100 cc)	251.3	59.5	242.0	51.5

Source: Veterans Administration Cooperative Study Group on Anti-hypertensive Agents (33). Reprinted from *The Journal of the American Medical Association,* 202:1028–1034, 1967, American Medical Association.

to follow-up with that obtained on those who remained in the study, and thus determine whether there are any differences between the groups. In these attempts to avoid bias, the investigator usually should assume the most conservative outcome for those patients who have withdrawn from the study or have been lost to follow-up. A broad estimate of the effect of these groups on the overall findings can be made by calculating the two extremes of a range, one based on assuming the most conservative outcome and the other based on assuming the best possible otucome. Of course, this determination depends on the endpoint used in a specific study.

A schematic outline of a clinical trial is given in Figure 10–2. Simply stated, the investigator specifies all aspects of the trial before it is started. He then follows that protocol rigidly. Perhaps the best advice on the conduct of a randomized experiment is that given by Cornfield: "Be careful" (11).

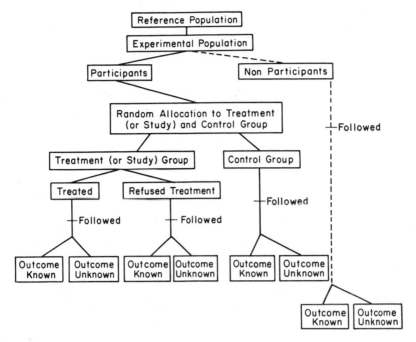

Figure 10–2. Outline of randomized clinical trial

C. ETHICAL CONSIDERATIONS

Clinical trials are similar in many ways to the observational studies discussed in Chapters 8 and 9. Because of the random allocation of subjects to the experimental and control groups, however, certain ethical questions naturally arise. These ethical issues have become of increasing concern to investigators, institutions, and sponsoring agencies. A detailed consideration of these issues is beyond the scope of this book. The reader is referred to Hill's and Chalmer's excellent discussions of this issue (9, 24). Hill has aptly stated the dilemma facing the investigator (24):

> The question at issue, then, is whether it is proper to withhold from any patient a treatment that might, perhaps, give him benefit. The value of the treatment is, clearly, not proven; if it were, there would be no need for a trial. But, on the other hand, there must be some basis for it—whether it be from evidence obtained in test tubes, animals or even in a few patients. There must be some basis to justify a trial at all.

Table 10–8. Ethical Considerations in a Clinical Trial

1. Is the proposed treatment safe for (unlikely to bring harm to) the patient?
2. For the sake of a controlled trial, can a treatment ethically be withheld from any patient in the doctor's care?
3. What patients may be brought into a controlled trial and allocated randomly to any of the different treatments?
4. Is it ethical to use a placebo or dummy treatment?
5. Is it proper for the trial to be in any way blind?

Source: Adapted from Hill (24).

It is clear that before a trial can be carried out, the consent of the subjects to participate must be obtained; it is important that the subjects be informed that they may be assigned to *either* the experimental or control groups. If the subjects, provided with this information, still decide to participate in the study, then they are said to have given their *"informed consent."* Such consent should be obtained in writing in accordance with regulations of governmental agencies (in the U.S.), or of the institution where the trial is to be conducted.

The investigator may, nonetheless, be troubled by the idea of withholding a possibly beneficial treatment from someone who is ill or at the risk of developing a disease. Green's statement is one of the better responses to this problem (24):

> Where the value of a treatment, old or new, is doubtful, there may be a higher moral obligation to test it critically than to continue to prescribe it year-in-year-out with the support merely of custom or wishful thinking.

Hill has provided some general criteria for the ethical conduct of clinical trials (Table 10–8). The investigator must also keep in mind whether it is ethical if *no trial* is conducted.

STUDY PROBLEMS

1. What are the differences and similarities between clinical trials and natural experiments? Between clinical trials and prospective studies?
2. Explain the concept of randomization.

3. A triple blind, multi-center randomized clinical trial of a newly discovered therapeutic drug was conducted recently. Ten centers, all in the same state, participated in this trial; in each center subjects were randomly assigned to either the experimental or control groups. All observations were sent to a central coordinating center, where they were analyzed. The trial indicated that the drug was clearly effective (using standard statistical techniques).
   a) List the various tabulations of the data that would be needed for a proper analysis of the drug's effectiveness.
   b) What inferences can be derived from such a trial?
   c) List the various problems that could occur during such a trial. How might they be handled?
   d) What questions should a physician ask himself about the trial before using the drug in his practice?
4. What types of research on a new agent should be done before using it in a clinical trial? Why?
5. What might be the advantages and disadvantages in conducting a sequential clinical trial in contrast to a nonsequential one?
6. In the discussion of "blinding," it was noted that there are certain advantages in conducting a trial in a double blind rather than a single blind manner, and in conducting a trial in a triple blind manner rather than a double blind one. What disadvantages might there be in using the double blind approach rather than the single blind one, and in using the triple blind approach rather than the double blind one?
7. What methods can one use to surmount the problems encountered by studying volunteers?
8. List several situations in which a randomized clinical trial could be considered unethical. What other methods could be used in these situations? Discuss the limitations of each of these methods.
9. What are the limitations of the randomized clinical trial?

REFERENCES

1. American Heart Association. 1968. *The National Diet–Heart Study: Final Report*. Amer. Heart Assoc. Monogr. No. 18, New York: The American Heart Association, Inc.
2. Anturane Reinfarction Trial Research Group. 1978. "Sulfinpyrazone in the prevention of cardiac death after myocardial infarction." *N. Engl. J. Med.* 298:289–295.

3. Armitage, P. 1971. *Statistical Methods in Medical Research*. Oxford: Blackwell.

4. ———. 1975. *Sequential Medical Trials,* 2nd ed., New York: John Wiley and Sons.

5. Ballintine, E.J. 1975. "Objective measurements and the double masked procedure." *Amer. J. Ophthalmol.* 79:763–767.

6. Bearman, J.E. 1975. "Writing the protocol for a clinical trial." *Amer. J. Ophthalmol.* 79:775–778.

7. Breslow, N.E. 1978. "Perspectives on the statistician's role in cooperative clinical research." *Cancer* 41:326–332.

8. Bury, K.V. 1975. *Statistical Models in Applied Science*. New York: John Wiley and Sons.

9. Chalmers, T.C. 1975. "Ethical aspects of clinical trials." *Amer. J. Ophthalmol.* 79:753–758.

10. Cochran, W.G., and Cox, G.M. 1957. *Experimental Designs*. 2nd ed. New York: John Wiley and Sons.

11. Cornfield, J. 1959. "Principles of research." *Amer. J. Mental Defic.* 64:240–252.

12. Council for International Organizations of Medical Sciences. 1960. *Conference on Controlled Clinical Trials*. Hill, A.B., Chairman. Springfield, Ill.: Charles C Thomas.

13. Crocetti, A.F. 1970. "An interview study of volunteers and nonvolunteers in a medical research project." Thesis, Dr.P.H., School of Hygiene and Public Health, The Johns Hopkins University.

14. Cutler, S.J., Greenhouse, S.W., Cornfield, J., and Schneiderman, M.A. 1966. "The role of hypothesis testing in clinical trials." *J. Chron. Dis.* 19:857–882.

15. Dimond, E.G., Kittle, C.F., and Crocket, J.E. 1958. "Evaluation of internal mammary artery ligation and sham procedure in angina pectoris (abstract)." *Circulation* 18:712.

16. Ederer, F. 1975. "Why do we need controls? Why do we need to randomize?" *Amer. J. Ophthalmol.* 79:758–762.

17. ———. ed. 1975. *The Randomized Controlled Clinical Trial*. National Eye Institute Workshop for Ophthalmologists, Washington, D.C.: U.S. Department of Health, Education and Welfare.

18. England, J.M. 1975. *Medical Research*. Edinburgh: Churchill Livingstone.

19. Fleiss, J.L. 1973. *Statistical Methods for Rates and Proportions*. New York: John Wiley and Sons.

20. Gilbert, J.P. 1974. "Randomization of human subjects." *N. Engl. J. Med.* 291:1305–1306.

21. Gross, A.J., and Clark, V.A. 1975. *Survival Distributions: Reliability Applications in the Biomedical Sciences*. New York: John Wiley and Sons.

22. Haynes, R.B., Taylor, D.W., and Sackett, D.L., eds. 1978. *Compliance in Health Care*. Baltimore: Johns Hopkins University Press.

23. Hill, A.B. 1951. "The clinical trial." *Brit. Med. Bull.* 7:278–282.

24. ———. 1977. *A Short Textbook of Medical Statistics*. 10th ed. Philadelphia: J.B. Lippincott Co.

25. Lancaster, H.O. 1974. *An Introduction to Medical Statistics*. New York: John Wiley and Sons.

26. Lasagna, L. 1955. "The controlled clinical trial: Theory and practice." *J. Chron. Dis.* 1:353–367.

27. Mann, N.R., Schafer, R.E., and Singpurwalla, N.D. 1974. *Methods for Statistical Analysis of Reliability and Life Data*. New York: John Wiley and Sons.

28. Multiple Risk Factor Intervention Trial Group. 1977. "Statistical design considerations in the NHLI multiple risk factor intervention trial (MRFIT)." *J. Chron. Dis.* 20:261–275.
29. Peto, R., Pike, M.C., Armitage, P., Breslow, N.E., Cox, D.R., Howard, S.V., Mantel, N., McPherson, K., Peto, J., and Smith, P.G. 1976. "Design and analysis of randomized clinical trials requiring prolonged observation of each patient: I. Introduction and Design." *Brit. J. Cancer* 34:585–612.
30. ———, Pike, M.C., Armitage, P., Breslow, N.E., Cox, D.R., Howard, S.V., Mantel, N., McPherson, K., Peto, J., and Smith, P.G. 1977. "Design and analysis of randomized clinical trials requiring prolonged observation of each patient: II. Analysis and examples." *Brit. J. Cancer* 35:1–39.
31. Reynolds, E., Joyce, C.R.B., Swift, J.L., Tooley, P.H., and Weatherall, M. 1965. "Psychological and clinical investigation of the treatment of anxious out-patients with three barbiturates and placebo." *Brit. J. Psychiat.* 111:84–95.
32. Uhlenhuth, E.H., Canter, A., Neustadt, J.O., and Payson, H.E. 1959. "The symptomatic relief of anxiety with meprobamate, phenobarbital and placebo." *Amer. J. Psychiat.* 115:905–910.
33. Veterans Administration Cooperative Study Group on Antihypertensive Agents. 1967. "Effects of treatment on morbidity in hypertension: Results in patients with diastolic blood pressure averaging 115 through 129 mm Hg." *JAMA* 202:1028–1034.
34. Zelen, M. 1974. "The randomization and stratification of patients to clinical trials." *J. Chron. Dis.* 27:365–375.

11 Experimental Epidemiology: II. Community Trials

> 1) That by experiment it might be ascertained in what excreta the poisons of certain of the epidemic diseases are located. . . .
> 3) Whether the virus of a disease in reproducing its disease in a healthy body, acts . . . by its own reproduction and presence, or by the evolution of another principle or product.
> 4) Whether climate, season, or other external influences modify the course of epidemics, by reproducing modifications of the epidemic poisons or modifications in the system of persons exposed to the poisons.
>
> "The Investigation of Epidemics by Experiments" B. W. RICHARDSON, 1858

Experimental epidemiology derives its strength from the investigator's ability to *control the conditions* under which a study is conducted. One of the principal means of control in a clinical trial is by randomly allocating individual subjects to the exposed and non-exposed groups, as discussed in Chapter 10. However, there are situations in experimental epidemiology that do not lend themselves to a randomized clinical trial. The determination of various factors that influence the course of an epidemic in a community (or group) can only be studied experimentally in an animal community. In fact, it should be noted that the term "experimental epidemiology" was originally used to describe these experimental animal epidemics, whereas in this book it is used in a broader sense (8).

Experiments that involve communities as a whole are known as "community trials," whether they are conducted in animals or humans. It should be emphasized that in a community trial, the group as a whole is collectively studied, while in a clinical trial it is the individual within a group (the experimental or control group) that is studied.

A. EXPERIMENTAL EPIDEMICS

Experimental epidemiology in animal communities took its classical form in the 1920s and 1930s from the work of Webster in the United States and Topley, Wilson, and Greenwood in England (7–9, 12, 13, 15). Greenwood summarized the aims of these experimental epidemics as (7):

> An attempt to simplify the study of general epidemiology by (1) limiting the number of variable factors (for example, rigorously excluding from the herd under observation all but one extraneous infection); (2) taking as the object of study a herd of short-lived animals, so that the time-scale of observations is magnified.

These investigations were conducted by selecting groups of mice, infecting them with an infectious agent, varying the host and environmental factors, and determining the effect of these factors on the development of epidemics in these animal populations. When these experiments were initiated in the 1920s, it was generally accepted that the rise and fall of epidemics in human populations, where the infectious agent was already established, was due to changes in the virulence of the microorganism and in the immunization of that portion of the population exposed to it by chance in small doses (15). These views changed radically as a result of the experimental production of epidemics in animals. Epidemics were found to result from changes in the proportion of susceptible individuals and the degree of contact between the susceptibles and the disease carriers in the population. The modern understanding of "herd immunity" can be traced to these findings (see Chap. 3, p. 61).

An important issue studied by these early investigators was the possible effect of a change from continuous to discontinuous contact within the animal community at the start and continuation of an epidemic. In one study, mice were placed in cages—one to a cage—and twenty-five were infected with mouse typhoid bacillus (*Salm. typhimurium*) while one hundred were not (12). Each Monday, Wednesday, and Friday, all the mice were assembled in a single large cage for a period of four hours, and each day, two normal, noninfected mice were added to the group. A small epidemic started among the normal mice, but quickly died down. After about 70 days, no deaths from mouse typhoid occurred, nor did any occur

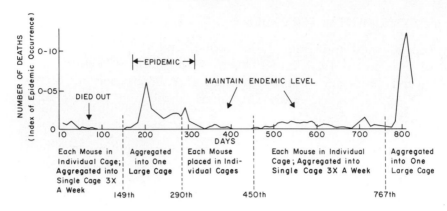

Figure 11–1. Diagrammatic representation of occurrence of epidemics among mice infected with mouse typhoid bacilli with changes in continuity of contact between mice

Source: Topley (12).

for a period of 149 days from the beginning of the experiment (Fig. 11–1). Since no deaths from mouse typhoid had occurred for about 80 days, it was decided to alter the experimental conditions. All the mice were aggregated into a single large cage and a major epidemic developed within a few days. After the 289th day, each mouse was removed and placed in a separate cage without being aggregated; the epidemic gradually declined and finally died out. Four hundred and fifty days after the experiment began, the mice were again re-aggregated three times a week, resulting in a low level of mortality. This level continued until the 767th day, when the mice were again put into a single cage, resulting in an acute major epidemic that reached a peak at about the 800th day, when the experiment was terminated. Thus continuous contact produced epidemics and discontinuous, infrequent, and short contacts generally led to a low level of mortality (endemicity). The absence of any contact terminated an acute major epidemic.

Among the findings from these experimental epidemics were the following:

1. If susceptible mice are added to infected mouse populations, recurrent epidemics develop and if the addition of susceptible mice is discontinued, the infection dies out in the population.

2. A high and constant immigration rate is associated with a relatively high death rate, a short interepidemic interval, and the regular occurrence of epidemics (following the usual epidemic curve).
3. Variation in the death rates of different inbred strains of mice showed that genetic factors influence resistance to infection.
4. Epidemics may not occur, even though less than 100 percent of the animal population has acquired immunity. This led to the concept of "herd" immunity (see Chap. 3, p. 61).
5. Dispersing the members of a population will affect the course of an epidemic if the total population is segregated into small enough groups. When the population was dispersed into a few relatively large groups, there was no effect; dispersal into many small groups, however, shortened the period of the epidemic. This latter effect was interpreted as being the result of decreasing contact between individual members of the animal population.

Christian has recently reinterpreted these classic experiments in terms of the influence of crowding, social behavior, and hormonal factors on the occurrence of disease (2). There is evidence that adrenocortical hormones suppress the immune mechanism of the host and, therefore, increase the pathogenicity of different infectious agents. Christian noted that new migrants into an animal population are usually in a socially subordinate position, leading to increased adrenocortical activity, which, in turn, inhibits immunological defense mechanisms. He therefore hypothesized that the mouse epidemics described by Topley and his colleagues may have been influenced by this sequence of events, rather than, or in addition to, representing a direct effect of increased contact.

Problems are encountered in extrapolating findings from animal experiments to man. Genetic, biochemical, and physiological factors that influence the occurrence of disease differ between animals and man; in many instances, they even vary between different species of animals. As Greenwood noted (7):

We can undoubtedly control many of the conditions of life of a herd of mice; but, on the other hand, our knowledge of the social biology of mice is more scanty than our knowledge of the social biology of men, and the conditions of life we can secure for our herds are no doubt very different from those appertaining to a colony of mice living . . . in the Sylvan world of mice. The application of our results to the elucidation of the problems of human epidemiology is therefore analogical at two removes. There is a gap between our mice and mice in general and men in general. We are, however, no rasher in this way than other experimental biologists are forced to be.

B. HUMAN COMMUNITY TRIALS

Human community trials have been conducted when particular circumstances required that the community as a whole serve as the experimental unit with regard to testing a specific etiological hypothesis or preventive procedure (3, 6, 11). The very nature of such trials does not usually allow the use of randomization. An example of this type of trial is the introduction of fluorides into the water supply in order to determine whether this would decrease the frequency of dental caries (see Chap. 1, p. 5) (1).

Classical community trials were conducted by Goldberger and his colleagues in studying the dietary etiology and prevention of pellegra (5, 6). Their human communities were closed ones—two orphanages and two wards of a state mental institution. In one of their earlier papers, these investigators described their approach as follows (5):

> Since the study was carried on throughout along the lines adopted at its beginning, and since, as stated, later results were in close harmony with those of the first year, it will be helpful to review at the outset the methods and results of the first year.
>
> *First year.*—The test of the preventive value of diet was begun at two orphanages at Jackson, Miss., in September, 1914, and in two wards of the Georgia State Sanitarium later that same year. These institutions had been endemic foci of the disease for some years. During the spring and summer of 1914, 79 cases of pellagra had been observed among the children of one orphanage and 130 among those of the other. . . .
>
> At the orphanages the diet of all the residents, and at the sanitarium that of a group of selected inmates of two wards set aside for the purpose, was modified in several respects, among others in that oatmeal almost entirely replaced grits as the breakfast cereal and the allowance of fresh animal protein foods (milk, meat, and, at the orphanages, eggs) and legumes was greatly increased. The allowance of maize was thus reduced but not abolished. . . .

At about the end of the first year following the inauguration of the modified diet, it was found that, at the orphanages, of an aggregate of 172 pellagrins who had completed at least the anniversary date of the 1914 attack under observation, only 1 had showed any evidence of a recurrence, and not a single case developed among an aggregate of 168 nonpellagrins who had been continuously under observation at least one year; and at the sanitarium of an aggregate of 72 pellagrins who had either remained continuously under observation up to October 1, 1915, or, at least, until after the anniversary date of the 1914 attack, not one presented recognizable evidence of a recurrence, although at the same time 47 per cent of a comparable group of 32 pellagrins not receiving the modified diet had recurrent attacks of the disease.

Second year.—The results of the first year . . . very clearly indicated that the disease could be prevented by an appropriate diet. Nevertheless by reason of the importance of the question involved, and in order to make the test and demonstration of preventability as convincing as possible, it seemed desirable to continue the investigation, as originally planned, for at least another year and, if possible, on a larger scale. . . .

The result of this more extensive test of the preventability of pellagra by dietary means was in the closest harmony with that of the first year. In not a single one of the individuals receiving the modified diet at the three orphanages and at the hospital for insane did pellagra develop either as an initial or a recurrent attack. So impressive was this outcome that it seemed unnecessary longer to continue the demonstration on so large a scale. Accordingly, the study at the orphanages was discontinued on September 1, 1916; but because of the much greater significance likely to attach to results of tests in the insane, that at the state Sanitarium was continued through a third year; that is, until December 31, 1917.

Third year.—. . . The result of the third year's study was exactly like that of the second year: no recurrence and no new case among those inmates taking the modified diet. . . .

At this point mention may be made of the history of pellagra at one of the institutions subsequent to the discontinuance of the foregoing study. Immediately following our withdrawal, there was a return to the unmodified and unsupplemented institution diet. During the period of from $3\frac{1}{2}$ to $9\frac{1}{2}$ months following this, approximately 40 per cent of those who were affected by the change in diet developed pellagra. Thereupon there were added to the institution diet, again under our direction, 4 ounces of fresh beef, about 7 ounces of sweet milk, and about 14 ounces of buttermilk per adult per day; and during an observation period of 14 months immediately succeeding the adoption of these supplements no evidence of pellagra developed in any of the group.

An interesting use of community trials was made by Watt and Lindsay in their studies of diarrheal diseases (14). One issue was to determine the effect of fly control on both the attack and death rates from diarrheal diseases including dysentery. In Hidalgo County, Texas, they selected one group of towns (Group A) for residual DDT application and another comparable group (Group B) in which no treatment was carried out. Fly counts were made using the same method in both the treated and untreated towns. Fly control activities using residual DDT were started in January 1946 in Group A, and by April the fly population was found to be smaller in the treated than in the untreated group of towns. Control activities were continued through August 1947 in these towns. In September 1947 treatment was discontinued in the originally treated Group A and was started in Group B. The result was that the fly counts were soon lower in Group B than in Group A towns.

One measure used to evaluate the efficacy of fly control was an A to B group comparison of reported death rates for Latin-American children under two years of age. This age and ethnic group was selected since it had the largest majority of all reported diarrheal disease deaths. The death rates for three cause groups are shown in Table 11–1. Up to the time fly control was started in January 1946, differences in the death rates in the two groups of towns for these causes of death were not statistically significant. Beginning with the first quarter in 1946, through August 1947, the death rates from diarrheal diseases in Group A towns were lower than those observed in Group B towns. When the change in treatment areas was made in September 1947, the death rates were essentially equal in Groups A and B in the quarter beginning in September, but in the following quarter the rate was higher in Group A. For those deaths from causes that were listed as unknown and ill-defined, a similar general pattern was observed but with greater variability because of smaller numbers, suggesting that at least some of these deaths were actually enteric infections. In contrast, no particular pattern of change was noted in death rates from all other causes of death. This pattern of change in death rates from acute diarrheal diseases was also observed with regard to the prevalence of infection and attack

Table 11–1. Reported Death Rates per 1,000 per Annum Under 2 Years of Age in Latin-American Children of Group A and Group B towns by Selected Causes and Quarters of the Year, 1945–1948

Quarters	Death Rates From					
	Diarrhea, dysentery, and related enteric infections in		Unknown and ill-defined causes in		All other causes in	
	Group A	Group B	Group A	Group B	Group A	Group B
1945						
Mar.–May	47.2	39.8	7.3	14.0	29.2	27.8
June–Aug.	46.8	49.2	17.9	15.8	34.1	19.7
Sept.–Nov.	8.8	15.6	15.9	15.6	24.7	35.2
1946						
Dec.–Feb.*	17.4	29.0	20.8	13.5	60.8	67.6
Mar.–May	13.7	40.4	0.0	17.2	54.8	53.6
June–Aug.	25.3	36.0	13.5	19.0	33.7	32.2
Sept.–Nov.	0.0	7.5	6.6	9.4	41.6	41.2
1947						
Dec.–Feb.	8.2	11.2	6.6	9.3	27.8	44.8
Mar.–May	12.9	35.0	9.7	16.6	38.7	16.6
June–Aug.	36.6	54.8	8.0	16.4	20.7	40.4
Sept.–Nov.†	20.4	19.9	12.6	7.2	22.0	29.0
1948						
Dec.–Feb.	26.3	1.8	29.4	14.4	44.8	46.8

* Fly control started this quarter in group A towns. No fly control in group B towns.
† Fly control started Sept. 1947 in group B towns. No fly control in group A towns.

Source: Watt and Lindsay (14).

Table 11–2. Poliomyelitis Attack Rates per 1,000 Population by Age Group in the Untreated and Treated Towns of Hidalgo County for Anglo-Americans and Latin-Americans

Age (years)	Attack Rates in	
	Untreated Towns	Treated Towns
Anglo-American		
<1	5.0	2.5
1–4	6.7	10.0
5–14	5.0	3.3
15+	0.0	0.6
Latin-American		
<1	4.5	3.3
1–4	2.6	2.7
5–14	0.3	0.5
15+	0.2	0.0

Source: Paffenbarger and Watt (10).

rates. The combined results of this human community trial indicated that fly control diminishes the occurrence of diarrheal diseases.

During February 1948, when this fly control program was terminating, some cases of poliomyelitis were reported in Hidalgo County (10). This provided an opportunity to evaluate the effect of fly control upon poliomyelitis incidence, which was desirable because of the then current belief that flies could serve as one means of spread of poliomyelitis virus through a community. Fly transmission was hypothesized because: 1) poliomyelitis epidemics usually occurred in the summer, 2) flies had been found to be contaminated with poliomyelitis virus under natural conditions, and 3) sources of virus had been found in human feces, in privy contents, and in sewage.

Fly control activities were continued and epidemiologic studies were initiated. In one of these studies, poliomyelitis attack rates by age and ethnic group were determined in treated and untreated towns for the period, Dec. 1, 1947, to Dec. 31, 1948. These are presented in Table 11–2, which shows that the attack rates in the treated and untreated towns were generally similar. Since the number of cases in each group was relatively small, the investigators used another method of comparison. The rates observed in each age-ethnic group in the untreated towns were used to calculate expected numbers of cases for the treated towns. These numbers were added for each age group and are shown in Table 11–3. The in-

Table 11–3. Comparison of Observed and Expected Number of Cases in Treated Towns by Age Group Corrected for Ethnic Differences, Hidalgo County, Texas

Age Group (years)	Observed Number of Cases	Expected Number of Cases
<1	6	4.1
1–4	15	17.3
5–14	8	7.4
15+	3	3.5
Total	32	32.3

Source: Paffenbarger and Watt (10).

vestigators concluded: "It is obvious from these figures that community fly control measures instituted some six months before the outbreak of poliomyelitis did not prevent the occurrence of paralytic cases of this disease, nor is there any suggestion that the number of cases was any less as a result of these measures."

Community trials are now being conducted with regard to diseases of current epidemiologic interest. A recent example is the attempt to determine whether community health education can decrease the risk of cardiovascular disease (4). In 1972 such a trial (termed by the investigators as a "field experiment") was initiated in three California communities in an attempt to modify three risk factors (cigarette smoking, elevated plasma cholesterol levels, and high blood pressure) by community education. In two of these communities, extensive mass-media campaigns were conducted over a period of two years. In one of these, face-to-face counseling was also provided for a small subgroup of high risk individuals. The third community served as a control.

In each community, people were interviewed and examined before the educational campaign began. One or two years later their knowledge and behavior with respect to diet and smoking were assessed. Physiological indicators of risk—blood pressure, relative weight, and plasma cholesterol—were also measured. The baseline values of the risk factors were remarkably uniform in these communities. The mass media and the combination of mass media plus face to face instruction had significant positive effects on all factors except relative weight after two years of campaigning. The comparison of the treated and control communities indicated an estimated decrease in risk in developing cardiovascular disease of approximately 25 percent. These results were sufficiently encouraging that the investigators have extended this community trial to five communities, which is currently in progress.

STUDY PROBLEMS

1. What are the major differences between clinical trials, reviewed in Chapter 10, and human community trials? Between natural experiments and human community trials?

2. Discuss the reasons for the differences in age-specific attack rates from poliomyelitis among Anglo-Americans and Latin-Americans shown in Table 11–2.

3. List the different reasons for conducting human community trials.

4. What are the limitations, if any, on the inferences that can be derived from the results of the California study of the effects of community education in the control of cardiovascular diseases?

5. In previous chapters, the problem of ecological fallacy was discussed. You will recall that it arose from deriving inferences from observations of groups, such as communities, or geographical or political units, rather than of individuals as in a clinical trial or observational study. Are human community trials subject to the ecological fallacy? Explain.

6. Discuss the limits of extrapolation from animal experiments, such as experimental epidemics, to the human situation.

7. In Chapter 10, the use of historical controls in clinical trials was discussed. If historical controls are used in human community trials, what factors must be taken into consideration in interpreting the findings of such a study?

8. Suppose that one randomly assigned 10,000 individuals to two communities, town A and town B. After the assignments had been made, iodine was added to the water supply of town A to prevent goiter, while the water supply of town B was left unchanged.
   a) What measurements would you make?
   b) What type of epidemiologic experiment is this study? Explain.
   c) What types of inferences can be derived from this experiment?
   d) What biases might be present in the study?

e) How might these biases be 1) eliminated or 2) corrected for in the analysis?

9. It is generally accepted that the design of a clinical trial is more important than the analysis of its results. Why? Is this also true of community trials? Explain.

10. List at least three situations in which one would conduct 1) an animal community trial and 2) a human community trial.

11. List some situations in which it would be preferable to conduct a human community trial rather than a clinical trial.

12. Discuss the ethical aspects of human community trials.

13. The housefly feeds on typhoid-bacilli infected excreta in the sickroom or privy and is able to carry such excreta from the sick to the well. In a city with a stable population, the privies in the city were often open and accessible to the housefly. In a period of a few months toward the end of one year, the privies were all made flyproof. The following number of cases of typhoid fever occurred in the city the year before and the year after the privies were made flyproof, by month.

	Typhoid cases occurring:	
Month	Year before privies were made flyproof	Year after privies were made flyproof
January	8	9
February	0	5
March	4	7
April	6	4
May	41	11
June	41	18
July	109	10
August	82	5
September	14	7
October	15	8
November	7	2
December	2	4
Total	329	90

a) What inferences could you derive from these data?

b) Are there any additional data you would like to have before deriving any inferences? If so, list the kinds of data.

REFERENCES

1. Ast, D.B., and Schlesinger, E.R. 1956. "The conclusion of a ten-year study of water fluoridation." *Amer. J. Pub. Health* 46:265–271.
2. Christian, J.J. 1968. "The potential role of the adrenal cortex as affected by social rank and population density on experimental epidemics." *Amer. J. Epid.* 87:255–266.
3. Cochrane, A.L. 1972. *Effectiveness and Efficiency: Random Reflections on Health Services.* London: The Nuffield Provincial Hospital Trust.
4. Farquhar, J., Wood, P.D., Breitrose, H., Haskell, W.L., Meyer, A.J., Maccoby, N., Alexander, J.K., Brown, B.W., Jr., McAlister, A.L., Nash, J.D., and Stern, M.P. 1977. "Community education for cardiovascular health." *Lancet* 1:1192–1195.
5. Goldberger, J., Waring, C.H., and Tanner, W.F. 1923. "Pellagra prevention by diet among institutional inmates." *Pub. Health Reps.* 38:2361–2368.
6. ———. 1964. *Goldberger on Pellagra.* M. Terris, ed. Baton Rouge: Louisiana State University Press.
7. Greenwood, M. 1931. "Observations on the factors determining the difference between an epidemic of one disease and that of another." *Brit. Med. J.* 2:231–234.
8. ———. 1932. *Epidemiology: Historical and Experimental.* Baltimore: The Johns Hopkins Press.
9. ———, Hill, A.B., Topley, W.W.C., and Wilson, J. 1936. *Experimental Epidemiology.* Medical Research Council Spec. Rep. Series No. 209. London: His Majesty's Stationery Office.
10. Paffenbarger, R.S., Jr., and Watt, J. 1953. "Poliomyelitis in Hidalgo County, Texas, 1948." *Amer. J. Hyg.* 58:269–287.
11. Rivlin, A.M. 1971. *Systematic Thinking for Social Action.* Washington, D.C.: The Brookings Institution.
12. Topley, W.W.C. 1942. The Croonian Lecture: "The biology of epidemics." *Proc. Roy. Soc. London,* Series B. 130:337–359.
13. ———, and Wilson, G.S. 1923. "The spread of bacterial infection: The problem of herd immunity." *J. Hyg.* 21:243–249.
14. Watt, J., and Lindsay, D.R. 1948. "Diarrheal disease control studies. I. Effect of fly control in a high morbidity area." *Pub. Health Reps.* 63:1319–1334.
15. Webster, L.T. 1946. "Experimental epidemiology." *Medicine* 25:77–109.

12 The Derivation of Biological Inferences from Epidemiologic Studies

> Louis' . . . method . . . is . . . the method of induction, the method of Bacon.
>
> JAMES JACKSON, Preface to
> *Effects of Bloodletting*
> by P.C.–A. LOUIS, 1836

The demonstration of a statistical relationship between a disease and biological or social characteristics is but the first step in the epidemiologic analysis of its etiology and/or natural history. The second step is to ascertain the meaning of the relationship. This chapter will deal with the inferences about the disease's etiology or natural history that can be derived from the pattern of the relationships and the reasoning by which the epidemiologist attempts to select the most plausible one. Several elements in this process have been discussed previously, but they need to be brought together into a meaningful whole. Although many of the examples in this chapter deal with noninfectious diseases, the ideas presented, as with other epidemiologic concepts (see Chap. 1), are equally valid for infectious diseases.

A. HYPOTHESES BASED ON STATISTICAL RELATIONSHIPS

Broadly speaking, a series of reported statistical associations can be explained as:

1. Artifactual (spurious)
2. Indirect, or
3. Causal or etiological.

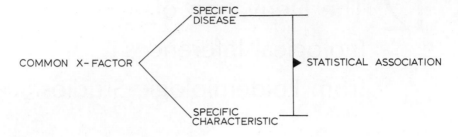

Figure 12–1.   Diagrammatic representation of an indirect statistical association between a specific disease and a specific characteristic resulting from a common "X" factor

Artifactual Associations

The possibility that an observed association represents a statistical *artifact* has been pointed out repeatedly in this book. As indicated in Chapter 8, an artifactual association can result from biased methods of selecting cases and controls. This point can be illustrated by the objections raised to certain retrospective studies of exogenous estrogens and endometrial cancer. It was argued that the users of exogenous estrogen, having had to see a physician for their prescriptions, would be more closely observed than the controls and, therefore, they would be more likely to have endometrial cancer diagnosed than the controls. A spurious association may also arise from biased methods of recording observations or obtaining information by interview. This is illustrated in its simplest form by a fictional example. Suppose that in a retrospective study of the possible relationship between automobile driving and "slipped discs" (herniated lumbar vertebral discs), an investigator, with a preconceived notion that automobile driving is of etiological importance, asks the patients "You frequently drive an automobile, don't you?" and the controls "You don't frequently drive an automobile, do you?" This difference in phrasing the question might easily lead to a difference in the response by cases and controls, resulting in an artifactual statistical association between automobile driving and slipped discs.

Indirect Association

The presence of a known or unknown factor common to both a characteristic and a disease may produce an indirect association between the two (Fig. 12–1). This can occur either in a population group (as a whole) or in individual persons. Suppose, for example, that a comparison between countries A and B reveals that there is a higher frequency of myopia ("nearsighted vision") in A than in B and that a larger proportion of the population of A than of B watches television. This, then, leads to a suspicion that television viewing and myopia are associated. However, it is possible that this suspected relationship between watching television and myopia is actually the result of another characteristic that is more prevalent in Country A than in Country B. The greater percentage of people who watch television in Country A than B may reflect, say, the higher economic status of that country. This, in turn, may affect another characteristic of the population, such as the educational system (including a lot of reading), which is causally related to myopia. The noncausal relationship between television viewing and myopia is the "ecological fallacy" referred to in Chapter 1 (p. 14). Since they are more likely to result from an ecological fallacy, associations established by studying characteristics of population groups have a greater chance of being indirect than those established by studying characteristics in individuals. In other words, it is preferable to have an association based on data obtained at the level of the individual and not at an "abstract" or "removed" level of a population or group. Conversely, an association between a disease and a characteristic observed in an individual person is more likely to be **biologically significant** than one observed in a population group. However, it is important to note that associations observed in individuals may *also* be indirect. For example, the observation that lung cancer patients have peptic ulcers more frequently than patients without lung cancer indicates that a relationship exists between peptic ulcers and lung cancer. But this relationship is an indirect one, as each disease is independently related to cigarette smoking.

Indirect associations have sometimes been called "self-selection" or "constitutional" relationships by investigators. The term "self-selection" evolved because it was hypothesized that persons predisposed to developing a certain disease have an unknown "X"-factor that automatically "selects" them for having the characteristic, particularly if it is a living habit such as diet, thereby resulting in a statistical association. Similarly, the "constitutional" hypothesis states that individuals who are predisposed to develop the disease are so physiologically constituted, possibly on a genetic basis, that they are also predisposed to having the characteristic. The difference between the two terms is purely semantic.

Causal Association

Before discussing causal associations, it is imperative to consider several issues concerning the meaning of "cause" in interpreting biological phenomena. Some investigators hold the view that a factor must be both necessary and sufficient for the occurrence of a disease before it can be considered the cause of that disease. This is the logician's definition of "cause." As one might intuitively guess, **necessary** refers to the fact that the factor *must* be present for the disease to occur, while **sufficient** indicates that if the factor is present, the disease *can* occur (but the factor's presence does not *always* result in the disease's occurrence). The concept of "necessary *and* sufficient" implies that there *must be* a one-to-one relationship between the factor and the disease; that is, whenever the factor is present, the disease must occur, and whenever the disease occurs, the factor must be present. Even in infectious diseases, however, a microorganism is not necessary and sufficient for the development of the disease; many environmental and host factors are also involved. For example, the tubercle bacillus is a necessary but not a sufficient factor in the development of tuberculosis; additional factors usually included under the term "susceptibility" are also important.

The classical rules for determining whether a microorganism can be regarded as a causal agent of an infectious disease are collectively known as the "Henle-Koch Postulates." Although the wording of these postulates varies, they can be simply stated as follows:

1. The organism must be found in all cases of the disease in question.
2. It must be isolated from patients with the disease and grown in pure culture.
3. When the pure culture is inoculated into susceptible animals or man, it must reproduce the disease.

To be considered a causal agent under these requirements, a microorganism must be a necessary condition for the occurrence of disease in man but need not be sufficient.

One wonders how rigorous the adherence has been even to the first postulate. Has the tubercle bacillus been found in 100 percent of patients with clinical manifestations of tuberculosis? No; it is found in perhaps 90 percent of clinically diagnosed cases. This does

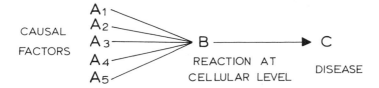

Figure 12–2. Diagrammatic representation of a causal relationship with multiple independent etiological factors

not preclude the statement that the tubercle bacillus causes tuberculosis. In actual practice, the clinician looks for another causative agent in the 10 percent of cases where the tubercle bacillus is not found. A related reason for regarding the first postulate with some suspicion is that it permits a degree of circular reasoning; the clinician does not decide that a disease with all the clinical signs and symptoms of tuberculosis is tuberculosis unless the tubercle bacillus is isolated.

Differences in causal thinking about infectious and noninfectious diseases—the latter being more likely to have multiple causal agents —depend upon the frame of reference within which the investigator operates, and reflect differences in our knowledge of the etiology of these two general categories of disease, rather than differences in logical reasoning. Cause and effect relationships, when multiple etiological factors (labeled A_1, A_2, A_3, and so on) each act independently, are illustrated in Figure 12–2. If this model is applied to carcinogenic or mutagenic agents, the etiological factors produce a change in B at a cellular level and this can lead to a change in the next level, C, the disease. Thus, each of the A factors produces a change at a cellular level, which becomes the necessary precondition of the disease.

That this sequence of events occurs in human biology is well recognized (12, 16, 29). X-radiation and a variety of chemicals and viruses, for example, may produce a neoplastic transformation of the cell resulting in clinical cancer. Many other agents may also produce cellular mutations resulting in clinical cancer. It is possible that as our knowledge of cancer increases, we may discover a common biochemical event that can be produced by each of the A factors at a molecular level. This molecular event would then be considered a necessary precondition or causal factor of cancer in conformity with the first Henle-Koch postulate. Another illustration is provided by epidemiologic investigations of coronary heart disease. A consistent, but unexplainable, sex difference has been demonstrated repeatedly. Although this difference in the incidence of this disease was discovered in the 1950s, only recently has a possible physiologic explanation (the effect of testosterone on blood clotting) been suggested by laboratory studies (42). Further, it is clear that testosterone is not *solely* responsible for the sex difference in the frequency of coronary heart disease. Similar chains of events can be postulated for other disease entities, such as congenital malformations.

This situation is similar to that of some infectious diseases. Outbreaks of typhoid fever, for instance, may result from contaminated milk, water, or food that serve as vehicles for the transmission of the disease agent, the typhoid bacillus. None of these vehicles should be regarded as a necessary cause of the disease since the others serve the same function, although the term "cause" can be applied to each. Similarly, with regard to lung cancer, cigarette smoke can be considered a "contaminated vehicle" as it has been found to be a mode of transmission for chemical carcinogens (48, 49).

Even the causal frame of reference where the typhoid bacillus is regarded as the cause of typhoid fever might be open to criticism. From a molecular biology viewpoint, the typhoid bacillus can be considered the vehicle of a specific biochemical agent, which is the "true" cause of the disease. Molecular differences, for example, have been found between the virulent and avirulent strains of the diphtheria bacillus. The virulent strain produces diphtheria toxin; the avirulent strain does not. The changing concepts of diphtheria from the microbial to the intracellular level are highly relevant in this regard (47).

It is important to remember that it was possible to control epidemics of diphtheria before the intracellular events were elucidated. In fact, even if knowledge of causative agents at a molecular level were complete, it would still be necessary, in most instances, to have information on the transmitting vehicles in order to apply the measures required for the prevention and control of many diseases. Thus, it is necessary to know that polluted water is a cause of typhoid fever; the knowledge that protein "X" in the typhoid bacillus is the causative agent at the molecular level does not directly suggest the method of control. Another illustration is provided by the results of the clinical trial of antihypertensive drug therapy for the prevention of strokes (17, 44, 45). Several studies had indicated that hypertension was one of the major causes ("risk factors") of strokes; logically, then, if one could "remove" the hypertension, (i.e., decrease the level of excess blood pressure) and then observe a decline in the incidence of stroke, the evidence that hypertension is a causal factor would be strengthened. Fries et al. conducted such a clinical trial to determine if the expected decline occurred; it did. Although the trial did not indicate why the antihypertensive drugs reduced blood pressure, at the cellular level, it did provide a means of preventing strokes.

In medicine and public health, it would appear reasonable to adopt a pragmatic concept of causality. *A causal relationship would be recognized to exist whenever evidence indicates that the factors form part of the complex of circumstances that increases the probability of the occurrence of disease and that a diminution of one or more of these factors decreases the frequency of that disease.* After all, the reason for determining etiological factors of a disease is to apply this knowledge to prevent the disease.

The model presented in Figure 12–2 is not the only multifactorial model of a causal relationship; others can be visualized. Figure 12–3 shows a model where each of the factors (A_1, A_2, and A_3) is necessary, but any individual one is not sufficient. It is also possible that each of several causative factors act independently, but when an individual is exposed to two or more, there is a synergistic effect. This sequence of events is apparent in leukemia (see Chap. 8, p. 212) and in the possible causal influence of both a familial factor and cigarette smoking in lung cancer (41). Additional and more detailed carcinogenic models are shown in Figure 3–9. Many of these issues have been discussed in a series of papers by Yerushalmy and Palmer, Lilienfeld, Sartwell, and Kempthorne (28, 32, 37, 51).

B. METHODS OF DISTINGUISHING BETWEEN HYPOTHESES

Evaluating observed statistical associations is essentially a matter of distinguishing among the three explanations discussed above. The *artifactual hypothesis* may be eliminated if the designs of the epidemiologic studies are determined to be adequate. If the studies were designed and conducted in accord with the principles that have

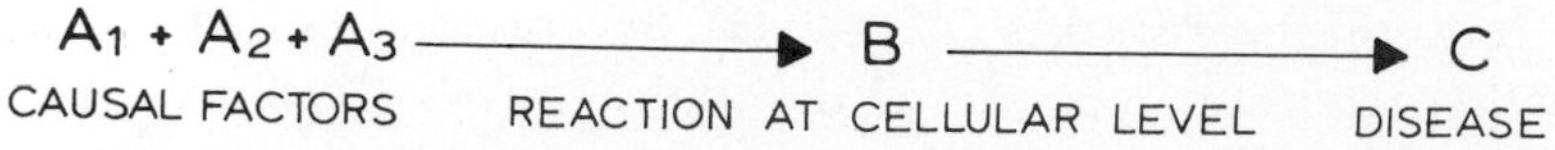

$$A_1 + A_2 + A_3 \longrightarrow B \longrightarrow C$$

CAUSAL FACTORS   REACTION AT CELLULAR LEVEL   DISEASE

Figure 12–3. Diagrammatic representation of a causal relationship with cumulative causal factors

been described in previous chapters, the artifactual hypothesis will probably be an unlikely explanation of an association. It becomes increasingly unlikely if the same statistical association is obtained from studies that are carried out in different geographical areas and population groups, and analyzed by a variety of statistical methods.

The major epidemiologic problem in evaluating a statistical relationship is to determine whether or not the association is indirect or of etiological significance. The following methods can be used to make this assessment.

Performing Controlled Randomized Experiments
in Human Population Groups

Several types of experiments can be performed in human population groups to distinguish causal from indirect associations (see Chaps. 10 and 11).

1. To study a possible relationship such as that between a diet high in saturated fat and cholesterol and the development of coronary heart disease, one might begin with the random selection of young persons (15–20 years of age) living under environmental conditions as nearly identical as possible. These individuals would be allocated at random to one group consuming a diet high in saturated fat and cholesterol and another consuming a diet low in saturated fat and cholesterol. Each group would be followed for several years to determine the incidence of coronary heart disease. If the incidence of coronary heart disease is higher in the high-fat diet group, the causal hypothesis would be proven. The underlying logic of this inference is that *randomly allocating* individuals to the two groups in the experiment makes these two groups comparable on all factors that might be assumed to be the basis for an indirect association (see Fig. 10–2). Hence, the possibility of an indirect association being responsible for any difference in the incidence of coronary heart disease between the groups is eliminated.

2. Experiments can be conducted to determine whether the ces-

sation of a living habit such as smoking or the diminution in exposure to an environmental factor of suspected etiological significance results in a decrease in the incidence of a disease. The selection and random allocation of people using oral contraceptives to groups that would continue or stop such use, followed by the observation of a decreased incidence of coronary heart disease in the oral contraceptive cessation group would strengthen the causal hypothesis for the same reasons cited earlier.

Positive results in these types of experiments essentially provide absolute proof of a causal hypothesis. It is obvious, however, that such experiments can be done only infrequently in human populations. If they are not feasible or ethical, it becomes necessary to carry out other types of studies whose collective results can provide the evidence necessary to discriminate between the indirect and causal associations.

Determining Pathogenetic Mechanisms

If the sequence of events from the time of exposure to the etiological agent through the pathogenetic mechanism to the manifestation of the disease can be elucidated, the causal hypothesis can be substantiated. This can be illustrated with cigarette smoking and lung cancer. If an isolated chemical from cigarette smoke, applied to a cell from the bronchus or lung in tissue culture, produces a neoplastic change, and if it is demonstrated that this chemical, in turn, produces a biochemical change within the cell known to be a precursor of the neoplastic transformation, then the causal hypothesis is far more credible. Although the present state of biological knowledge rarely permits such a set of observations, it is possible to determine some of the biological links in the chain of causation for many diseases; also, the addition of each link to the chain increases the biological plausibility of a causal hypothesis. In the case of oral contraceptives and thromboembolism, for example, the determination of the specific actions of estrogens on the coagulation process represents one such link (39). Similarly, for cigarette smoking, the identification of approximately fifteen chemical carcinogens in tobacco smoke and the finding that the application of tobacco tar to the tissues of several animal species produces cancer, indicate that tobacco tar contains carcinogenic agents (49). Inhalation of cigarette smoke through a tracheostomy tube in beagle dogs has resulted in carcinoma *in situ* (2). In addition, laryngeal papillomata have been produced in hamsters, thereby strengthening the links in the chain of causation. The data in Table 5–14 (p. 124), indicating that the bronchial mucosa of cigarette smokers show histological changes considered to be precancerous more frequently than that of nonsmokers, provides yet another link.

The ability to produce a particular disease in animals by exposing them to possible etiological agents considerably enhances the causal hypothesis. Though one must be cautious in generalizing from the results of animal experiments to the human condition, this may be a relatively minor problem if the results of both animal experiments and epidemiologic studies in human population are consistent (see Chaps. 10 and 11). Animal experiments can also be valuable in determining the intermediate biological mechanisms that are involved in a disease, thereby providing the basis for seeking similar mechanisms in humans. Of course, the opportunities afforded by human natural experiments should not be ignored. For example, the Coronary Drug Project, a randomized controlled clinical trial of various drugs for the prevention of reinfarction in patients with previous myocardial infarction, broke its protocol and discontinued the use of the 5 mg dose of conjugated estrogens (8). It was later found that this high estrogen dosage group also had a fourfold relative risk of pulmonary embolism compared to the placebo group.

Obtaining Additional Epidemiologic Evidence

To assess the causal nature of a statistical association, additional epidemiologic evidence should be collected. This may include information on various aspects of the association and data from different studies that makes it possible to determine the relative degree of the biological plausibility of the causal or indirect association hypotheses. The following approaches can be used:

ASSESSMENT OF VARIOUS ASPECTS OF THE ASSOCIATION

Consistency of Association. The distribution of a possible etiological factor in the population should be determined by age, color, sex, occupation, and as many other population characteristics as possible. The distribution of the disease by the same population characteristics should be ascertained. These two patterns should then be analyzed to determine whether the population distribution of the disease is consistent with that of the etiological factor. Consistency between the two strengthens a causal hypothesis, for it is unlikely that an indirect association would operate to the same degree in all subgroups of a population. Of course, complete consistency is unusual if a disease is caused by multiple factors; it will then be necessary to evaluate the degree of consistency between the two distributions in the population subgroups. Finding such consistency is logically equivalent to the replication of results in laboratory experiments under a variety of environmental or biological conditions.

The analysis of consistency of association can be illustrated by data from many studies of the relationship of oral contraceptives to cardiovascular disease in which the following observations were made:

1. An increase in pulmonary embolism mortality in women of childbearing age shortly after the introduction of oral contraceptives. Further, the increase began to slow down and, finally, reverse itself after the type of oral contraceptive was switched to those of lower-estrogen dosage (3, 34, 38).
2. Age consistency in mortality. The consistency of the relationship between oral contraceptive use and myocardial infarction

Table 12-1. Estimated Relative Risk of Death from Myocardial Infarction Among Different Categories of Oral Contraceptive Use

	Age of patients (years)	
Use of oral contraceptives	30–39	40–44
"Never users"	1.00	1.00
Current users	3.36	4.38
24 months or less	1.91	2.19
25 months or more	5.06	6.57
Ex-users	2.18	0.55
"Ever users"	2.92	1.82
"Never users" and ex-users	1.00	1.00
Current users	2.80	4.55

Source: Jain (25). Reprinted from *The American Journal of Obstetrics and Gynecology,* "Cigarette smoking, use of oral contraceptives and myocardial infarction," 126: 301–307, 1976.

Table 12–2. Mortality Rates per 100,000 Women-Years from Cardiovascular Disease (I.C.D. 390–458) by Smoking Habit at Entry and Oral-Contraceptive Use (Standardized for Age, Social Class, and Parity)

Cigarette Smoking Status	Cause of Death	Mortality Rate Users	Mortality Rate Nonusers	Relative Risk
Nonsmokers				
	Cardiovascular disease	13.8	3.0	4.7
	All causes	49.8	36.3	1.4
Smokers				
	Cardiovascular disease	39.5	8.9	4.4
	All causes	76.8	57.9	1.3

Source: Adapted from Royal College of General Practitioners' Oral Contraception Study (36).

in younger and older women is compatible with the hypothesis that oral contraceptives are etiologically related to myocardial infarction (Table 12–1) (25).

3. Smoker-nonsmoker differences in cardiovascular disease mortality. Several studies in the United States and other countries have shown a higher mortality from cardiovascular diseases among cigarette smokers. However, even when cigarette smoking is taken into account, the effect of oral contraceptive use remains. Note that in Table 12–2 the relative risks for oral contraceptive users, compared to nonusers, is the same for smokers and nonsmokers (36).

4. Confirmation by *repeated* findings of an association in retrospective and prospective studies in different population groups and different countries strengthens an inference of a causal connection. Over ten retrospective and four prospective studies of oral contraceptives and cardiovascular disease have shown similar findings (43).

Strength of the association. If all cases of the disease under study, but none of the controls, have a history of exposure to the suspected etiological factor (or characteristic)—that is, a one-to-one correspondence between the disease and the factor exists—a causal hypothesis would then be most credible. But most diseases have many etiological factors, so that a one-to-one correspondence would be unex-

Table 12-3. Retrospective Studies of Oral Contraceptives and Thrombo-embolism

Investigator	Source of Data	Type of Disease Studied*	Relative Risk (Contraceptive Users to Nonusers)
Royal College of General Practitioners (1967)	British general practices (1961–66)	Superficial VT	3
		Other VT or PE	2
Inman & Vessey (1968)	British deaths (1966)	Idiopathic PE	8
Vessey & Doll (1968, 1969)	British hospital admissions (1964–67)	Idiopathic PE	6
Sartwell et al. (1969)	U.S. hospital admissions (1963–67)	Idiopathic superficial VT	3
Vessey et al. (1960)	British hospital admissions (1964–67)	Idiopathic deep VT	4
		Post-op deep VT or PE	4
Bottiger Westerholm (1971)	Swedish hospital admissions (1964–67)	Idiopathic deep VT	11
Greene & Sartwell (1972)	U.S. hospital admissions (1963–67)	Post-op deep VT or PE	6
Boston Collab. Drug Surveillance Program (1973)	U.S. hospital admissions (1970)	Idiopathic deep VT	11
Stolley et al. (1975)	U.S. hospital admissions (1970–73)	Idiopathic deep VT or PE	7

*VT = Venous thrombosis;   PE = Pulmonary embolism

Source: Adapted from Vessey and Mann (43).

pected. Therefore, it becomes necessary to be satisfied with a degree of association that is somewhat less than complete.

Measuring the strength of an association in terms of relative risks indicates the relative importance of the possible etiological factor in producing the disease. It has been estimated that oral contraceptive users, on the average, have a risk of developing various forms of cardiovascular disease four to six times greater than nonusers (Tables 12–3 to 12–6) (43). To account for such a high degree of relative risk in terms of an indirect association between oral contraceptive use and an unknown causative factor, "X," it would be necessary for that factor to be present at least four times more frequently among users than nonusers. Since no such factor has been demonstrated, the finding of such a strong association makes a causal hypothesis more probable.

Similarly, with regard to the cigarette smoking–lung cancer relationship, the relative risks that have been observed are sufficiently high to indicate that a strong association exists (26).

Specificity of Association. If a given factor is related to other diseases, its association with the disease being studied is less likely to be interpreted as causal, a position taken by Yerushalmy and Palmer (51). In considering this concept of specificity, several points must be kept in mind.

First, the concept of specificity cannot be entirely divorced from the degree of association. It can be seen in Figure 12–4, for example, that the association of lung cancer mortality with smoking is outstanding when compared with other causes of death among smokers. In fact, when the quantitative aspect of the association is considered, this association can be regarded as being specific (13).

With regard to the association between oral contraceptive use and stroke, the specificity of the relationship is very clear: only thrombotic stroke has been associated with oral contraceptive use; hemorrhagic stroke has not been so associated (Table 12–7) (7). This is quite consistent with the hypothesis that oral contraceptives interfere with the clotting mechanism of the circulatory system, thereby causing intimal proliferation and thromboses to form, which in turn cause various types of cardiovascular disease (1, 14, 24).

Second, many diseases have multiple causes. Congenital malformations, for example, result from prenatal radiation as well as from drugs administered during pregnancy, and there are probably other

Table 12-4. Prospective Studies of Oral Contraceptives and Venous Thrombosis

Investigator	Source of Data	Type of Disease Studied*	Relative Risk (Users to Nonusers)
Royal College of General Practitioners (1977)	British general practices (1968–72) and deaths (1968–75)	Idiopathic superficial VT Idiopathic deep VT Other VT	1.5 5.7 2.1
Vessey et al. (1976, '77, '78)	British hospital referrals (1968–75) and deaths (1968–77)	Idiopathic VT Post-op VT	6.3 2.0

* VT = Venous Thrombosis.

Source: Adapted from Vessey and Mann (43).

Table 12–5. Retrospective and Prospective Studies of Oral Contraceptives and Stroke

Investigator	Data Source	Relative Risk (Users to Nonusers)
	Retrospective Studies	
Vessey & Doll (1968, '69) Collaborative Group (1973)	British hospital admissions (1964–67) U.S. hospital admissions (1969–71)	6 (thrombotic) 9 (thrombotic) 2 (hemorrhagic)
	Prospective Studies	
Royal College of General Practitioners (1977)	British general practices (1968–72) and deaths (1968–76)	>10 (thrombotic stroke) 1.8 (hemorrhagic stroke) 3.5 (other stroke) >10 (fatal subarachnoid hemorrhagic stroke) 1.0 (other fatal stroke)
Vessey et al. (1976, '77)	British hospital referrals (1968–75) and deaths (1968–77)	4.1 (thrombotic stroke) 1.5 (hemorrhagic stroke) >10 (other stroke) >10 (any fatal stroke)

Source: Adapted from Vessey and Mann (43).

Table 12–6. Retrospective Studies of Oral Contraceptives and Myocardial Infarction (MI) and Prospective Studies of Oral Contraceptives and Non-rheumatic Heart Disease

Investigator	Source of data	Relative Risk (Users to Nonusers)
	Retrospective Studies	
Inman & Vessey (1968)	British deaths (1966)	2
Vessey & Doll (1968, '69)	British hospital admissions (1964–67)	1
Mann et al. (1975, '76)	British hospital admissions (1968–72)	4 (any MI)
		2 (idiopathic MI)
		5 (MI in smokers—no other risk factors)
Mann & Inman	British deaths (1973)	3
Jick et al. (1978)	U.S. hospital admissions (1975)	14
	Prospective Studies	
Royal College of General Practitioners (1977)	British deaths (1968–76)	4
Vessey et al. (1977)	British deaths (1968–77)	>10

Source: Adapted from Vessey and Mann (≤3).

Table 12–7. Type of Stroke, Control Subject, and Use of Oral Contraceptive Agents (OCA)

	Thrombosis		Hemorrhage	
	OCA Nonuser	OCA User	OCA Nonuser	OCA User
No. of stroke cases	81	59	152	44
Comparison with hospital controls				
Control subjects	340	53	340	53
Relative risks	1.0	4.4	1.0	2.0
Confidence limits (95%)	0.7–1.5	2.8–6.9	0.7–1.4	1.3–3.2
Comparison with neighbor controls				
Control subjects	382	69	382	69
Relative risks	1.0	4.1	1.0	1.9
Confidence limits (95%)	0.7–1.5	2.6–6.6	0.7–1.5	1.2–2.9

Source: Collaborative Group for the Study of Stroke in Young Women (7). Reprinted from *The Journal of the American Medical Association*, 231:718–722, 1975. Copyright 1975, American Medical Association.

Table 12–8. Death Rates among Male Workers at Chromate-producing and Control Plants by Cancer Site: United States

| | Annual Number of Cancer Deaths per 1,000 Males for All Ages | | | | | | |
| | | Respiratory System | | | | | |
Plant	All Sites	Bronchus and Lung	Oral Region	Diges-tive Tract	Other	Person-years	Period
Total chromate-producing plants	4.17	2.63	0.27	1.18	0.09	11,019	1930s–1940s
Control group (oil refining company)	0.78	0.09	0.05	0.59	0.05	60,000	1933–1938

Source: Machle and Gregorius (33).

as yet unknown factors (19, 30). The greater the number of causal agents producing a given disease, the weaker will be the association between any one of them and the disease. It has been shown that lung cancer can result from occupational exposures to a variety of substances. Table 12–8 compares the death rate from

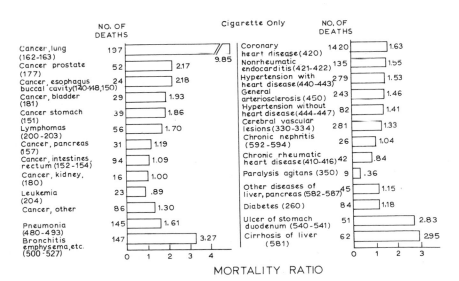

Figure 12–4. Mortality ratios of observed-to-expected number of deaths among cigarette smokers by selected causes of deaths*
Source: Dorn (13).

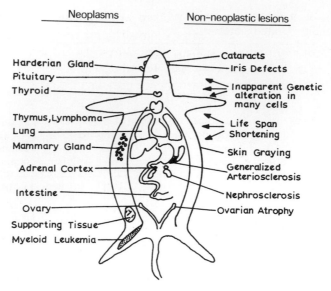

Neoplasms   Non-neoplastic lesions

Figure 12–5. Events triggered in mice by a single exposure to ionizing radiation

Source: Furth (18).

cancer by site for employees of six chromate-producing plants for periods varying from 4 to 17 years during the 1930s and 1940s to similar rates for workers in an oil refinery (33). These data, together with additional analyses for different age groups and causes of death indicated that the death rate from lung cancer for all ages was twenty-five times higher in the workers at the chromate plant. Table 12–9 summarizes the results of studies of several occupations that

Table 12–9. Summary of Occupations Associated with Increased Risk of Lung Cancer

Occupations	Assessment of Excess Risk of Lung Cancer
Uranium mining	Definite
Nickel refining	Definite
Chromate manufacture	Definite
Asbestos manufacture	Definite
Gas and tar workers	Definite
Arsenic	Definite
Iron (metal workers and hematite miners)	Suggestive
Typographers	Suggestive

are associated with an increased risk of lung cancer, describing the evidence for each association as definite, probable, or suggestive mainly on the basis of the number of studies, the degree of association, and the quality of the control groups used. Again, the greater the number of causal agents producing a given disease, the weaker will be the association between any one of them and the disease. But, it may be possible to combine the multiple etiological factors to show a strong association between this combination and the disease.

Third, a single pure substance in the environment may produce a number of different diseases. The experimental production of a variety of diseases in mice by exposure to X-ray is a good example of this (see Fig. 12–5) (18).

Fourth, a single factor may be a vehicle for several different substances. Tobacco contains a complex of substances with possible additive and synergistic actions. It would not be surprising to find that these diverse substances are able to produce more than one disease.

Fifth, there is no reason to assume that the relationships between one factor and each of a variety of diseases have similar explanations. The association between cigarette smoking and lung cancer, for example, is considered causal, whereas that between cigarette smoking and cirrhosis of the liver is probably an indirect one, reflecting the association of cigarette smoking and alcohol consumption.

In summary, despite the fact that the demonstration of specificity in an association makes a causal hypothesis more acceptable, many biological and epidemiologic aspects of an association must be considered when a factor is found to be related to several diseases.

Degree of exposure to a factor. If a factor is of causal importance in a disease, then the risk of developing the disease should be related to the degree of exposure to the factor; that is, a *dose-response relationship* should exist. The dose-response relationship between the cholesterol level and the relative risk of coronary heart disease illustrates this important aspect of assessing such relationships (see Chap. 9, p. 232, and Table 9–2). Another illustration can be found in Table 8–8, which shows the dose-response effect for estrogen use and endometrial cancer. The risk of developing lung cancer increases with an increasing number of cigarettes smoked, as

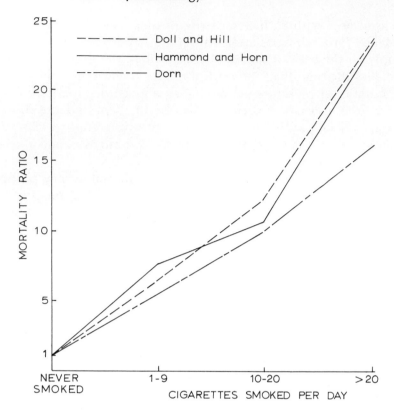

Figure 12–6. Mortality ratios of deaths from malignant neoplasm of lung by number of cigarettes smoked daily in three prospective studies

Source: Doll and Hill (10); Dorn (13); Hammond and Horn (21). Reprinted from *The Journal of the American Medical Association,* 166:1159–1308, 1958. Copyright 1958, American Medical Association.

shown by three prospective studies summarized in Figure 12–6 and confirmed in five additional prospective studies (4, 6, 10, 11, 20–22, 27, 46). Studies of those who stop smoking cigarettes show that ex-smokers have a lower risk of developing lung cancer than smokers and that the risk decreases as the length of time since cessation increases.

Recent studies also suggest that low-dose estrogen contraceptives have a lower risk of venous thromboembolism than do higher dose estrogens. This has been shown in two studies and is consistent with the Coronary Drug Project's findings regarding estrogen and thromboembolism, which has also been confirmed (5, 8, 9).

Table 12–10. Summarized Assessment of Studies Showing Association of Tobacco Use with Cancers of Various Sites

Tobacco Use	Cancer Site	Assessment
Cigarettes	Lung	Definite
	Larynx	Definite
	Bladder	Definite
	Oral cavity*	Definite
	Esophagus	Definite
	Kidney	Probable
Pipe	Oral cavity	Definite
	Larynx	Probable
	Esophagus	Probable
Cigars	Oral cavity	Definite
	Larynx	Probable
	Esophagus	Suggestive
Chewing tobacco	Oral cavity	Definite

* Oral cavity includes lip, tongue, tonsil, mouth, and pharynx.

An observed dose-response relationship makes a causal hypothesis more plausible. Unfortunately, it is sometimes impossible to obtain quantitative estimates of the degree of exposure to an etiological agent.

STUDY OF THE RELATIONSHIP BETWEEN A SUSPECTED ETIOLOGICAL FACTOR AND DIFFERENT FORMS OR SITES OF DISEASE

When the disease under study is part of a family of diseases with common clinical and biological characteristics occurring in different forms or sites, additional types of studies can be conducted. Cancer is a good example of this; the causal hypothesis receives additional support if cancers develop in several parts of the body exposed to the suspected etiological agent. Tobacco use, for example, is related to cancers of organs other than the lungs. With the same type of assessment as presented in Table 12–9, Table 12–10 summarizes evidence from many studies that strengthens the likelihood that tobacco contains substances that the carcinogenic to human tissues. It must, however, be recognized that differences do exist in the response of different organs or tissues to noxious agents.

Another example is that of the widespread effect of oral contraceptive use (Tables 12–3 to 12–6).

COMPARISONS OF THE CHARACTERISTICS OF PERSONS WITH OR
WITHOUT THE SUSPECTED ETIOLOGICAL FACTOR

To evaluate an indirect association hypothesis regarding, say, lung cancer and cigarette smoking, one could select a sample of the population, obtain a history of cigarette smoking among those in the sample, and then compare the cigarette smokers and nonsmokers for as many characteristics as possible. Such a study essentially attempts to identify the "X" factor to the extent that existing biological and sociological knowledge permits. If the indirect association hypothesis is true, the cigarette smokers should differ from the nonsmokers in one or more characteristics.

This type of study was conducted in 1956 with a sample of the adult population of Buffalo, New York, who were interviewed to determine whether cigarette smokers differ from nonsmokers in their emotional status and other selected characteristics (31). Cigarette smokers and nonsmokers drawn from the sample were matched by age, sex, color, and social class. Their emotional status was assessed by neuropsychiatric screening, consisting of a series of thirty-one questions that had been developed to differentiate "normal" from "neurotic" persons, some of which are shown in Table 12–11 (40). Smokers responded to a vast majority of the questions in the neurotic direction. These findings have been confirmed in other studies (23, 35).

Smokers and nonsmokers were also compared on more objective characteristics (Table 12–12). Clearly, smokers differed from nonsmokers in the number of times they were employed, married, and hospitalized. They also moved more frequently and participated in sports to a greater extent than did nonsmokers. The excesses observed for smokers in variables such as employment and marital experience are consistent with the results on the emotional-status questionnaire.

These differences between smokers and nonsmokers found in a cross-sectional study are subject to different interpretations. It is possible that cigarette smoking could be responsible for the traits observed among the smokers. This hypothesis would have to be evaluated in a prospective study in which nonsmoking teenage children were given a battery of psychological tests and followed for a number of years to determine whether those with neurotic traits tend to smoke more, less, or equally as often as those without the traits. On the other hand, it may be that neurotic traits lead to

Table 12–11. Selected Responses to a Questionnaire on Emotional Status of Matched Groups of Cigarette Smokers and Nonsmokers, Buffalo, 1956

Question	Percent Distribution of Response of		Percent of Responses in Which Cigarette Smokers and Non-smokers Agreed	Chi-Square (one degree of freedom)	P
	Cigar-ette Smokers	Non-smokers			
1. Do you ever feel like smashing things for no good reason?					
Almost never	75.5	84.4	66.4	21.3	<.001
Sometimes	22.5	14.9			
Very often	2.0	0.8			
2. How often does it make you sore to have people tell you what to do?					
Almost never	33.4	42.7	43.7	20.7	<.001
Sometimes	56.0	51.6			
Very often	10.5	5.7			
3. Do your hands ever tremble enough to bother you?					
Never	80.6	88.4	72.3	20.33	<.001
Sometimes	17.1	10.2			
Often	2.3	1.4			
4. Are you bothered with nervousness?					
Never	29.7	40.1	44.2	19.96	<.001
Sometimes	56.2	50.3			
Often	14.1	9.6			
5. How often do people get on your nerves so that you want to do just the opposite of what they want you to do?					
Almost never	39.4	48.0	47.2	14.5	<.001
Sometimes	53.8	48.5			
Very often	6.8	3.5			
6. Do you find that you often have to tell people to mind their own business?					
Almost never	63.7	72.2	55.6	14.5	<.001
Sometimes	31.5	25.7			
Very often	4.8	2.0			

Source: Lilienfeld (31).

Table 12–12. Comparison of Cigarette Smokers and Nonsmokers with Respect to Selected Characteristics, Buffalo, 1956

| | Total Group | | |
| | Cigarette Smokers Minus Nonsmokers: Mean | | |
Characteristic	Difference	t	P
Number of times employed	+.39	5.54	<.001
Number of times married	+.10	5.01	<.001
Number of hospitalizations	+.26	4.17	<.001
Number of different residences	+.16	1.83	.10>P>.05
Number of X-ray fluoroscopic examinations during twelve months preceding interview	−.002	0.03	>.95
Number of X-ray or radium treatments during lifetime	−.20	0.83	.40
Number of sports	+.10	2.33	.02

Source: Lilienfeld (31).

smoking. It is also possible that smoking and neurotic traits both result from the same underlying emotional or social factors.

The results of this study could be interpreted as supporting an indirect association between cigarette smoking and lung cancer, suggesting that emotional factors are etiologically important in lung cancer. However, the degree of association between emotional factors and cigarette smoking is not sufficiently high to explain the marked association between cigarette smoking and lung cancer. Relative risks were computed for the items in the questionnaire that represent the most neurotic response (see Chap. 8). The highest figure obtained was 2.6, which is not sufficient to explain the relative risk of ten obtained in studies of the relationship between cigarette smoking and lung cancer. Another way of evaluating the relevance of this relationship would be to determine if neurotic factors are related to lung cancer independently of cigarette smoking. If this strategy of comparing smokers and nonsmokers is used to evaluate an indirect association hypothesis and no differences between the two groups are found, the hypothesis still cannot be entirely dismissed. The characteristics that can be used in such a comparison are limited by contemporary biological knowledge. Thus, it is possible that the characteristic representing the common "X" factor may have been omitted from these comparisons.

STUDIES OF SPECIAL GROUPS THAT MAY OR MAY NOT HAVE
BEEN EXPOSED TO THE FACTOR

It may be possible to find special population groups whose living habits and exposures to possible etiological agents differ from those of the general population because of their religious and social beliefs. Among practicing Seventh Day Adventists, who do not smoke, low mortality rates from lung cancer would be expected. Early studies show that this is the case (50). Among strictly practicing Roman Catholic women, who have not used oral contraceptives, a lower rate of cardiovascular disease would be expected. Similarly, to study the relationship of diet to disease, it would be useful to compare those who do not eat various substances with those who do. Mormons, who do not consume alcoholic beverages, would comprise a large nonexposed group in a study of the relationship between alcohol consumption and liver cancer, liver cirrhosis, and esophageal cancer. Of course, the problems of deriving inferences from comparisons of special population groups discussed in Chapters 5 through 7 must be considered.

THE NATURAL EXPERIMENT

Occasionally, a natural experiment closely simulates the conditions of a randomized, controlled study and thus offers a unique opportunity to establish a causal inference. Such natural experiments were discussed in Chapters 1 and 2.

Biological Plausibility of the Observed Association

A causal hypothesis must be viewed in the light of its biological plausibility. A causal association between ingrown toenails and lung cancer, to take an absurd example, would be highly improbable. On the other hand, an association that does not appear biologically credible at one time may eventually prove to be so; indeed the observation of a seemingly implausible association may actually represent the beginning of an extension of our knowledge. The established statistical association between circulatory diseases and oral contraceptive use is an excellent example of such a relationship. At first, there was no known physiologic mechanism by which hormones could so profoundly affect the circulatory system. Yet the statistical association was present and later, possible physiological mechanisms were ascertained, such as the production of a hypercoagulable state, increased platelet adhesiveness, and direct effects on the arterial wall. It becomes important, therefore, to further investigate such biologically implausible associations. On the other hand, the cigarette smoking–lung cancer relationship is clearly biologically plausible in the light of our current knowledge of carcinogenesis, for it is not unreasonable to visualize the inhalation and deposition of a chemical carcinogen from cigarette smoke, which initiates and/or promotes a neoplastic transformation. Two other clear examples of biologically plausible relationships are estrogen consumption and endometrial cancer, and alcohol use and esophageal cancer.

Furthermore, the necessity that a biologically plausible association must exist before the association can be regarded as causal indicates the fine distinction between statistical significance and biological significance in epidemiologic studies. For though the statistical association (resulting in statistical significance) must be present before *any* relationship can be said to exist, only biologically plausible associations can result in "biological significance" (recall the definition of epidemiology in Chap. 1, p. 3).

C. GENERAL COMMENT

Experimentation and the determination of biological mechanisms provide the most direct evidence of a causal relationship between a factor and a disease. Epidemiologic studies usually provide very strong support for hypotheses of either a causal or indirect association. However, inferences from such studies are not made in isolation; they must take into account all relevant biological information. Epidemiologic and other evidence can accumulate to the point where a causal hypothesis becomes highly probable. Unfortunately, it is not yet possible to quantitate the degree of probability achieved by all the evidence for a specific hypothesis about the cause of a disease, so an element of subjectivity remains. Nevertheless, a causal hypothesis can be sufficiently probable to provide a reasonable basis for preventive and public health action.

Following the principles discussed in this chapter and in the papers by Yerushalmy and Palmer, and by Lilienfeld, Evans has developed a unified concept of causation that parallels the Henle-Koch postulates and is generally applicable to both infectious and noninfectious diseases (15). Evans's criteria, with some modifications, effectively serve as a summary of the methods and reasoning presented in this and previous chapters:

1. Prevalence of the disease should be significantly higher in those exposed to the hypothesized cause than in controls not so exposed (the cause may be present in the external environment or as a defect in host responses).
2. Exposure to the hypothesized cause should be more frequent among those with the disease than in controls without the disease—when all other risk factors are held constant.
3. Incidence of the disease should be significantly higher in those exposed to the cause than in those not so exposed, as shown by prospective studies.
4. Temporally, the disease should follow exposure to the hypothesized causative agent with a distribution of incubation periods on a log-normal-shaped curve.
5. A spectrum of host responses should follow exposure to the hypothesized agent along a logical biologic gradient from mild to severe.
6. A measurable host response following exposure to the hypothesized cause should have a high probability of appearing in those lacking this before exposure (e.g., antibody, cancer cells), or should increase in magnitude if present before exposure; this response pattern should occur infrequently in persons not so exposed.
7. Experimental reproduction of the disease should occur more frequently in animals or man appropriately exposed to the hypothesized cause than in those not so exposed; this exposure may be deliberate in volunteers, experimentally induced in the laboratory, or demonstrated in a controlled regulation of natural exposure.
8. Elimination or modification of the hypothesized cause or of the vector carrying it should decrease the incidence of the disease (e.g., control of polluted water, removal of tar from cigarettes).

9. Prevention or modification of the host's response on exposure to the hypothesized cause should decrease or eliminate the disease (e.g., immunization, drugs to lower cholesterol, specific lymphocyte transfer factor in cancer).
10. All of the relationships and findings should make biologic and epidemiologic sense.

STUDY PROBLEMS

1. In 1852, William Farr noted that mortality from cholera for different localities in London was inversely related to the localities' elevation above sea level, i.e., residents at higher levels above sea level had lower death rates from cholera than those at sea level. This finding was interpreted as providing evidence in support of the "miasma" theory of disease causation for cholera (see Chapter 2, p. 25), since those at higher elevations would be less exposed to the miasms than those at lower ones.
   a) What are the major flaws in this inference?
   b) What studies should be done to confirm or refute the hypothesis that elevation is causally related to cholera?
   c) Although Farr's observations are more than 100 years old, they remain valuable as an illustration of epidemiologic reasoning. Discuss this example in terms of the ideas presented in this chapter.
2. To show how the concepts of sufficiency and necessity apply to the epidemiologic study of disease, give examples of: (1) a factor that is sufficient but not necessary; (2) a factor that is necessary but not sufficient; (3) a factor that is both necessary and sufficient; (4) a factor that is etiologically related to a disease but is neither necessary nor sufficient for that disease.
3. What is the difference between biological significance and statistical significance? Why are *both* important in deriving biologic inferences? List some situations in which the results would be: (a) statistically significant, but not biologically, (b) biologically but not statistically significant.
4. Assume that a retrospective study showed a statistical relationship between factor F and disease D, with a relative risk of 10. Outline the different types of studies that would be needed to show that a biologic relationship existed between F and D.

5. Apply Evans's Postulates to Snow's data (p. 36). Was Snow justified in his inference? If not, list other data that you would require to arrive at the same conclusion.
6. Discuss the relationship between the concepts of "time, person, place" (p. 3) and deriving a biologic inference.
7. How is the attributable risk (p. 217) related to making a biologic inference?
8. What problem does one encounter when trying to make a biologic inference using only population-based data?
9. Provide a justification for each of Evans's Postulates. Do they apply differently for infectious and noninfectious diseases?

REFERENCES

1. Astedt, B., Issacson, S., Nilsson, I.M., and Pandolfi, M. 1973. "Thrombosis and oral contraceptives: Possible predisposition." *Brit. Med. J.* 4:631–634.
2. Auerbach, O., Hammond, E.C., Kirman, D., and Garfinkel, L. 1970. "Effects of cigarette smoking on dogs: II. Pulmonary neoplasms." *Arch. Environ. Health* 21:754–768.
3. Beral, V. 1976. "Cardiovascular disease mortality trends and oral contraceptive use in young women." *Lancet* 2:1047–1052.
4. Best, E.W.R., Josie, H.G., and Walker, C.B. 1966. *A Canadian Study of Smoking and Health.* Ottawa, Canada: Department of Health and Welfare.
5. Blackard, C.E., Doe, R.P., Mellinger, G.T., and Byar, D.P. 1970. "Incidence of cardiovascular disease and death in patients receiving diethylstilbestrol for carcinoma of the prostate." *Cancer* 26:249–256.
6. Cederlof, R., Friberg, L., Hrubec, Z., and Lorich, U. 1975. *The Relationship of Smoking and Some Social Covariables to Mortality and Cancer Morbidity. A Ten Year Follow-up in a Probability Sample of 55,000 Swedish Subjects Age 18 to 69.* Stockholm, Sweden: The Karolinska Institute.
7. Collaborative Group for the Study of Stroke in Young Women. 1975. "Oral contraceptives and stroke in young women." *JAMA* 231:718–722.
8. Coronary Drug Project Research Group. 1970. "The coronary drug project. Initial findings leading to modifications of its research protocol." *JAMA* 214:1303–1313.
9. Daniel, D.G., Campbell, H., and Turnbull, A.C. 1967. "Puerperal thromboembolism and suppression of lactation." *Lancet* 2:287–289.
10. Doll, R., and Hill, A.B. 1964. "Mortality in relation to smoking: Ten year's observation of British doctors." *Brit. Med. J.* 1:1399–1410; 1460–1467.
11. ———, and Peto, R. 1976. "Mortality in relation to smoking: 20 years observation on male British doctors." *Brit. Med. J.* 2:1525–1536.
12. ———, Vodopija, I., and Davis, W., eds. 1973. *Host Environment Interactions in the Etiology of Cancer in Man.* Lyon: International Agency for Research on Cancer.

13. Dorn, H.F. 1959. "Tobacco consumption and mortality from cancer and other diseases." *Pub. Health Reps.* 74:581–593.

14. Dugdale, M., and Masi, A.T. 1969. "Effects of the oral contraceptive on blood clotting." In *Second Report on the Oral Contraceptives.* Advisory Committee on Obstetrics and Gynecology, Food and Drug Administration. Washington, D.C.: Government Printing Office, pp. 43–51.

15. Evans, A.S. 1976. "Causation and disease: The Henle-Koch postulates revisited." *Yale J. Biol. Med.* 49:175–195.

16. Fraumeni, J.F., Jr., ed. 1975. *Persons at High Risk of Cancer.* New York: Academic Press.

17. Freis, E.D. 1971. "Medical treatment of chronic hypertension." *Modern Concepts of Cardiovascular Disease* 40:17–22.

18. Furth, J. 1959. "A meeting of ways in cancer research: Thoughts on the evolution and nature of neoplasms." *Cancer Res.* 19:241–258.

19. Goldstein, L., and Murphy, D.P. 1929. "Etiology of the ill-health in children born after maternal pelvic irradiation. Part II. Defective children born after postconception pelvic irradiation. *Amer. J. Roentgenol.* 22: 322–331.

20. Hammond, E.C. 1966. "Smoking in relation to the death rates of one million men and women." In *Epidemiological Approaches to the Study of Cancer and Other Chronic Diseases,* W. Haenszel, ed. Washington, D.C.: United States Public Health Service, Natl. Cancer Inst. Monogr. No. 19, pp. 127–204.

21. ———, and Horn, D. 1958. "Smoking and death rates—Report of forty four months of follow-up of 187,783 men. Part II. Death rates by cause." *JAMA* 166:1294–1308.

22. Hirayama, T. 1972. "Smoking in relation to the death rates of 265,118 men and women in Japan. A report on 5 years of follow-up." Presented at the American Cancer Society's 14th Science Writers' Seminar, Clearwater Beach, Florida, March 24–29, 1972.

23. Horn, D. 1963. "Behavioral aspects of cigarette smoking." *J. Chron. Dis.* 16:383–395.

24. Irey, N.S., and Norris, H.J. 1973. "Intimal vascular lesions associated with female reproductive steroids." *Arch. Pathol.* 96:227–234.

25. Jain, A.K. 1976. "Cigarette smoking, use of oral contraceptives, and myocardial infarction." *Am. J. Obst. Gyn.* 126:301–307.

26. Jarvik, M.E., Cullen, J.W., Gritz, E.R., Vogt, T.M., and West, L.J. 1977. *Research on Smoking Behavior.* NIDA Monograph 17. DHEW Publication No. (ADM) 78–581. Department of Health Education and Welfare, Washington, D.C.: Government Printing Office.

27. Kahn, H.A. 1966. "The Dorn study of smoking and mortality among U.S. veterans: Report on 8½ years of observation." In *Epidemiological Approaches to the Study of Cancer and Other Chronic Diseases.* W. Haenszel, ed. Washington, D.C.: United States Public Health Service, Natl. Cancer Inst. Monogr. No. 19, pp. 1–125.

28. Kempthorne, O. 1978. "Logical, epistemological and statistical aspects of nature-nuture data interpretation." *Biometrics* 34:1–23.

29. Lee, D.H.K., and Kotin, P., eds. 1972. *Multiple Factors in the Causation of Environmentally Induced Disease.* New York: Academic Press.

30. Lenz, W. 1966. "Malformations caused by drugs in pregnancy." *Am. J. Dis. Child.* 112:99–106.

31. Lilienfeld, A.M. 1959. "Emotional and other selected characteristics of cigarette smokers and nonsmokers as related to epidemiological studies of lung cancer and other diseases." *J. Natl. Cancer Inst.* 22:259–282.

32. ———. 1959. "On the methodology of investigations of etiologic factors in chronic diseases: Some comments." *J. Chron. Dis.* 10:41–46.

33. Machle, W., and Gregorius, F. 1948. "Cancer of the respiratory system in the United States chromate-producing industry." *Pub. Health Reps.* 63: 1114–1127.

34. Markush, R., and Seigel, D. 1969. "Oral contraceptives and mortality trends from thromboembolism in the United States." *Am. J. Public Health* 59:418–434.

35. Matarazzo, J.D., and Saslow, G. 1960. "Psychological and related characteristics of smokers and nonsmokers." *Psychol. Bull.* 57:493–513.

36. Royal College of General Practitioners' Oral Contraception Study. 1977. Mortality among oral contraceptive users. *Lancet* 2:727–731.

37. Sartwell, P.E. 1960. "On the methodology of investigations of etiologic factors in chronic diseases: Further comments." *J. Chron. Dis.* 11:61–63.

38. ———, and Anello, C. 1969. "Trends in mortality from thromboembolic diseases." In *Second Report on the Oral Contraceptives.* Advisory Committee on Obstetrics and Gynecology, Food and Drug Administration. Washington, D.C.: Government Printing Office, pp. 37–40.

39. Stolley, P.D. 1977. "The use of epidemiologic methods in the elucidation of the relationship between oral contraceptives and cardiovascular disease." In *Epidemiological Evaluation of Drugs,* F. Colombo, S. Shapiro, D. Slone, and G. Tognoni, eds. Littleton, Mass.: PSG Publishing Company, pp. 85–92.

40. Stouffer, S.A., Guttman, L., Suchman, E., Lazarsfeld, P.F., Star, S.A., and Clausen, J.A. 1950. *Measurement and Prediction (Studies in Social Psychology in World War II)* Vol. IV, New York: John Wiley and Sons.

41. Tokuhata, G.K., and Lilienfeld, A.M. 1963. "Familial aggregation of lung cancer in humans." *J. Natl. Cancer Inst.* 30:289–312.

42. Troen, P. 1978. "Physiology and pharmacology of testosterone." In *Proceedings, Hormonal Control of Male Fertility,* D.J. Patanelli, ed. DHEW Publication No. (NIH) 78–1097. United States Department of Health, Education and Welfare, pp. 1–12.

43. Vessey, M.P., and Mann, J.I. 1978. "Female sex hormones and thrombosis: Epidemiological aspects." *Brit. Med. Bull.* 34:157–162.

44. Veterans Administration Cooperative Study on Antihypertensive Agents. 1967. "Effects of treatment on morbidity in hypertension: Results in patients with diastolic blood pressures, averaging 115 through 129 mm Hg." *JAMA* 202:1028–1034.

45. ———. 1970. "Effects of treatment on morbidity in hypertension: II. Results in patients with diastolic blood pressure averaging 90 through 114 mm Hg." *JAMA* 213:1143–1152.

46. Weir, J.M., and Dunn, J.E., Jr. 1970. "Smoking and mortality: A prospective study." *Cancer* 25:105–112.

47. Wood, W.B., Jr. 1961. *From Miasmas to Molecules.* New York: Columbia University Press.

48. Wynder, E.L. 1972. "Etiology of lung cancer: Reflections on two decades of research." *Cancer* 30:1332–1339.

49. ———, and Hoffmann, D. 1967. *Tobacco and Tobacco Smoke: Studies in Experimental Carcinogenesis.* New York: Academic Press.

50. ———, Lemon, F.R., and Bross, I.D.J. 1959. "Cancer and coronary artery disease among Seventh-Day Adventists." *Cancer* 12:1016–1028.

51. Yerushalmy, J., and Palmer, C.E. 1959. "On the methodology of investigations of etiologic factors in chronic diseases." *J. Chron. Dis.* 10:27–40.

APPENDIX 1
Selected Statistical Procedures

This appendix describes some of the statistical tools and concepts that epidemiologists use. The methods selected are limited to those that can be applied to most studies and that do not require elaborate computing devices. The discussion is condensed and certain technical aspects have been omitted or only briefly described. More detailed expositions of these methods can be found in many textbooks of biostatistics.

A. SAMPLING OF AREAS AND GROUPS

Some General Considerations

In most epidemiologic studies, it is necessary to deal with a sample of the population or a subgroup of a population about whose members certain information is desired. The population may be an entire community, the male members of the community, or another subgroup of the community that has a certain characteristic such as sex, color, or religion. Hospital inpatients can also be regarded as a population from which a sample may be taken. The sample does not have to be individuals, but may consist of households, families, or blocks in a city.

When a list of all members of the population is available, the selection of a representative sample is relatively simple. However, it is important to make certain that any available list of names, households, or addresses is indeed complete. The investigator should determine how the list was obtained and maintained, to make sure that duplicates and mistaken entries were removed and that necessary additions were made. Most routinely obtained lists that have not been developed for specific research purposes will reveal one or more deficiencies.

The members of the population list from which a sample is selected will be referred to as the sampling unit. If it is a list of names of individuals, each name is the sampling unit; if of addresses, each address is the sampling unit.

Samples are selected from a population and their characteristics are studied so that one can make inferences from the sample about the population from which it is derived. In other words, the investigator wants the sample to be representative of the population.

Samples may be selected in a variety of ways: the recommended method is known as *probability sampling,* in which each sampling unit has a known probability of being selected. This allows one to derive inferences from the sample about the population with a measurable degree of precision. There are various methods of probability sampling, and they will be discussed below.

Other sampling procedures are of limited or no value in epidemiology since the probability by which a sampling unit enters the sample is not known. Therefore, no statistical assessment can be made of the accuracy of the characteristics of the selected sample in representing the population. Also, unlike probability sampling, there is no objective assurance that potential biases have not entered into the method of selecting the sample. The following are some examples of these sampling procedures:

1. The sample is chosen haphazardly, as in many laboratory experiments where experimental animals are chosen as the investigator can catch and remove them from a cage.

2. An investigator may select individuals who, in his opinion, are typical of the population being studied. The disadvantage of this method is that one really does not know if there are differences between these "typical" or "representative" individuals and the population, so that generalizations made from the sample may be incorrect.

3. The sample consists of self-selected individuals such as those who have volunteered for an experiment, series of measurements, or interview.

Such methods may be used in exploratory epidemiologic studies to obtain a "quick and dirty" look at the problem being investigated. They could provide some information about the population, serving as a basis for planning more adequate studies.

Selecting a Probability Sample

For probability sampling it is necessary to have a complete list of the sampling units of the total population, whether the units are individual persons, households, addresses, blocks, etc. as the specific study requires. If some type of list is available, it may have to be revised; if not available, it is necessary to prepare a list and this usually requires ingenuity and work.

The simplest form of probability sampling is simple random sampling in which each unit in the population list has an equal probability of being selected for the sample. To select a simple random sample the investigator: 1) makes a numbered list of the units in the population that he wants to sample; 2) decides on the size of the sample, a matter which is beyond the scope of this book but is discussed in most texts on statistics and sampling, e.g., Cochran (5); and 3) selects the required number of sampling units using a table of random numbers. Such tables of random numbers are found in most books of statistical tables or texts on statistics. Table A1-1 is a table of 1,000 random digits from Snedecor and Cochran (19) for illustrative purposes.

If such a table is not available and the size of the population to be sampled is not too large, one can write the numbers 1 to N on small cards or discs, place them in a bowl, and mix them thoroughly. If the size of the sample to be selected is n, the cards or discs are selected from the bowl in succession until n cards are drawn. These cards are not returned to the bowl after being drawn. The different numbers are recorded and the correspondingly numbered sampling units in the population are then selected. Mixing the cards provides equal probability of selection and assures randomness. However, since mixing and selection may not be done properly, it is better to use a table of random numbers.

To illustrate the use of these tables, assume that the investigator has a population of 900 case records and a simple random sample of 250 records is desired for a study. He will number the records from 1 to 900. He can enter a table such as A1-1 in a variety of ways,

Table A1–1.   One Thousand Random Digits

	00–04	05–09	10–14	15–19	20–24	25–29	30–34	35–39	40–44	45–49
00	54463	22662	65905	70639	79365	67382	29085	69831	47058	08186
01	15389	85205	18850	39226	42249	90669	96325	23248	60933	26927
02	85941	40756	82414	02015	13858	78030	16269	65978	01385	15345
03	61149	69440	11286	88218	58925	03638	52862	62733	33451	77455
04	05219	81619	10651	67079	92511	59888	84502	72095	83463	75577
05	41417	98326	87719	92294	46614	50948	64886	20002	97365	30976
06	28357	94070	20652	35774	16249	75019	21145	05217	47286	76305
07	17783	00015	10806	83091	91530	36466	39981	62481	49177	75779
08	40950	84820	29881	85966	62800	70326	84740	62660	77379	90279
09	82995	64157	66164	41180	10089	41757	78258	96488	88629	37231
10	96754	17676	55659	44105	47361	34833	86679	23930	53249	27083
11	34357	88040	53364	71726	45690	66334	60332	22554	90600	71113
12	06318	37403	49927	57715	50423	67372	63116	48888	21505	80182
13	62111	52820	07243	79931	89292	84767	85693	73947	22278	11551
14	47534	09243	67879	00544	23410	12740	02540	54440	32949	13491
15	98614	75993	84460	62846	59844	14922	48730	73443	48167	34770
16	24856	03648	44898	09351	98795	18644	39765	71058	90368	44104
17	96887	12479	80621	66223	86085	78285	02432	53342	42846	94771
18	90801	21472	42815	77408	37390	76766	52615	32141	30268	18106
19	55165	77312	83666	36028	28420	70219	81369	41943	47366	41067

Source: Snedecor and Cochran (19). Reprinted by permission from *Statistical Methods* by George W. Snedecor and William G. Cochran, 6th ed. © 1967 by The Iowa State University Press, South State Avenue, Ames, Iowa 50010.

either from the beginning, or arbitrarily placing a pencil at any number in the table, or selecting certain columns. Since $N = 900$, it is only necessary to select random numbers composed of three digits. The investigator can go down columns 15–17, for instance, selecting the numbers between 001 and 900 until 250 have been selected. Any number greater than 900 is discarded, as well as any number that is repeated. Since these three columns will not provide all the 250 numbers, he can skip to another set of three columns, e.g., 30–32, and repeat the procedure. If large sample sizes are required, the most practical method is to use a larger table and select all eligible numbers. The Rand Corporation has published a table of one million digits, and Kendall and Smith one of 100,000 digits (11, 17). Books with smaller tables usually provide instructions as to the most convenient method of using the table.

Simple random sampling may become tedious if the sample and population are large. Suppose an investigator has a list of 250,000 inhabitants or file cards and wants to choose a sample of 1,000. A method of sampling that is used more frequently than simple random sampling in such cases is systematic sampling. To select a systematic sample, two things are needed: a sampling interval and a random start. For example, if $N = 250,000$ and $n = 1,000$, one divides 250,000 by 1,000, which equals 250. Beginning with a random number between 1 and 250 (random start), one selects every 250th number thereafter. Thus if the random number is 125, the next number would be 375, then 625, etc. If n does not divide evenly into N, one selects the nearest whole number. One advantage of systematic sampling is that it spreads the sample more evenly over the population. It is conceivable, however, that the systematic sample may be biased if there is a periodicity or systematic ordering in the population list, e.g., it may always be a corner household.

Certain assumptions must be made about the characteristics of the population to be sampled in order to estimate the sampling error. A full discussion of these problems and their solutions can be found in Cochran (5).

It should be emphasized that the listings of the population must have the same units as the desired sample, e.g., samples of individuals from lists of persons and samples of households from household lists. If a household list is available to the investigator but a simple random sample of persons is desired, there are additional considerations. If the investigator selects a simple random sample of n households and interviews or examines one person per household, the resulting sample of n persons will not be a simple random sample since individuals in smaller households will have a greater chance of being selected than those in larger households. Thus, each individual would not have had an equal probability of being selected for the sample. If the factor being studied is related to the size of the household, a biased sample will result. More complex methods can be used to obtain an unbiased sample in such situations and some of these will be mentioned below, but again the interested reader should consult Cochran (5).

The population to be sampled can be divided into subgroups or *strata* by one or more characteristics, such as age, sex, or severity of disease, and within each stratum a random sample can be selected. This procedure is known as *stratified sampling* and it has several advantages. It reduces sampling variability by eliminating variation with respect to the characteristic by which the *strata* are constructed and/or if the *strata* are more uniform than the total population with respect to other factors. It also has the advantage of allowing one to use different sampling fractions (percent of individuals in the strata that is being selected for the sample) in the different strata since it is possible to obtain larger fractions in strata with a smaller number of units.

Sampling Where No Population Lists Exist

In many areas where epidemiologic studies are needed, there is no satisfactory population list of individuals. Frequently, lists of various groupings of individuals are available or can be compiled. These groups are socially or politically defined clusterings of individuals, such as households, addresses of buildings, city blocks, or census enumeration districts. When such lists are available or when they can be readily compiled, two methods may be used to select the desired sample of individuals:

1. A random sample of clusters is selected and all individuals in the cluster are included in the study. This is known as single-stage cluster sampling.

2. A random sample of clusters is selected as in 1., a list is made of all the individuals in each cluster, and a random sample of individuals is then selected independently within each cluster. This is known as two-stage cluster sampling with subsampling.

If a list of households is available and a random sample of individual persons is desired, a random sample of households may be selected and all individuals in the household may be interviewed or studied. This represents single-stage cluster sampling as in 1. If, after selecting the households, a roster of all individuals in each household is made and a random sample of one or more individuals is randomly selected from each roster, one has performed two-stage cluster sampling as in 2.

There may be more than two stages of sampling. For example, a list of blocks in a city may be available from the population census. A sample of blocks may be randomly selected. Each of the selected blocks may be cruised to obtain a list of households. A sample of households may then be selected and for each household a roster of household members compiled. This procedure results in a three-stage sample with subsampling at all stages.

If not available, lists of such clusters can be constructed by the investigator. In addition, aerial photographs or maps can be used to divide a geographical area into smaller areas with definable boundaries and then samples of areas and subareas can be selected.

Cluster sampling is convenient not only when no population lists are available but also when the investigator wants to study people living in a small number of households or villages rather than individuals in more scattered populations.

Cluster multistage samples have larger sampling errors than simple random samples of the same size. A cluster is composed of individuals who are likely to be more similar to each other than those selected at random from the population. For example, individuals in the same household have similar dietary and smoking habits (generally known as "intra-class correlation"). In addition, fewer large clusters will be available for sampling and the sample will be concentrated in a smaller number of clusters. It is therefore preferable to have a large number of small clusters than a small number of large clusters. It should be emphasized that biases can result if a cluster sample of individuals is analyzed as if it were a random sample of individuals. It should also be noted that clusters, like individuals, can be grouped into more homogeneous strata and a certain percentage of clusters selected from within each stratum. Thus, the methods used in analyzing stratified sampling can be applied. Again, the reader is referred to Cochran for a detailed discussion of these methods (5).

B. SAMPLING VARIABILITY

Drawing a sample so that biases of selection are avoided does not guarantee that it will be completely representative of the population from which it was derived. The sampling procedure itself (unless it is a sample of 100 percent of the population) will eliminate individuals with certain characteristics. If many different samples are drawn from the same population by random sampling or by one of its variants, different values or estimates will be obtained of the same characteristic from each sample selected. If all the possible samples of a certain size drawn from a population vary considerably, the investigator has less assurance that his particular selection is representative of the population characteristic to be estimated. However, if there is little variation from sample to sample and no biases are present, either in the method of selecting the sample or in the way the population characteristic is estimated, the investigator has more assurance that his particular sample is a representative one. Random sampling provides the means of measuring the degree of assurance from the particular sample selected. It can be shown theoretically or by experimental sampling that the amount of variation in the frequency of a characteristic from one sample to another depends upon the amount of variation of the characteristic (whether quantitative or qualitative) in the population. Random sampling allows one to obtain from any selected sample an unbiased estimate of the population variation. This estimate is then used to set limits within which the population value being estimated will lie, with varying degrees of confidence. A numerical value for these degrees of confidence can be calculated by making some assumptions, or preferably by having some knowledge about the distribution of the estimated characteristic in the population.

Assessing Sampling Variability

As already mentioned, when random sampling is used, the variability of samples drawn from a population can be measured in terms of the variability found in the population itself, which can be estimated from the selected sample. For example, if the average age at menarche is estimated from a sample, the variation in the estimate from that sample reflects the variation in the age of menarche in the population, which can be estimated in a randomly selected sample.

Variation of individuals in a population can be measured in several ways. Most frequently it is measured by its variance or the square root of the variance, the standard deviation. The variance of a characteristic or measurement is defined as the mean of the sum of squared deviations of individuals from the population's arithmetic mean. The standard deviation of a characteristic is usually denoted by the Greek lower case letter sigma (σ) and the variance as σ^2. Symbolically, the variance may be defined as:

$$\sigma^2 = \frac{1}{N}\left[(x_1 - \overline{X})^2 + (x_2 - \overline{X})^2 + \ldots + (x_N - \overline{X})^2\right]$$

where N is the size of the population, x is the particular characteristic being measured, and x_i is the value of the characteristic for the ith individual in the population. In the equation

$$\overline{X} = \frac{1}{N} \ (x_1 + x_2 + \ldots + x_N)$$

$\overline{X}$ is the arithmetic mean of the xth characteristic in the population. If the characteristic being examined is dichotomous (i.e., present or absent) rather than a measurement, the arithmetic mean reduces to the population proportion, P, of individuals having that characteristic and the variance to $P(1 - P)$.

If a simple random sample of n persons is chosen from a population of persons and the sample arithmetic mean, or sample proportion, is to be estimated, it can be shown that the sampling variation of the mean can be computed in terms of the variance of the population as

$$\sigma_{\overline{x}}^2 = \frac{\sigma^2}{n} \left(1 - \frac{n}{N}\right).$$

The terms in parenthesis represent the reduction in the variance due to the proportion of the population (n/N) that has been sampled, i.e., the sampling fraction; if there were 100 percent sampling, then $(n/N) = 1$, and samples would not vary from each other. For small sampling fractions, $(n/N) < .05$, this factor is usually ignored. The important point to note is that the sampling variation depends essentially on two quantities: the variance of the population (σ^2) and the sample size (n). Populations with more variable characteristics of interest require larger sample sizes to compensate for this fact. With a qualitative characteristic, the formula is $\sigma^2 = P(1 - P)$, where P is the frequency of the characteristic in the population. Therefore, the greatest amount of variation in the population occurs when P equals 0.50, and this decreases as P is higher or lower than 0.50. Thus, when sampling from a population where the characteristic occurs 50 percent of the time, much larger samples are necessary to provide the same degree of assurance one has in a population where the characteristic occurs only 10 percent of the time.

Study results are usually assessed in terms of the standard deviation. The formula used to determine the precision of the sample mean or proportion is

$$\sigma_{\overline{x}} = \frac{\sigma}{\sqrt{n}}.$$

It should be noted that a change in the sample size affects the standard deviation. To reduce the standard deviation by one-half, for example, it is necessary to quadruple the sample size. Thus it is possible to achieve any desired reduction in the standard deviation, but the necessary increase in the sample size may be prohibitively costly.

Rarely does the investigator have knowledge of the variance or standard deviation of the population being studied. When the sample is a probability sample, an estimate of the sampling variation is obtained from the sample itself. For a simple random sample, the estimated variance of a sample mean is:

$$\frac{s^2}{n}\left(1 - \frac{n}{N}\right)$$

where s^2 is the sample estimate of the variance defined by:

$$s^2 = \frac{1}{n-1}\left[(x_1 - \bar{x})^2 + (x_2 - \bar{x})^2 + \ldots + (x_n - \bar{x})^2\right]$$

where $x_1, x_2, \ldots, x_n$ are the sample values of the xth characteristic and $\bar{x} = \dfrac{x_1 + x_2 + x_3 + \ldots + x_n}{n}$. The estimate of the variability of the sample proportion is

$$\left(1 - \frac{n}{N}\right)\frac{p(1-p)}{n}$$

where p is the proportion of individuals in a sample of size n with the characteristic being studied.

Thus, if a simple random sample of 100 individuals is selected from a large population, among whom 40 persons have a certain characteristic, the estimated proportion of people with this characteristic in the population is $p_0 = \dfrac{40}{100} = 0.40$ (p_0 will be used as the sample estimate of P). Assuming the finite population correction, $\left(1 - \dfrac{n}{N}\right)$, is ignored, the estimated sampling variability is

$$s = \sqrt{\frac{p_0(1 - p_0)}{n}} = \sqrt{\frac{(.40)\,(1 - .40)}{100}} = \sqrt{.0024} = .049$$

or approximately .05. This can be interpreted to mean that while the estimated frequency of the characteristic in the population as derived from this sample was 40 percent, other samples of the same size, drawn similarly from the same population, would vary from each other on the average by about 5 percent.

However, the value of .049 was also derived from sample values so that another sample would likely give a different estimate of the precision or standard deviation of the sample. The estimates of precision are not likely to vary as much as the estimated proportions themselves. If only ten (or even ninety persons) had been found to have the characteristic rather than forty, the estimated precision would have changed from 5 to 3 percent.

The formula:

$$s = \sqrt{\frac{P(1-P)}{n}}$$

is known as the standard error of a proportion. It refers to the variability of a sample proportion p_0 from one sample to another. It is estimated from the sample itself by:

$$s = \sqrt{\frac{p_0(1-p_0)}{n}}.$$

Confidence Intervals

The estimation of variation represents the average amount of sampling variability. Under certain conditions, however, it can be shown that for reasonably large samples [large enough so that $n(1-p) > 10$], the proportion estimated from approximately 95 percent of samples of a given size will lie within ± 1.96 standard errors of the true population proportion P.

If the value of P is known, it can then be stated that 95 percent of the samples of size n selected from this population have a proportion that will fall in the interval

$$P - 1.96\sqrt{\frac{P(1-P)}{n}}, \ P + 1.96\sqrt{\frac{P(1-P)}{n}}.$$

If, for example, random samples of size 100 are selected from a population in which 50 percent of the persons have a certain characteristic, 95 percent of the samples will provide estimates of this percentage that will lie between

$$0.50 - 1.96\sqrt{\frac{0.5(1-0.5)}{100}} \text{ and } 0.50 + 1.96\sqrt{\frac{0.5(1-0.5)}{100}}$$

or between 40 and 60 percent (the multiplier 2.0 can be used rather than 1.96 for convenience). Thus, estimates that are less than 40 percent or greater than 60 percent will occur in only 5 percent of the samples of size 100 selected from such a population. It can be further shown that 99 percent of the samples will lie within the interval.

$$P - 2.58 \sqrt{\frac{P(1-P)}{n}} \text{ and } P + 2.58 \sqrt{\frac{P(1-P)}{n}}.$$

Using data from the above example, 99 percent of the estimates from samples of size 100 will lie between 38 and 62.9 percent.

Then, what can be inferred from any particular random sample of size n that is selected from this population? From the sample, first compute p_0, and then the following expression:

$$p_0 \pm 1.96 \sqrt{\frac{P(1-P)}{n}},$$

$$\text{i.e., } \left(p_0 + 1.96 \sqrt{\frac{P(1-P)}{n}} \right) - \left(p_0 - 1.96 \sqrt{\frac{P(1-P)}{n}} \right).$$

This interval will include P only if p_0 is one of the 95 percent of all possible estimates that fall within the interval

$$P \pm 1.96 \sqrt{\frac{P(1-P)}{n}}.$$

In the numerical example above, if p_0 were one of the estimates between 0.40 and 0.60, the interval formed by adding and subtracting

$$2 \sqrt{\frac{0.5(1-0.5)}{100}} = 0.10$$

will contain the population proportion, 0.50. This interval will not contain 5 percent of the samples that have estimates of p_0 greater than 0.60 or less than 0.40, and therefore will not contain the population proportion, 0.50. Thus, 95 percent of the samples will provide intervals that contain the population percentage, while 5 percent will not. Before selecting a particular sample of size n, the investigator is thus assured in 95 times out of 100 that the interval calculated from his sample will contain the population proportion he is interested in estimating.

The investigator will not know before (or after) selecting the sample whether or not his particular estimate is one of the 95 percent lying within the two standard error range of the true proportion or if it is one of the 5 percent outside this range. If the investigator's sample is one of the latter 5 percent, then the statement that the interval

$$p_0 \pm 2 \sqrt{\frac{P(1-P)}{n}}$$

contains the population proportion will be wrong; otherwise, it will be a correct statement. For these reasons the interval

$$p_0 \pm 2 \sqrt{\frac{P(1-P)}{n}}$$

is called a 95 percent confidence interval, the word "confidence" referring to the investigator's assurance that the sample he has selected is one of 95 percent of all samples that will provide a correct statement based on the interval.

It should be noted that in order to calculate these confidence intervals the unknown population proportion P has been used in the standard error formula. Since the investigator is either attempting to estimate P or to test some hypothesis about it, he will not know its value. The obvious solution is to substitute the sample value of p_0 in the formula for the standard error and calculate the interval

$$p_0 \pm 1.96 \sqrt{\frac{p_0(1-p_0)}{n}}.$$

This increases the variation of the interval since the standard error will vary from sample to sample. Fortunately, as was pointed out earlier, the standard error changes little from sample to sample, even though the sample proportion p_0 might. Thus, the statements that were made using P in the standard error hold fairly well when the sample estimate p_0 is used in place of P.

In summary: if a simple random sample of size n is selected from a population and the sample proportion p_0 is calculated, a 95 percent confidence interval for P, the population proportion, is given by

$$p_0 \pm 1.96 \sqrt{\frac{p_0(1-p_0)}{n}}.$$

If a 99 percent confidence interval is desired, the multiplier 1.96 is replaced by 2.58. (For most practical applications, 1.96 can be replaced by 2.0 and 2.58 by 2.6 with little loss of accuracy.) For example:

Suppose in a simple random sample of 400 persons from a large population of smokers, 80 are found to be "heavy" smokers (smoking more than one pack of cigarettes a day). The proportion of "heavy" smokers in the population can be estimated by the 95 percent confidence interval

$$p_0 \pm 2 \sqrt{\frac{p_0 (1 - p_0)}{n}} = \frac{80}{400} \pm 2 \sqrt{\frac{\frac{80}{400}(1 - \frac{80}{400})}{400}} = 0.20 \pm .04,$$

or 16 percent to 24 percent. Thus, it can be stated that there is a 95 percent probability that the percentage of "heavy" smokers in the population lies between 16 and 24 percent.

The confidence interval can be made as small as desired by increasing the sample size, but the decrease is proportional to the square root of the increase rather than to the increase itself. In the example, in order to decrease the confidence interval from 16–24 percent to 18–22 percent, the sample size would have to be quadrupled from 400 to 1,600 persons. Thus, beyond a certain level, reductions in the confidence interval can only be achieved at higher cost.

NINETY-FIVE PERCENT CONFIDENCE INTERVAL
FOR RARELY OCCURRING EVENTS

We have seen that for a percentage or rate, good approximations for 95 percent confidence intervals are easily computed when the condition $n(1 - p) > 10$ is satisfied. But many diseases, such as cancer, have annual incidence, prevalence, or mortality rates ranging from 1 to 100 per 100,000 population so that sample sizes of 10,000 to 1,000,000 would be necessary before the above calculations of confidence limits could be used safely. In practice, rates must often be estimated from smaller samples.

In calculating confidence intervals for rarely occurring events, different methods must be used. These are based on the Poisson rather than the normal (Gaussian) distribution used earlier. With these methods, unfortunately, it is not possible to use multipliers for the standard error that are analogous to 1.96 and 2.58, which are derived from the normal curve. To simplify matters, a table of 95 percent confidence interval factors was prepared by Haenszel, Loveland, and Sirken and is reproduced as Table A1-2 (7). The au-

Table A1–2. Tabular Values of 95 Percent Confidence Limit Factors For Estimates of a Poisson-Distributed Variable

Observed number on which estimate is based (n)	Lower limit factor (L)	Upper limit factor (U)	Observed number on which estimate is based (n)	Lower limit factor (L)	Upper limit factor (U)	Observed number on which estimate is based (n)	Lower limit factor (L)	Upper limit factor (U)
1	0.0253	5.57	21	0.619	1.53	120	0.833	1.200
2	0.121	3.61	22	0.627	1.51	140	0.844	1.184
3	0.206	2.92	23	0.634	1.50	160	0.854	1.171
4	0.272	2.56	24	0.641	1.49	180	0.862	1.160
5	0.324	2.33	25	0.647	1.48	200	0.868	1.151
6	0.367	2.18	26	0.653	1.47	250	0.882	1.134
7	0.401	2.06	27	0.659	1.46	300	0.892	1.121
8	0.431	1.97	28	0.665	1.45	350	0.899	1.112
9	0.458	1.90	29	0.670	1.44	400	0.906	1.104
10	0.480	1.84	30	0.675	1.43	450	0.911	1.098
11	0.499	1.79	35	0.697	1.39	500	0.915	1.093
12	0.517	1.75	40	0.714	1.36	600	0.922	1.084
13	0.532	1.71	45	0.729	1.34	700	0.928	1.078
14	0.546	1.68	50	0.742	1.32	800	0.932	1.072
15	0.560	1.65	60	0.770	1.30	900	0.936	1.068
16	0.572	1.62	70	0.785	1.27	1000	0.939	1.064
17	0.583	1.60	80	0.798	1.25			
18	0.593	1.58	90	0.809	1.24			
19	0.602	1.56	100	0.818	1.22			
20	0.611	1.54						

Source: Haenszel et al. (7).

thors tabulated factors necessary to calculate 95 percent confidence limits for standardized mortality ratios (SMRs). The following calculation of 95 percent confidence limits for low incidence rates exemplifies the method used.

If, in a simple random sample of 5,000 adult males, 2 new cases of stomach cancer had occurred during a year of observation, which projects to an incidence rate of 40 per 100,000 population, in order to calculate 95 percent confidence limits, enter Table A1-2 at $n = 2$ (observed number of cases on which the estimate is based). A lower limit factor (L) of 0.121 and an upper limit factor (U) of 3.61 are found corresponding to $n = 2$. To convert these numbers to a rate per 100,000, multiply both lower and upper limits by the sample rate per 100,000 (i.e., by 40).

Thus, L = 40 × 0.121 = 4.84, and U = 40 × 3.61 = 144.40.

The 95 percent confidence interval for the incidence of stomach cancer is therefore 4.84–144.40 cases per 100,000 of population. This interval is wide, reflecting the uncertainties based on estimates involving only two cases.

If, in a sample of any size, no cases are found, an upper 95 percent confidence limit can be estimated by using $n = 3$ as the upper limit. Thus, if in a sample of 10,000 persons, $n = 0$ cases of a disease were found, the upper 95 percent confidence limit would be calculated as 3 per 10,000 cases, or 30 per 100,000.

This method is also applicable to subclasses of the sample population. If simple random sampling is not used, or if the numerators and denominators of the rates are not derived from the same survey, then certain complications can arise from using Table A1-2. Some of these complications are discussed by Haenszel et al. (7).

C. TESTS OF HYPOTHESES FOR PROPORTIONS

Samples are often selected not only to estimate frequencies or proportions but also to test certain hypotheses. It is often desirable to know if an incidence or prevalence rate for a certain group of the population has decreased or increased over a period of time. The new rate p_0 can be estimated from a simple random sample and the investigator wants to determine ("test the hypothesis") whether the sample with this rate may have come from a population with a certain hypothesized rate. Is the difference between the observed and hypothesized rate large enough to exclude sampling variation as an explanation? For example, it might be known that the yearly survival rate from a certain group of diseases is 30 percent. After a new method of treatment is introduced, it is observed in a random sample of 100 persons with the disease, that 50 have survived one year. Is this difference of 20 percent due to sampling variation or must one hypothesize another explanation of the difference? (This issue is hypothetical since, as discussed in Chapter 10, a randomized clinical trial is the best method for determining whether a new treatment has an effect.)

In the previous section, it was noted that for samples which are large enough $[n(1 - p) > 10]$, the 95 percent confidence interval is

$$p_0 - 2.0\sqrt{\frac{P(1-P)}{n}} \leq P \leq p_0 + 2.0\sqrt{\frac{P(1-P)}{n}}.$$

This relationship would be true for 95 percent of the samples selected from that population. This can be rewritten in the form

$$|p_0 - P| \leqq 2.0 \sqrt{\frac{P(1-P)}{n}}.$$

The vertical strokes on either side of a quantity refer to the absolute value of the quantity regardless of algebraic sign.

Thus, if a sample with a proportion p_0 comes from a population with proportion P, the difference (either in a positive or negative sense) can be expected to exceed twice the standard error *only* 5 percent of the time. If the observed difference does, indeed, exceed twice the standard error, it can be concluded that this sample belongs to that group that occurs infrequently (less than 5 percent of the time), or that it has in fact been derived from some other population. If the latter explanation is accepted, then there is a 5 percent chance of being wrong.

In the hypothetical survival rate problem, $p_0 = \dfrac{50}{100} = .50$, $P = .30$, and

$$\sqrt{\frac{P(1-P)}{n}} = \sqrt{\frac{(.30)(.70)}{100}} = .046;$$

$1.96(.046) = .0902$ and $|p_0 - P| = |.50 - .30| = .20$. Since the difference of .20 is greater than .090, one can conclude that, either there was no increase in survival and a rather rare event was observed, or that there really was an increase in survivorship, resulting in the observed difference. If the investigator is unwilling to accept the possibility that the study sample is one that occurs rarely, he can state that the difference is statistically significant at the 5 percent probability level. If he is reluctant to accept a sample that occurs less than 5 percent of the time as being rare, he may specify a higher level of statistical significance; for example, by classifying as rare those samples that occur less than 1 percent of the time. It is then necessary that the difference $|p_0 - P|$ exceed

$$2.6 \sqrt{\frac{P(1-P)}{n}}.$$

This will occur less than 1 percent of the time if the hypothesis is true that p_0 was derived from a population with proportion P. If this hypothesis is rejected, there is a 1 percent chance of having rejected a true hypothesis.

The test appears in its simplest form if the following quantity is calculated:

$$\frac{|p_0 - P|}{\sqrt{\dfrac{P(1-P)}{n}}} = \frac{\text{difference}}{\text{standard error (S.E.)}}.$$

If this difference exceeds 2.0, the difference is said to be statistically significant at the 5 percent level; if it exceeds 2.60 the difference is said to be statistically significant at the 1 percent level.

Testing Hypotheses About Two Sample Proportions

It can be shown that the standard error of the difference between two sample percentages p_1 and p_2 from the same population will have a standard error of

$$\sqrt{\frac{P(1-P)}{n_1} + \frac{P(1-P)}{n_2}},$$

where P is the proportion of the population with the characteristic, $(1 - P)$ is the proportion of the population without the characteristic, n_1 is the size of one sample, and n_2 is the size of the other sample. If one wants to test the hypothesis that the two samples have been independently selected from a population having the common population proportion P, a ratio is calculated that is similar to the one given in the previous section, namely,

$$\frac{\text{difference between proportions}}{\text{standard error of difference}} = \frac{|p_1 - p_2|}{\sqrt{\dfrac{P(1-P)}{n_1} + \dfrac{P(1-P)}{n_2}}}.$$

This provides a satisfactory method of testing the hypothesis that there is no difference between p_1 and p_2 at the 5 percent or 1 percent significance level, if an estimate of P and $(1 - P)$ is available. Up to this point we have assumed that the values of P and $(1 - P)$ were provided or known. The hypothesis to be tested here states that the two samples come from a population with a common population proportion without specifying the value of the proportion. Thus, it is necessary to estimate the value of P from the two samples by taking a weighted average of their proportions,

$$\hat{p} = \frac{n_1 p_1 + n_2 p_2}{n_1 + n_2} = \frac{\text{total number in both samples}}{\text{total number of observations}}.$$

Table A1–3. Determination of Percentage Cured for Patients Receiving Treatments A and B

Treatment	Number of Patients		
	Cured	Not Cured	Total
A	10	30	40
B	65	95	160
Total	75	125	200

The cure rate for those receiving treatments A and B are $p_a = \frac{10}{40} = .25$, $p_b = \frac{65}{160} = .406$, respectively. The difference in cure rates is $p_a - p_b = .156$.

The test criterion then becomes:

$$\frac{\text{difference in proportions}}{\text{standard error of difference}} = \frac{|p_1 - p_2|}{\sqrt{\dfrac{\hat{p}(1 - \hat{p})}{n_1} + \dfrac{\hat{p}(1 - \hat{p})}{n_2}}}.$$

If this value exceeds 1.96 (or 2.0), then the hypothesis, that the observed difference is due to sampling alone, is rejected at the 5 percent level of statistical significance. If it exceeds 2.58 (or 2.6), the hypothesis is rejected at the 1 percent level.

For a simple example of the procedure, assume an investigator has observations on the number of patients who have and have not been cured after receiving one of two treatments, A and B, as shown in Table A1-3. He wants to test whether the observed cure rate of those who had received treatment A is significantly different from those who had received treatment B. This can be restated as follows: would one frequently observe a difference of .156 (or 15.6 percent) in these cure rates if these two samples being compared were derived from a population with the same cure rate? The estimate of the population cure rate is given by $\hat{p} = \frac{75}{200} = .375$.

The statistical test can now be calculated as

$$\frac{.156}{\sqrt{\dfrac{(.375)\,(.625)}{40} + \dfrac{(.375)\,(.625)}{160}}} = \frac{.156}{.0866} = 1.8.$$

Since this value is less than 1.96, it is concluded that either the difference observed is due to sampling (or chance) variation in the two groups or that the sample sizes used in this comparison are not large enough to detect differences of this size.

Table A1–4. Symbolic Representation for Determining Cure Rates for Receiving Treatments A and B

Treatment	Number of Patients		Total
	Cured	Not Cured	
A	a	b	a + b
B	c	d	c + d
Total	$a + c = n_1$; $b + d = n_2$		$N = a + b + c + d = n_1 + n_2$

The test can be put into another form that allows simpler computations. If the observations in the fourfold table (Table A1-3) are expressed in a more general form, as in Table A1-4, it is possible to obtain, after some algebraic manipulation, the following:

$$\text{(test criterion)}^2 = \frac{N(ad - bc)}{(a + c)\,(b + d)\,(a + b)\,(c + d)} = \chi^2 \text{ (chi square)}.$$

This last quantity is often given as the computational form when data are expressed in a fourfold table such as A1-3 or A1-4. Rather than comparing the observed value with 1.96 to determine the significance, χ^2 is compared with $(1.96)^2 = 3.84$. If χ^2 is greater than 3.84, the difference in the observed proportions is said to be significantly different at a probability level of .05. Equivalently, there is said to be a significant association between the method of treatment and cure of the disease. For a further explanation of χ^2 tests and examples of their extension to other situations involving qualitative data, the reader is referred to Hill (9) and Snedecor and Cochran (19).

D. RELATIVE AND ATTRIBUTABLE RISKS: DERIVATION, TESTS OF SIGNIFICANCE, VARIANCE, AND CONFIDENCE LIMITS

Relative Risk

In Chapter 8, Section B, the method of calculating the relative risk as a measure of association in retrospective studies was presented. The derivation of the formula for the relative risk is useful in order to indicate the assumptions upon which it is based. Using the relationship of cigarette smoking to lung cancer as an example:

Let: P = Frequency of lung cancer in population
        p_1 = Frequency of smokers among lung cancer patients

$(1 - p_1) =$ Frequency of nonsmokers among lung cancer patients

$p_2 =$ Frequency of smokers among non–lung-cancer cases (controls)

$(1 - p_2) =$ Frequency of nonsmokers among non–lung-cancer cases (controls).

In a population, the lung cancer cases and controls are distributed by smoking habits according to Table A1-5.

Table A1–5.   Distribution of Lung Cancer Patients and Controls by Smoking Habits

	Lung Cancer Patients	Controls	Total
Smokers	p_1P	$p_2(1 - P)$	$p_1P + p_2(1 - P)$
Nonsmokers	$(1 - p_1)P$	$(1 - p_2)(1 - P)$	$(1 - p_1)P + (1 - p_2)(1 - P)$
Total	P	$(1 - P)$	1

Therefore:

1. The lung cancer rate among smokers $= \dfrac{p_1 P}{p_1 P + p_2(1 - P)}$

2. The lung cancer rate among nonsmokers $= \dfrac{(1 - p_1)P}{(1 - p_1)P + (1 - p_2)(1 - P)}$

The Relative Risk is

$$RR = \frac{\text{Lung cancer rate among smokers}}{\text{Lung cancer rate among nonsmokers}} = \frac{\dfrac{p_1P}{p_1P + p_2(1 - P)}}{\dfrac{(1 - p_1)P}{(1 - p_1)P + (1 - p_2)(1 -P)}}$$

$$= \frac{p_1P}{p_1P + p_2(1 - P)} \times \frac{(1 - p_1)P + (1 - p_2)(1 -P)}{(1 - p_1)P}$$

and, *if P is small,* this reduces to $\dfrac{p_1(1 - p_2)}{p_2(1 - p_1)}$, which is an estimate of the relative risk. In terms of the symbols used in Table 8-1, this expression is equivalent to $\dfrac{ad}{bc}$.

TEST OF SIGNIFICANCE, VARIANCE AND CONFIDENCE LIMITS

When the relative risk equals one, then $\dfrac{ad}{bc}$ as an approximation of the relative risk (RR) is exact. This is the case when the risk of disease for those with and without the characteristic under study is the same $\left(\dfrac{ad}{bc} = 1 \text{ or } ad = bc\right)$; one can therefore say that the disease and the characteristic are unrelated.

A test of whether or not the observed difference between ad and bc is due to sampling variation is provided by the χ^2 test for fourfold tables:

$$\chi^2 = \frac{(|ad - bc| - \dfrac{N}{2})^2 N}{N_1 N_2 M_1 M_2}$$

where $N = a + b + c + d$; $N_1 = a + c$; $N_2 = b + d$; $M_1 = a + b$; $M_2 = c + d$, as shown in Table 8-1, with one degree of freedom. The term $\dfrac{N}{2}$, which is subtracted from the difference, is the correction factor that is needed to make the test valid for small sample sizes. If the value of χ^2 is greater than 3.84, one may conclude that it is unlikely that the difference in risk between the group with and the group without the characteristic is a result of chance, at a probability level of .05.

A more useful method of testing the hypothesis of equal relative risks, which at the same time provides an estimate of the confidence limits of the relative risk, is that recommended by Haldane (8). Confidence limits of the logarithm (to the base e) of a corrected relative risk are computed and the logarithmic confidence intervals are then reconverted to the original scale. The addition of 0.50 to each of the values a, b, c, and d corrects for a bias that can occur with small numbers of observations.

Using the log-relative risk rather than the relative risk itself simplifies calculations of standard errors necesssary for computing confidence intervals. If the reconverted confidence interval does not contain the value 1.0, the hypothesis that there is no difference in risk between the two groups (cases and controls) is rejected. The risk of falsely rejecting the hypothesis depends upon the level of confidence interval selected. If, for example, a 95 percent confidence interval is selected, there will be a 5 percent chance of falsely rejecting the hypothesis of equal relative risk. If the hypothesis is rejected, an interval within which the investigator is confident the "true" relative risk lies is then provided.

For an example of the above procedure, consider the data of Breslow et al. (2) presented in Table A1-6.

Table A1–6. Distribution of Smokers and Nonsmokers Among Lung Cancer Patients and Controls

	Lung Cancer Patients	Controls	Totals
Smokers	a = 499	b = 462	$M_1 =$ 961
Nonsmokers	c = 19	d = 56	$M_2 =$ 75
Total	$N_1 = 518$	$N_2 = 518$	N = 1036

Source: Breslow et al. (2).

The relative risk of lung cancer of smokers to nonsmokers $= \dfrac{ad}{bc} \quad \dfrac{(499)\,(56)}{(462)\,(19)} = 3.18.$

The χ^2 test of equal risk is:

$$\chi^2 = \frac{(|ad - bc| - \dfrac{N}{2})^2 N}{N_1 N_2 M_1 M_2} = \frac{(|(499)\,(56) - (462)\,(19)| - \dfrac{1036}{2})^2 \, 1036}{(518)\,(518)\,(961)\,(75)} = 18.63$$

with one degree of freedom. The value of χ^2 is statistically significant at the 1 percent level, indicating that there is less than one chance in one hundred that such a relative risk could occur by chance alone if the two risks were equal.

While the χ^2 test shows that the risks are significantly different at the 1 percent level of significance, no indication is given of the limits within which the "true" relative risk might lie in the population from which these two samples have been selected. The first step is to calculate $\log_e$ (corrected relative risk):

$$\log_e \frac{(a + 0.50)\,(d + 0.50)}{(b + 0.50)\,(c + 0.50)} = \log_e \frac{(499.5)\,(56.5)}{(462.5)\,(19.5)}$$

$$= \log_e (3.129)$$

$$= 1.1408.$$

One should note that the correction of 0.50 added to each cell made little difference in the relative risk calculated in this example (3.13 versus 3.18). When the sample size is of the order of 50 rather than 500 in each of the disease groups, the correction will be more important.

The formula given by Haldane for the variance of the $\log_e$ (RR) is

$$\text{Var}\,(\log_e \text{RR}) = \frac{1}{(a + \frac{1}{2})} + \frac{1}{(b + \frac{1}{2})} + \frac{1}{(c + \frac{1}{2})} + \frac{1}{(d + \frac{1}{2})}.$$

Using the data in Table A1-6:

$$\text{Var}(\log_e \text{RR}) = \frac{1}{499.5} + \frac{1}{462.5} + \frac{1}{19.5} + \frac{1}{56.5} = .073145;$$

the standard error is the square root of this quantity, 0.2705. A 95 percent confidence interval for the $\log_e$ of the corrected relative risk is calculated as

$$\log_e (\text{corrected RR}) \pm 1.96 \text{ S.E.} (\log_e \text{RR}) = 1.1408 \pm 1.96 \,(0.2705)$$
$$= 0.6101 \text{ to } 1.6705.$$

Upon reconverting to the original measurement scale by takmg antilogs of the upper and lower limits, one finds that tne 95 percent confidence interval for the relative risk is 1.8406 to 5.3148, which means that one is approximately 95 percent confident that the risk of developing lung cancer is between 1.84 and 5.31 times as great in smokers as in nonsmokers.

Additional statistical methods for the use of the relative risk in both retrospective and prospective studies may be found in Fleiss (6). Katz et al. recently discussed methods of obtaining confidence intervals for relative risks in prospective studies (10).

Attributable Risk

The calculation of attributable risk was presented in Chapter 8. It was derived in the following manner by Levin (14).

Let:
- X = Incidence or a disease in those without the characteristic
- r = Relative risk
- rX = Incidence of disease in those with the characteristic
- b = Proportion of total population with the characteristic
- $1 - b$ = Proportion of total population without the characteristic.

Then:

1. $brX + X(1 - b)$ = The incidence of disease in the total population and

2. $\dfrac{rX - X}{rX} = \dfrac{X(r - 1)}{Xr} = \dfrac{r - 1}{r}$ = Proportion of disease attributable to the characteristic among those with the characteristic

3. $\dfrac{brX\left(\dfrac{r - 1}{r}\right)}{brX + X(1 - b)} = \dfrac{b(r - 1)}{b(r - 1) + 1}$ = The proportion of disease in the population that is attributable to the characteristic, that is, the attributable risk (AR).

A simpler form was reported by Levin and Bertell, using the symbols of Table 8-2 (15). Since $r = \dfrac{ad}{bc}$, $d = (1 - b)$ and $c = (1 - a)$. Then

$$\frac{ad}{bc} = \frac{a(1 - b)}{b(1 - a)} = \frac{(a - ab)}{(b - ab)}, \text{ and } AR = \frac{b(r - 1)}{b(r - 1) + 1} = \frac{a - b}{1 - b}.$$

Walter has derived a formula from which the variance of the attributable risk can be estimated from a retrospective study (20). Using the symbols of Table 8-2, the variance of $\log_e(1 - AR)$ is

$$\frac{a}{c(a + c)} + \frac{b}{d(b + d)}.$$

Walter showed that $\log_e (1 - AR)$ is normally distributed, and tests of significance and approximate confidence intervals can therefore be calculated using the normal distribution.

E. CONTROLLING EXTRANEOUS FACTORS

We have been assuming that the groups being compared were homogeneous with respect to all characteristics other than the specific ones for which the strength of association was being measured. Thus, when measuring the association between lung cancer and cigarette smoking, we assumed that the individuals with lung cancer and those without the disease were similar in all respects (age, sex, socioeconomic status) except for the factor being studied, namely, their cigarette-smoking status.

If the samples of diseased and nondiseased persons are randomly selected from the populations of diseased or nondiseased persons, they may be similar with regard to the distribution of some extraneous factors if the populations from which they were derived are similar with respect to these factors. However, any population differences would be reflected in these samples. If, for example, lung cancer patients differ in age and sex from the population from which the controls are selected, the samples will also differ in these characteristics. To avoid biases that can arise from such differences, various methods of selection or analysis are available to the investigator. The adjustment procedure described in Chapter 4 is useful when comparing incidence or mortality rates as well as other sets of data.

It is also possible to make a series of specific comparisons for each level of the extraneous factor; for example, age- and sex-specific comparisons of the frequency of lung cancer in smokers and nonsmokers. One disadvantage with factor-specific comparisons is that they separate the total sample into many segments, and some of these may contain too few observations or none at all to make a factor-specific comparison within these segments. Even when a particular segment contains both cases and controls, there may be a large number of cases but only a small number of controls, or vice versa. Generally speaking, the precision of the comparison varies with the factor

$$\frac{1}{\sqrt{\dfrac{1}{n_1} + \dfrac{1}{n_2}}}$$

where n_1 is the number of cases in a particular segment and n_2 is the number of controls. For a fixed total $n = n_1 + n_2$, the precision will be greater when $n_1 = n_2$. If n_1 happens to be small, an increase in the size of n_2 will not necessarily compensate for this. If a random sample is drawn from both the case and control populations, the factor-specific comparisons will vary in their degrees of precision and the comparisons that have the lowest precision may be in those segments where the greatest interest lies.

Group Matching

One means of assuring equal numbers of disease and control samples for each factor level is to "group match" the samples by stratification of one of the groups, using each factor level as a stratum. Usually the cases are self-selected in terms of the disease, with the investigator having no control over the number of cases at each factor level. The investigator then attempts to select controls with the same characteristics as the cases have. If the characteristics of the cases are known in advance, the best method of group matching is to stratify the control population on the levels of the factor to be controlled. Simple random samples of the same size as found in the disease sample at each factor level are then selected independently from the corresponding stratum of the population controls.

If the comparisons are to be made on a factor-specific basis, the percentage with and without the characteristic can be compared at each factor level by the simple binomial test described earlier. However, a useful method of combining the comparisons for each factor level has been developed by Cochran (4). It takes into account the variation in the number of observations in both cases and controls at each factor level and the variation in the proportion of individuals (cases and controls combined) having the characteristic of interest at each level. The method and its limitations are reviewed by Snedecor and Cochran (19).

For the ith factor level, let

$n_{i1}, n_{i2} =$ sample sizes of cases and controls, respectively

$p_{i1}, p_{i2} =$ observed proportion with the characteristics of interest in the two groups

$$\hat{p}_i = \text{combined proportion} = \frac{n_{i1}\, p_{i1} + n_{i2}\, p_{i2}}{n_{i1} + n_{i2}}$$

$$\hat{q}_i = 1 - \hat{p}_i$$

$$d_i = p_{i1} - p_{i2} = \text{observed difference in proportions}$$

$$w_i = \frac{n_{i1}\, n_{i2}}{n_{i1} + n_{i2}}; \; w = \Sigma w_i.$$

The weighted mean difference is first computed:

$$\bar{d} = \frac{\Sigma w_i d_i}{w}$$

which has a standard error of

$$\text{S.E.} = \frac{\sqrt{\Sigma w_i \hat{p}_i \hat{q}_i}}{w}.$$

As in the binomial test, the criterion for testing the hypothesis of no difference in proportions is:

$$\frac{\bar{d}}{\text{S.E.}} = \frac{\Sigma w_i d_i}{\sqrt{\Sigma w_i \hat{p}_i \hat{q}_i}}.$$

This is referred to in the tables of normal distribution. If it is greater than 1.96, it is concluded that the over-all difference is statistically significant at a probability level of 5 percent.

An example of the computations is presented in Tables A1-7 and A1-8. These are derived from a study of the possible relation-

Table A1–7. Number and Percent of Mothers With History of Previous Infant Loss Among Cases and Controls by Birth Order (Birth Certificate Data)

Birth Order	Children's Status	No. of Mothers with History of		Total	Percent with History of Loss
		Losses	No Losses		
2	Cases	14	86	$100 = n_{11}$	$14.0 = p_{11}$
	Controls	7	67	$74 = n_{12}$	$9.5 = p_{21}$
	Total	21	153	$174 = n_1$	$12.1 = p_1$
3–4	Cases	22	44	$66 = n_{21}$	$33.3 = p_{21}$
	Controls	7	35	$42 = n_{22}$	$16.7 = p_{22}$
	Total	29	79	$108 = n_2$	$26.9 = p_2$
5+	Cases	22	14	$36 = n_{31}$	$61.1 = p_{31}$
	Controls	10	7	$17 = n_{32}$	$58.8 = p_{32}$
	Total	32	21	$53 = n_3$	$60.3 = p_3$

Source: Rogers et al. (18).

Table A1–8. Computations for the Combined Test

Birth Order	d_i	p_i	$p_i q_i$	w_i^*	$w_i d_i$	$w_i p_i q_i$
2	+ 4.5	12.1	1,063.6	42.5	+191.3	45,203.0
3–4	+16.6	26.9	1,996.4	25.7	+426.6	51,307.5
5+	+ 2.3	60.3	2,393.9	11.6	+ 26.68	27,769.2

$$* w_i = \frac{n_{i1} \, n_{i2}}{n_{i1} + n_{i2}}$$

$\Sigma w_i d_i = 644.6$

$\Sigma w_i p_i q_i = 124{,}279.7$

$$\text{Test Criterion} = \frac{\Sigma \, w_i \, d_i}{\sqrt{\Sigma \, w_i \, \hat{p}_i \, \hat{q}_i}} = \frac{644.6}{\sqrt{124{,}279.7}} = 1.83$$

ship between prenatal and paranatal factors and childhood behavior disorders by Rogers et al. (18). The cases were those children referred by their teachers as behavior problems and the controls were those not so referred. A factor of interest was the history of previous infant loss prior to the birth of the study children as reported on the birth certificates of the study children among the mothers of case and control children. Since this is influenced by the birth order of the child, and its distribution may vary in the cases and controls, it was necessary to take the birth order into account in comparing the cases and controls. The criterion for the significance test in the example is 1.83, which is referred to the table of the normal distribution. This indicates a P value of .07, which is slightly higher than the usually accepted value of .05 for statistical significance. However, one can regard the difference as having borderline significance.

Relative risks can also be calculated for group matching with the method developed by Mantel and Haenszel (16). This and other methods are more fully discussed by Fleiss (6).

Individual Case-Control Matching

As an alternative to group matching, individual cases and controls can be matched for various factors so that each case in the study will have its own pairmate. Ideally, pairmates should be as much alike as possible in all characteristics except the one being studied. If many factors are selected for matching, it becomes difficult to find matches for each of the cases. In epidemiologic studies there is usually a limited number of cases and a large number of controls. Each case is then classified according to the factor to be controlled, and a search is made for a control with the same characteristics. If the number of factors and their levels are not too great and there is a large enough number of controls from which to select, matching may be carried out with little effort. Matching becomes difficult and time-consuming if a large number of factors and levels are considered and the number of potential controls is of a magnitude similar to the number of cases. It is likely that there will be many cases for which no control can be found. Therefore, it becomes necessary either to eliminate some of the factors or to reduce the number of levels of some factors. If age is a factor, for example, it is unlikely that pairs can be formed readily using six-month or one-year age intervals; but with five- or ten-year age intervals, matching becomes feasible.

While matching is probably desired to reduce biases, the number of factors or levels on which it is practical is rather small. There should be good reasons for including a factor as a matching variable in any study. Matching should usually be limited to a small number of factors, rarely more than 4, each consisting of a small number of levels or categories.

In addition to eliminating bias, matching also increases the precision of the comparisons by providing more homogeneous groups within which the comparisons are made. The increased precision is largely dependent on the degree of association of the matching factor with the variable of interest. Rather strong associations must exist before substantial increases in precision can be expected. Therefore, the major aim of matching in retrospective studies should be to provide comparisons that are relatively free from bias that might arise from the dissimilarities of the case and control populations.

When cases and controls are individually matched, the fourfold table assumes the form presented in Table 8.10. For matched pairs where $RR = \frac{s}{t}$ (13), (using the symbols in Table 8-10), reference (6) shows that the estimated variance $= (1 + RR)^2 \left(\dfrac{RR}{s + t}\right)$ and the estimated standard error $= (1 + RR) \sqrt{\dfrac{RR}{(s + t)}}$.

A useful test of significance for matched pairs, when s and t are not small (> 3), is the McNemar test:

$$\chi^2 = \frac{(|t - s| - 1)^2}{t + s}, \text{ with one degree of freedom.}$$

In this section we have dealt only with factors that are qualitative and dichotomous. The reader is referred to Fleiss (6) for a more detailed discussion of these issues, including the use of multiple controls in such studies. When the study characteristics are quantitative, other methods of controlling for extraneous factors are available. Extraneous effects often can be eliminated more efficiently in the analysis of the data by the method of co-variance analysis. This allows the investigator to select simple random samples of case and control groups without first matching pairs for the factors to be controlled. The reader is referred to Snedecor and Cochran (19) for details of this technique.

F. AGE-ADJUSTED MORTALITY RATES: VARIANCE AND STANDARD ERRORS

The direct method of age adjustment of death rates and the standardized mortality ratio (SMR) were described in Chapter 5. It is often useful to calculate the variance and standard error of these rates, and therefore the formulas for these statistics will be presented. For a more detailed discussion, the reader may consult Chiang (3), Keyfitz (12), and Armitage (1).

Age Adjustment by the Direct Method

Let $r_i =$ the age specific death rate in the ith age group
$N_i =$ the number of people in the ith age group of the standard population
$n_i =$ the number of people in the ith age group of the population which is being age-adjusted

The age-adjusted death rate is then $R = \Sigma \left(\dfrac{N_i}{\Sigma N_i} \right) r_i$, the

Variance of $R = \Sigma \left(\dfrac{N_i}{\Sigma N_i} \right)^2 \dfrac{r_i(1 - r_i)}{n_i}$ and the

Standard Error $= \sqrt{ \Sigma \left(\dfrac{N_i}{\Sigma N_i} \right)^2 \dfrac{r_i(1 - r_i)}{n_i} }.$

Standardized Mortality Ratio (SMR)

The SMR $= \dfrac{O \text{ (Observed number of deaths per year)}}{E \text{ (Expected number of deaths per year)}} \times 100$, and is usually expressed as a percentage.

Assuming that the standard population from which the expected numbers are calculated is much larger than the population being studied, and that the age-specific death rates in the standard population are small, which is usually the case, the Variance of SMR $\left(\text{or } \dfrac{O}{E} \right)$ is approximately $\dfrac{O}{E^2}$, and the Standard Error $= \dfrac{\sqrt{O}}{E}$.

REFERENCES

1. Armitage, P. 1971. *Statistical Methods in Medical Research.* New York: John Wiley and Sons.
2. Breslow, L., Hoaglin, L., Rasmussen, G., and Abrams, H.K. 1954. "Occupations and cigarette smoking as factors in lung cancer." *Amer. J. Public Health* 44:171–181.
3. Chiang, C.L. 1961. *Standard error of the age-adjusted death rate. Vital Statistics-Special Report, Selected Studies, No. 9;* Washington, United States Department of Health, Education and Welfare; Public Health Service.
4. Cochran, W.G. 1954. "Some methods of strengthening the common χ^2 tests." *Biometrics* 10:417–451.
5. ———. 1977. *Sampling Techniques.* 3rd ed. New York: John Wiley and Sons.
6. Fleiss, J.L. 1973. *Statistical Methods for Rates and Proportions.* New York: John Wiley and Sons.

7. Haenszel, W., Loveland, D., and Sirken, M.G. 1962. "Lung-cancer mortality as related to residence and smoking histories." *J. Natl. Cancer Instit.* 28: 947–1001.

8. Haldane, J.B.S. 1956. "The estimation and significance of the logarithm of a ratio of frequencies." *Ann. Hum. Genet.* 2:309–311.

9. Hill, A.B. 1977. *A Short Textbook of Medical Statistics.* 10th ed. Philadelphia: J.B. Lippincott.

10. Katz, D., Baptista, J., Azen, S.P., and Pike, M.C. 1978. "Obtaining confidence intervals for the risk ratio in cohort studies." *Biometrics* 34:469–474.

11. Kendall, M.G. and Smith, B.B. 1938. "Randomness and random sampling numbers." *J. Roy. Stat. Soc.* 101:147–166.

12. Keyfitz, N. 1966. "Sampling variance of standardized mortality rates." *Human Biology* 38:309–317.

13. Kraus, A.S. 1958. "The use of family members as controls in the study of the possible etiologic factors of a disease." Sc.D. Thesis, Graduate School of Public Health, University of Pittsburgh.

14. Levin, M.L. 1953. "The occurrence of lung cancer in man." *Acta Unio. Internat. Contra Cancrum* 9:531–541.

15. ———, and Bertell, R. 1978. "Re: Simple estimation of population attributable risk from case-control studies." *Amer. J. Epid.* 108:78–79.

16. Mantel, N., and Haenszel, W. 1959. "Statistical aspects of the analysis of data from retrospective studies of disease." *J. Natl. Cancer Inst.* 22:719–748.

17. Rand Corporation. 1955. *A Million Random Digits.* Glencoe, Ill.: Free Press.

18. Rogers, M.E., Lillienfeld, A.M., and Pasamanick, B. 1959. *Prenatal and Paranatal Factors in the Development of Childhood Behavior Disorders.* Baltimore, Md.: The Johns Hopkins University School of Hygiene and Public Health.

19. Snedecor, G.W., and Cochran, W.G. 1967. *Statistical Methods.* 6th ed. Ames, Iowa: Iowa State University Press.

20. Walter, S.D. 1975. "The distribution of Levin's measure of attributable risk." *Biometrika* 62:371–374.

APPENDIX 2
Theoretical Epidemiology

As a scientific discipline matures, a desire develops among scientists in the field to express the phenomena they are studying in mathematical terms. A major appeal is the precision in mathematical symbols that can rarely be achieved in verbal descriptions of biological phenomena. Mathematical models of the relationships between agent, host, and the environment, for example, are essentially a symbolic description of a scientific hypothesis (5, 6). Such descriptions may represent valuable exercises since the models can be manipulated by a variety of methods to deduce relationships that can then be compared with actual observations. If the deductions from the mathematical model correspond to the observations, the underlying hypothesis is strengthened, resulting in a better understanding of the phenomenon. When the deductions do not correspond with the observations, the mathematical model or concept used as a basis for the model will need revision. The discrepancies between the deductions and observations will indicate areas for such revisions.

When the deductions do correspond to the observations, an epidemiologic model may:

1. Provide insight into the mechanisms of a disease that is not clearly understood.
2. Shed light on the relationships between factors that influence the occurrence of a disease in the population.
3. Suggest additional observations that should be made.
4. Help clarify the meaning of some of the underlying concepts.

Despite the considerable appeal of mathematical models in scientific disciplines, the contribution of this approach to epidemiology is not clear beyond refining some concepts and facilitating some aspects of teaching. Models should be judged mainly by their ability to stimulate a change in the concepts or methods of a discipline. They have not yet had this influence in epidemiology, but it is too early to pass final judgment.

It should be emphasized that this discussion of "mathematical models" does not include a consideration of those statistical models that have been devised for the summarization and analysis of data. These have been very valuable and widely used in epidemiologic studies.

A. EPIDEMIC THEORY

Attempts have been made to describe the causes of epidemics by mathematical equations (4, 26), one of the simpler methods being that developed by Reed and Frost. This is a "deterministic" model, meaning that the future state of an epidemic is determined when the initial set of conditions is established. Probabilistic concepts do not enter into the equations. The assumptions made in formulating this model were few and simple (1). In a closed, freely mixing population of susceptible and immune individuals, a single case of disease is introduced. The infection spreads from infected persons to others by "adequate contact," defined as contact between an infected and a susceptible individual that results in the transmission of the infectious agent to the latter, who is then called a "case." A case is only considered a source of infection for a brief period of time, after which he becomes immune. Each person has a fixed probability of coming into adequate contact with any other individual during the period of time a case is infectious, which is the same for each member of the group. The concept of adequate contact includes the effect of several factors such as population density, season of the year, climate, hygienic conditions, and those that influence the transfer of infectious material from one individual to another, including host susceptibility or resistance, length of exposure, infectivity of the parasite, variability of dose, and infective period. If "p" is defined as the probability of contact between any two specified individuals in a given time period, then

"q" is the probability of escaping contact, and equals $1 - p$. If the number of contacts can b ecounted, then $p = k/(N - 1)$ where k is the average number of individuals with whom a person has an adequate contact and N represents the total number of individuals in the closed population. $N - 1$ is used in the denominator since p represents the probability of a person having contact with another person, exclusive of himself.

When C_t represents the number of cases at time t, then q^{C_t} is the probability that a given individual will not have adequate contact with any of the C_t cases and $(1 - q^{C_t})$ is the probability that a given individual will have contact with at least one case. If S_t represents the number of susceptible persons in the population at time t, then the number of new cases that will occur in the next time interval $(t + 1)$ is expressed as $C_{t+1} = S_t (1 - q^{C_t})$. This relationship permits calculating the number of cases in successive time periods, that is, the epidemic curve or "wave." This equation can be mathematically reduced to $C_{t+1} = C_t (1 - e^{-rC_t})$ where r is a proportionality constant (26).

Abbey has provided a numerical example of an epidemic based on this model, assuming a contact rate of $p = .05$ and a population of one hundred susceptibles and one hundred immunes. Her calculations made it clear that the number of new cases increases because of the increasing number of new sources of infection to which the susceptibles are exposed. A point is reached, however, at which the number of susceptibles is not sufficient to maintain the development of new cases and then the epidemic declines.

The Reed-Frost model has been modified to account for the effects of inapparent infections; variations in the duration of the infectiousness of cases, incubation periods, and immunity; stratification of the population into subgroups with different probabilities of contact; and the competition between viral agents in the presence of interference (10, 14–16, 21).

The Reed-Frost model has shown that if the probability of contact is high, the epidemic is explosive and short and does not leave any residual susceptibles. If it is low, the epidemic is prolonged and susceptibles are still present when it ends. The model has shown that the course of an epidemic is essentially a function of the relationship between susceptibles and their contacts with infected cases in the population rather than the result of changes in virulence of the infectious agent.

Attempts to determine whether the Reed-Frost model corresponds to actual epidemics have had varying results. Abbey fitted the model to epidemics of measles, chickenpox, and German measles (1). The observations did not conform to the model, which could be explained by errors in estimating the number of reported susceptible persons or by a declining contact rate as the epidemic progressed.

B. AGE-SPECIFIC PREVALENCE OF CERTAIN SEROLOGICAL AND SKIN TESTS

Attempts have been made to develop models that explain the age distribution of such characteristics as serum levels of antibodies to a specific disease, the results of skin tests, and the history of previous infectious diseases. In their simplest form, these models assume that:

1. The population is susceptible at birth.
2. The risk of infection is constant over time and at all ages.
3. Migration is negligible in the population studied.
4. The test used to indicate prior infection is perfect.
5. The results of the test do not change with the passage of time.
6. Mortality due to the infection is negligible.

Let:

$$p = \text{probability of becoming infected in one year,}$$
$$y = \text{age in years, and}$$
$$(1 - p)^y = \text{probability of not having become infected by age } y \text{ (i.e., in } y \text{ years), and}$$
$$I_y = \text{proportion of the population who have become infected by age } y.$$

Then $I_y = 1 - (1 - p)^y$.

The values of I_y at various ages can be determined for different levels of p. If an investigator measures I_y by serological or skin test surveys in a population at different ages, then applying elementary algebra to the above equation simplifies it so that he can estimate the probability of a person becoming infected in a year:

$$\log (1 - p) = \frac{\log (1 - I_y)}{y}.$$

This model as well as several more complex ones have been reviewed by Muench (22).

C. AGE-SPECIFIC INCIDENCE CURVE OF CANCER IN MAN

Models have been hypothesized stating that there are a number of "targets" in each cell or organism, and cellular changes can occur from a random "hit" on these targets by an external agent. These concepts are relevant in considering the effects of ionizing radiation. Similar theories have been developed to explain senescence and the damaging effects of agents other than radiation, including those that are mutagenic (27). These concepts have provided a basis for the development of models to fit the age distribution of several forms of cancer. One such model was proposed by Burch (8):

Let:

$P_{r,t}$ = age-specific prevalence at t years of age of a condition that is initiated by r random events, and

S_o = percent of the population that is genetically predisposed (i.e., susceptible to the condition), and

$k_r = Lm^r$, where L = number of cells and m = the mutation rate per cell per year,

then, $P_{rt} = S_o (1 - e^{-k_r t^r})$.

Unexpectedly, this model was very similar to the following reduced form of the Reed-Frost model:

$C_{t+1} = S_t(1 - e^{-rC_t})$.

It is important to note the underlying biological similarities between these two models. A hit represents the effect of an environmental agent on a cell and is similar to a contact. The conversion of a susceptible to a case by contact is similar to a mutation which converts a normal cell to a malignant cell.

Other models have been proposed for the different patterns of age-specific incidence rates of cancer observed in man (see Chap. 7), which have been used to construct different theories of carcinogenesis (2, 3, 7, 9, 11–13, 17–20, 23–25, 28). Interest has been focused on cancer sites that progressively increase with age. For many sites, the increased incidence rates between thirty to seventy-nine years of age can be represented by:

$I_t = bt^k$

where I_t is the incidence rate at age t, and b and k are constants.

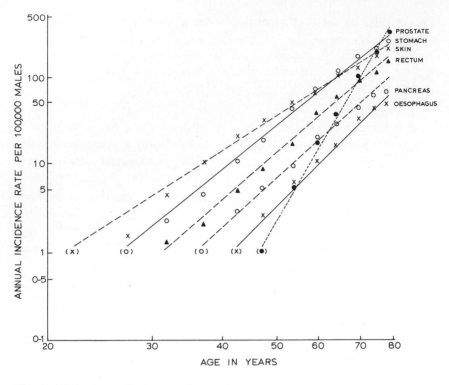

Figure A2-1 Annual age-specific incidence rates for cancer of selected sites among men, on logarithmic scale, England and Wales
Source: Cook, Doll, and Fellingham (9).

Recently, Cook and associates used data collected by the International Union Against Cancer for twenty-two cancer sites in men and nine in women in eleven countries to test this model (9). The previous equation reduces to:

$$\log (I_t) = \log b + k \log (t)$$

so that a plot of the age-specific incidence rates on a double logarithmic scale should result in a straight line. Plotting the incidence rates for several cancer sites shown in Figure A2-1 indicates that the correspondence between observed rates and theoretical expectancy is not perfect. The observed rates tend to fall below the theoretical rates in the older age group.

Visual inspection of all the data (thirty-one sites in eleven countries) showed that only 21 percent of these site-country combinations seemed to fit the model adequately. The incidence rates were not linear but curved downward in 54 percent of the combinations and an upward curvature of observed rates was noted in 25 percent. The results varied from one type of cancer to another, and sex differences were also present. To account for the presence of the curvatures, the mathematical model was modified to:

$$\log (I_t) = \log b + k \log (t) + c \log^2 (t).$$

The simple power relationship between cancer incidence and age did not adequately explain the greater part of the observations.

The model was then modified according to a variety of possible biological assumptions. One modification was made to account for the possibility that the incidence rate is related to a period of effective exposure to some carcinogen and not age. This model was found to be consistent with evidence from both animal experiments and human observations.

The major interest in determining whether these models actually represent the observed age distribution of cancer has been stimulated by speculation on different mechanisms of carcinogenesis, as previously shown by the model proposed by Burch. Among mechanisms that have been considered to result in cancer are:

1. A series of five to seven mutations or other changes of state because some of the age-specific incidence rates can be fitted with an equation with age raised to the fifth or seventh power.
2. A smaller number of changes with a relative advantage of growth for the malignantly transformed cells, which increase at an exponential rate or as a function of a square or cube of time.
3. The production of a critical mass of five to seven cells in contact with one another, all of which have been similarly transformed.

Doll has succinctly summarized the efforts at developing these models (11):

Some investigators have used the power relationship between incidence and age as a basis for the belief that cancer is the end product of a series of successive nuclear changes or mutations. Nordling assumed that the true value of k, the power of age in the equation relating incidence and age, was an integer and pointed out that the relationship of this type would be obtained if man was exposed to mutagenic agents throughout life and $k + 1$ mutations were needed to produce the disease [24]. In Nordling's data, which were confined to mortality, the rates increased approximately in proportion to the sixth power of age and he, therefore, postulated that 7 mutations were needed to produce the disease.

Others have developed this hypothesis and introduced several major modifications. The number of mutations required has been reduced by postulating a prolonged development time for the tumour or a period of freedom before exposure begins, or by postulating that one or more of the mutations gives rise to a clone of susceptible cells that increase in size exponentially or in proportion to the second or third power of its age [2, 17, 28]. Burch has shown that in some of these circumstances the mutation rate required could be of the same order of frequency as is observed with genetic mutations, and I suspect that by the judicious choice of appropriate ancillary hypotheses we could derive the observed relationship with any given number of mutations from 2 to 7 [7]. . . . The single mathematical relationship is in fact an inadequate basis on which to build a theory of the mechanism of cancer ab initio. Given the limiting conditions under which a disease can be produced by changes in one of a large number of cells and in which the individual cells behave independently, Pike has shown that a wide class of mathematical relationships will lead to this same result [25]. . . . All we can properly conclude is that no mechanism that fails to lead to this relationship can possibly be valid; but by itself it provides little indication of what that mechanism may be.

REFERENCES

1. Abbey, H. 1952. "An examination of the Reed-Frost theory of epidemics." *Hum. Biol.* 24:201–233.
2. Armitage, P., and Doll, R. 1957. "A two-stage theory of carcinogenesis in relation to the age distribution of human cancer." *Brit. J. Cancer* 11:161–169.
3. ———. 1961. "Stochastic models for carcinogenesis." In *Proceedings of the Fourth Berkeley Symposium on Mathematical Statistics and Probability.* Berkeley and Los Angeles: University of California Press 4:19–38.
4. Bailey, N.T.J. 1957. *The Mathematical Theory of Epidemics.* London: Charles Griffin and Company, Ltd.
5. Bross, I.D.J. 1970. "The role of mathematical models in clinical research." *Amer. Stat.* 24:53–56.
6. ———. 1975. *Scientific Strategies in Human Affairs: To Tell the Truth.* Hicksville, New York: Exposition Press.
7. Burch, P.R.J. 1965. "Natural and radiation carcinogenesis in man. I. Theory of initiation phase. II. Natural leukaemogenesis: Initiation. III. Radiation carcinogenesis." *Proc. Roy. Soc. B.* 162:223–287.
8. ———. 1966. "Age and sex distributions for some idiopathic non-malignant conditions in man. Some possible implications for growth-control and natural and radiation-induced ageing." In *Radiation and Ageing.* P.J. Lindop and G.A. Sacher, eds. London: Taylor and Francis, pp. 117–155.
9. Cook, P.J., Doll, R., and Fellingham, S.A. 1969. "A mathematical model for the age distribution of cancer in man." *Int. J. Cancer* 4:93–112.

10. Cooke, K.L. 1975. "A discrete-time epidemic model with classes of infectives and susceptibles." *Theoretical Pop. Biol.* 7:175–196.
11. Doll, R. 1968. "The age distribution of cancer in man." In *Thule International Symposia*. A. Engel and T. Larsson, eds. Stockholm: Nordiska Bokhandelns Forlag, pp. 15–40.
12. ———. 1971. "The age distribution of cancer: Implications for models of carcinogenesis." *J. Roy. Stat. Soc. A.* 134:133–166.
13. ———. 1973. "Age." In *Host Environment Interactions in the Etiology of Cancer in Man*. R. Doll, I. Vodopija, and W. Davis, eds. Lyon: International Agency for Research on Cancer, pp. 39–48.
14. Elveback, L.R., Ackerman, E., Young, G., and Fox, J.P. 1968. "A stochastic model for competition between viral agents in the presence of interference. I. Live virus vaccine in a randomly mixing population, model III." *Amer. J. Epid.* 87:373–384.
15. ———, Fox, J.P., and Varma, A. 1964. "An extension of the Reed-Frost epidemic model for the study of competition between viral agents in the presence of interference." *Amer. J. Hyg.* 80:356–364.
16. ———, and Varma, A. 1965. "Simulation of mathematical models for public health problems." *Pub. Health Reps.* 80:1067–1076.
17. Fisher, J.C. 1958. "Multiple mutation theory of carcinogenesis." *Nature* 181:651–652.
18. Hakama, M. 1971. "Epidemiologic evidence for multistage theory of carcinogenesis." *Int. J. Cancer* 7:557–564.
19. Iversen, S., and Arley, N. 1950. "On the mechanism of experimental carcinogenesis." *Acta Pathol. Microbiol. Scand.* 27:773–803.
20. Lilienfeld, A.M., and Johnson, E.A. 1955. "The age distribution in female breast and genital cancers." *Cancer* 8:875–882.
21. Maia, J.D.O.C. 1952. "Some mathematical developments on the epidemic theory formulated by Reed and Frost." *Hum. Biol.* 24:167–200.
22. Muench, H. 1959. *Catalytic Models in Epidemiology*. Cambridge, Massachusetts: Harvard University Press.
23. Neyman, J., and Scott, E.L. 1967. "Statistical aspect of the problem of carcinogenesis." In *Proceedings of the Fifth Berkeley Symposium on Mathematical Statistics and Probability*. Berkeley and Los Angeles: University of California Press 4:745–776.
24. Nordling, C.O. 1953. "A new theory on the cancer inducing mechanisms." *Brit. J. Cancer* 7:68–72.
25. Pike, M.C. 1966. "A method of analysis of a certain class of experiments in carcinogenesis." *Biometrics* 22:142–161.
26. Serfling, R.E. 1952. "Historical review of epidemic theory." *Hum. Biol.* 24:145–166.
27. Smith, J.M. 1968. *Mathematical Ideas in Biology*. Cambridge, England: The University Press.
28. Stocks, P. 1953. "A study of the age curve for cancer of the stomach in connection with a theory of the cancer producing mechanisms." *Brit. J. Cancer* 7:407–417.

Author Index

Subject Index

Actuarial or life tables, 9, 245, 250–51
Age
  and biological factors, 110–13
  and cohort analysis, 117–22
  and environmental factors, 97, 110
  and maternal age, 179–80
  and mathematical models, 358–62
  at migration, 97
  patterns, 110–13, 177–79
  See also Rates
Age-adjustment
  by direct method, 76–78, 353
  by indirect method, 78–80, 353
  See also Standardized mortality ratios
Agent of disease, 46–47
Age-specific rate, definition, 73
Age-standardized rate and standardized
    mortality ratios, 78–80. *See also*
    Age-adjustment
Alcohol, 149
Angina pectoris and sex, 180–81
Animal experiments
  and causal hypothesis, 297–98
  and endemicity, 277–80
Ankylosing spondylitis, 54, 56
Antihypertensive agents, 268–70
Arsenic, 5, 242
Arteriosclerotic heart disease
  and international differences, 95–96
  and risk factors, 96
  See also Cardiovascular disease
Arthritis, 148, 150
Artifactual factors. *See* Mortality
Association
  and animal experiments, 297–98
  artifactual, 290

biological plausibility of, 315–16
causal, 292–95
consistency of, 298–300
indirect, 290–91
measurement of, 209–17
specificity of, 302–9
spurious, 199–202, 289
statistical, 13–20, 216
strength or degree of, 210–11, 215–16,
    300–302
Asthma
  and corticosteroids, 91
  and isoprenaline, 92
  mortality, 91
  and pressurized aerosols, 91–92
Atherosclerosis. *See* Cardiovascular
    disease
Atomic bomb exposure, 52–54
Attack rate. *See* Rates
Attributable risk, 217–18
  derivation, 346–47
  variance of, 347
Autopsy studies, 39, 89, 122–25, 203–4

Benign breast disease, 241–42
Bias
  Berksonian, 199
  and blinding, 264–66
  and follow-up studies, 242–44
  interviewers', 207–9
  and lost to follow-up, 267
  selection, 199–202, 204–5, 248
  subjective, 246–48
  and volunteers, 266
  and withdrawals, 267